SENSORY FUNCTIONS
OF THE
SKIN OF HUMANS

SENSORY FUNCTIONS
OF THE
SKIN OF HUMANS

EDITED BY

DAN R. KENSHALO

Florida State University
Tallahassee, Florida

PLENUM PRESS · NEW YORK AND LONDON

Library of Congress Cataloging in Publication Data

International Symposium on the Skin Senses, 2d, Florida State University, 1978.
   Sensory function of the skin of humans.

   Includes index.
   1. Senses and sensation – Congresses. 2. Skin – Innervation – Congresses.
I. Kenshalo, Dan R. II. Title.
QP450.I57 1978   612'.88   79-22582
ISBN 0-306-40321-8

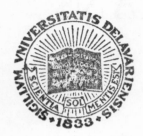

Proceedings of the Second International Symposium on Skin Senses, held at
Florida State University, Tallahassee, Florida, June 5–7, 1978.

© 1979 Plenum Press, New York
A Division of Plenum Publishing Corporation
227 West 17th Street, New York, N.Y. 10011

Printed in the United States of America

Preface

This volume represents the Proceedings of the Second International Symposium on Skin Senses held on the campus of Florida State University, Tallahassee, Florida. The symposium was held on June 5 through 7, 1978, in honor of Professor Yngve Zotterman to commemorate his 80th birthday and his more than 50 years of energetic involvement in physiological and psychophysical problems of cutaneous, gustatory, and olfactory sensitivities.

The First International Symposium on Skin Senses was intended to stimulate dialogues between electrophysiologists and psychophysicists in order to examine the mechanisms of cutaneous sensitivity by way of a multi-disciplinary approach. The 12 years since that meeting has seen much progress in the morphology, electrophysiology, and taxonomy of cutaneous receptors. There has been a growing awareness among psychophysicists that, not only are psychometric threshold functions of importance, but descriptions of the growth of sensations to suprathreshold stimuli are of at least equal importance. One of the most exciting recent events has been the development of a technique that permits recording activity in single primary afferent nerve fibers by poking a microelectrode through the skin into a nerve bundle--microneurography. This development allows one to conduct psychophysical measurements of sensation and, at the same time, to sample the primary neural activity associated with the same stimuli. The aim of this symposium was to bring together psychophysicists and microneurographers in order to explore the power and the limitations of such an approach when applied to the cutaneous senses.

This symposium was supported by National Institutes of Mental Health Grant MH11218 and Florida State University.

Dan R. Kenshalo

August 13, 1979

v

Contents

WELCOMING SPEECH

Robert Spivey, Dean, College of Arts and Sciences

Florida State University, Tallahassee, Florida 32306

It is good to see you this morning. I would like to welcome
you officially on behalf of the University and on behalf of
President Sliger. When we first began thinking about this symposium,
it was quite late and I did not think it would be possible to pull
it off. I am glad to see actual people here.

We are proud of our Psychobiology program here at the University, and we are looking forward to your conversations during this
conference that will help to make it even better.

In my judgement there is a crisis in the colleges and universities throughout the world today--a crisis of values. On the one
hand, there are pressing demands by students; on the other hand,
there are traditional ways of doing things in higher education.
The two often result in conflict.

There are a number of things we could say about what the universities ought to be doing in order to meet the crisis in values
of our societies, but one small point I want to make this morning
is particularly relevant coming from a person who has been educated
in the humanities, rather than the sciences.

One image of the excellence of universities that we have tra-
ditionally used is the name of the college of which I serve as
Dean--that is, Arts and Sciences. This title has been a traditional
image to connote excellence to the world, students, and to the pub-
lic. In the original meaning of "arts and sciences" the arts were
the skills that were necessary for human knowledge. Included in the
arts was, for example, number. That was one of the skills that was
taught in the medieval university under the arts. The sciences were

1

the subjects taught; included in the subjects taught in the medieval
university were, for example, literature and philosophy. But today,
or at least in our College of Arts and Sciences, these words have
changed meaning such that we think of the arts as the humanities or
the humanistic subjects of knowledge, whereas we think of the
sciences as the quantifying subjects of knowledge which deal with
the physical world in a particular way.

In my judgment this is an unfortunate development within the
modern university and is part of the reason for the present confusion about values. There are two camps as in C.P. Snow's famous
"Two Cultures"; these two camps, the sciences and the humanities,
rarely speak to each other effectively and never the twain shall
meet.

One way of thinking about the two camps is to imagine first the
scientific person. One picture that comes to mind is the person
in the white jacket--the cool professional, detached, value free,
dealing only in that which can be quantified. The second image,
on the other hand, of the arts person, not even called a professional, is of the passionate, involved, temperamental person, who
is not cool, detached, or in control.

This kind of division is characteristic of our society and
mirrors an inability to communicate. One indication of this difficulty in communication (at least in the United States) is a per-
vasive speech pattern which people use, not just young people, but
professionals too--and that is the speech pattern of peppering
every sentence with a phrase like "you know." "You know" creeps
into every sentence, and the reason according to Paul Goodman is
that people know that you do not know, and therefore they put in a
"you know" because they know they are not communicating, because
there is no solid world from which to communicate.

People do miscommunicate with each other. I do not have any
magnificant solution to this division in our culture between the
arts and the sciences, but I think that if we got to know each
other better we would find that a lot of humanities scholars are
very much of the cool, professional, detached type, and we would
find also that a lot of scientist scholars are of the passionate,
involved type. The thing that has amazed and impressed me, as
dean of arts and sciences for the last four years, is the tremendous
devotion and passion which scientists carry to their work. As a
group, they stay at the tasks much longer than the humanities
people do, or maybe that perception simply mirrors the fact the
grass is always greener on the other side. At any rate, there is a
passion involved in good science that is terribly important.

The other observation, coming from an outsider, that seems to
me crucial to science is that in the best science there is a

recognition of the limits of our knowledge. Scientism, or popular science, has a view of science that anything or everything is possible. But true science seems to recognize its limits, seeks to know only what it can know, and that provides a basis for speaking across one area to the other, from the sciences to the humanities.

I have one final bit of advice that I would like to give the sessions coming up. It was suggested to me by an English professor. One summer I was teaching at the University of North Carolina at Chapel Hill and there was a little article in the local newspaper about an English professor's class experience. He came into his class one day and said that he had just read the most beautiful line of poetry of his life. He got a piece of chalk and wrote on the blackboard, "Walk with light". The students pondered and one remarked, "You know, that is beautiful," and someone else said, "Who wrote it?" The professor replied, "Well, I'm not sure; I read it on a traffic light while crossing the street." That story says something about how the more practical, or at least the technological, and the humanities can speak with each other, and it is also pretty good advice for beginning a conference--"Walk with light."

We welcome you here. We hope that it is a good meeting. If there is anything that we can do to help make it a better one, please let us know. Thank you.

HOW IT STARTED: A PERSONAL REVIEW

Yngve Zotterman

Wenner-Gren Center

Sveavägen, 166, S-113 46 Stockholm, Sweden

Life is full of unexpected happenings. Who could predict that
one April morning in 1919 I happened to be in the entrance hall of
the Institute of Physiology of the old Karolinska Institute when
Professor Johansson came out of his room with a volume of Journal
of Physiology of 1908 open in his hand. He handed over the book
to me and said: "Read this paper; it is very interesting". The
paper was about the all-or-none principle in skeletal muscle and
the author was Keith Lucas of Cambridge (Lucas, 1908).

It was indeed a very interesting story. After reading the paper
I went to the library and looked through more recent volumes of the
Journal and found a series of papers by Adrian and Keith Lucas
(Adrian and Lucas, 1912) and finally only by Adrian. And the latest
papers were about the all-or-none principle and nervous condition.
Keith Lucas was killed in an air accident in 1917 but Adrian carried
on his work and even prepared a monograph about nervous conduction
in the name of his beloved senior friend and teacher, Keith Lucas.

These early experiments were mostly performed on the conduction
in the sciatic nerve of the frog using the muscle twitch as a
criterion or indication of what had occurred in the motor nerve
fibers. These experiments were quite fundamental as they gave us
information of the absolute and relative refractory period in the
nerve fiber as well as the time course of what they called the
"recovery curve" during the relative refractory period.

I learned all this directly from the lips of Adrian during
October and November of 1919 when I attended his, A. V. Hill's,
and other lectures and demonstrations to the advanced class at
Cambridge. I returned to Cambridge in 1920 and made a small bit

of research on the conductivity of the motor end plates when the
muscle was kept in solutions of different pH's and later went on
testing ammonia, etc., on the end plates. Returning to my classmates and clinical studies, I remember how my classmates pulled my
leg for doing such research -- pure nonsense which never could come
to any clinical use. Well, 30 years later curare-like acting substances were introduced and are of great value in surgery.

After 5 years of clinical studies I returned to Cambridge and
Adrian in September 1925 thanks to the great generosity of an
American institution, The Rockefeller Foundation. Adrian had just
got a 3-stage amplifier for the Lucas capillary electrometer and
the previous spring he had used this set-up to record the electrical response of sensory nerves. These preliminary experiments
were very promising, and now he wanted to go further and see what
was signalled in single sensory nerve fibers. So we started in the
middle of October 1925. Fortunately, he turned his attention to
the sensory fibers which terminate in muscles. These had been
discovered and their important function in the control of muscular
movement had been described some twenty years earlier by Sir
Charles Scott Sherrington at Oxford and by Hoffman at Freiburg in
Germany. The Master of Caius and Gonville College, Dr. Anderson,
a keen anatomist, had told Adrian that the sterno-cutaneous muscle
in the chest of the frog contained only one sensory ending, one
single spindle. Thus we set out to dissect the nerve running to
this tiny muscle. It was my special task to make this dissection
and slowly I acquired a certain skill in the work. However, we
soon found out that this muscle, the sternocutaneous, had several
muscle spindles. When we recorded from the nerve while stimulating
the spindles by stretching the muscle our records showed that the
electrical response derived from quite a few sensory nerve fibers.
Before abandoning this preparation however, one day I made cuts
from the medial side of the muscle, successively cutting away one
muscle spindle after the other from its connection with the nerve.
Finally, as can be seen in Fig. 1, we were left with a tiny strip
of muscle which obviously contained only one functioning spindle,
signalling in one single afferent nerve fiber.

November 2, 1925, was a red letter day for both of us. Under
strong emotional stress we hurried on, recording the response to
different degrees of stimulation. Adrian ran in and out controlling
the recording apparatus in the dark-room and developing the photo-
graphic plates. We were excited, both of us quite aware that what
we now saw had never been observed before and that we were dis-
covering a great secret of life, how the sensory nerves transmit
their information to the brain. In the following weeks we went on
collecting more and more data, but the principal idea about the
conduction in sensory nerves, the relation between the strength of
stimulation and nervous response, we conceived that very day of

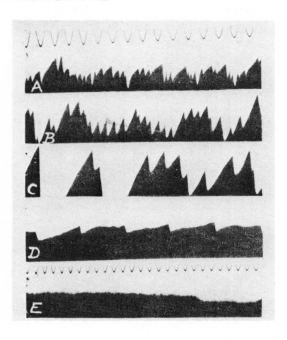

Fig. 1.   Experiment on the sternocutaneous muscle in the frog
          November 2, 1925. Afferent responses from the nerve when
          the muscle is stretched by a weight applied 10 sec. before
          record is made. Capillary electrometer with 3-valve am-
          plifier, magnification 490. The marker gives .01 sec.
          Responses vary in size as electrodes are adjusted between
          each record. A. Muscle intact, 2 g weight. B. First
          strip removed 2 g weight. C. Second strip removed 1 g
          weight. Impulses in four regular series. D. Third strip
          removed 1 g weight. Single regular series. E. Fourth
          strip removed 1 g weight. Slower plate. No impulses.
          (Adrian and Zotterman, 1926).

November 2, 1925. We had found that the transmission in the nerve
fiber occurred according to impulse frequency modulation, twenty
years before FM was introduced in teletechnique.

    In the modest way, characteristic of a highly cultured Cam-
bridge don, Adrian presented these results at a meeting at University College in London in December 1925. I still remember how he
started: "In these days anybody can buy an amplifier in the next
garage and put any sensory nerve on the electrodes, connect them
to the amplifier and record". This was of course a gross

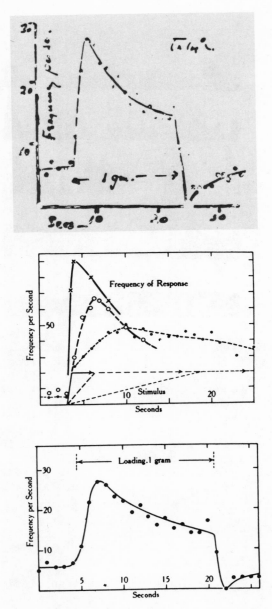

Fig. 2.   The upper diagram is the original hand drawn graph made by
           Adrian in 1925. The middle diagram shows the frequency
           of discharge of a single muscle spindle at various rates
           of loading the muscle, showing effect of adaptation. Low-
           er diagram shows frequency before, during and after load-
           ing. (Adrian and Zotterman 1926a).

overstatement and 20 years later I still met trained and skilled physiologists who complained that they were not able to record the impulses from single sensory fibers.

On the new year 1926 Adrian suggested that we should try to tap off the optic nerve of the cat. It was a difficult task. I tried hard to cut the thick nerve stem in small strips but none of these finer strands worked when the eye was illuminated. So after a week of negative results, Adrian decided to change over to the cutaneous nerves of the cat. So at the end of January 1926 we started the first electrophysiological work on the sensory functions of the skin using the plantar nerves of the cat. Adrian, who was exceptionally handy, built up the stimulating apparatus himself using odd tools in his large room (an oil dash pot (D) working on a series of levers (L_1, L_2 and L_3) and a spring balance (S) (see Fig. 3). It resulted in the discovery of rapidly ("touch") and slowly adapting ("pressure") mechanoreceptors.

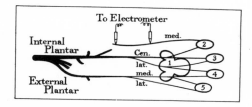

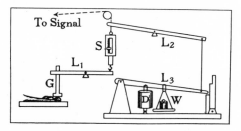

Fig. 3. The upper diagram shows the digital nerve to plantar surface of cat's foot. The lower diagram shows the stimulating apparatus. (Adrian and Zotterman 1926b).

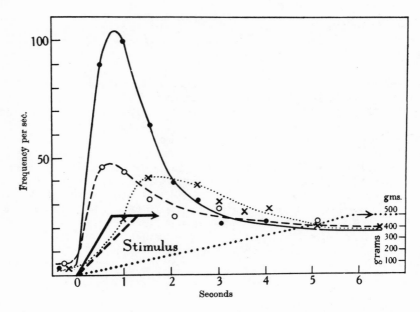

Fig. 4. Diagram showing frequency with different rates of in-
          crease of pressure on cat's pad. Every impulse counted.
          (Adrian and Zotterman 1926b).

        In 1927, when I returned to Stockholm from 2 years research
work in Cambridge and London, I started immediately to construct a
gadget enabling me to record impulses from single sensory fibers.
The old mechanic of the lab helped me to make a copy of Lucas's
apparatus for drawing fine glass tubes to make a capillary electrometer. An old French microscope (the very instrument with which
Christian Lovén, in 1875, had discovered the taste buds of the
tongue) was adapted to it on an optic bench. The thermionic valves
available at that time were very strongly microphonic. I therefore had to build a special box shielded by heavy lead plates to
house the amplifier.

        As soon as I got my recording set-up in order, I started to
lead off from tiny plantar nerves. When I touched the pads I got
good responses but to my great disappointment there was hardly any
response at all when I burned the pad with radiating heat, carefully avoiding any mechanical stimulation. I repeated my experiments for months in 1927 - 28 with increasing amplification but
with no success. A burning stimulation leads to strong avoiding
reflexes and intense sensations of pain, and yet I saw hardly any
response at all from the nerve. How could this be? What a dilemma.

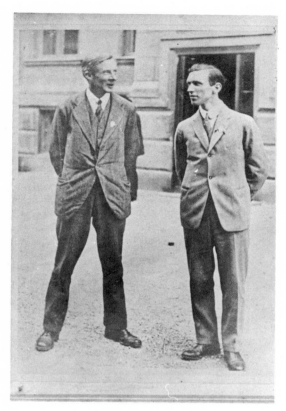

Fig. 5.   Edgar Douglas Adrian and Yngve Zotterman outside the
Physiology Lab of Karolinska Institutet during the 12th
International Congress of Physiology, Stockholm 1926.

It puzzled me for several years. Was it possible that pain was
mediated by means other than volleys of impulses in the nerve
fibers; or could it be that pain fibers conducted in the usual way
but gave too small spikes to be detected by the present recording
technique? I was more inclined to believe the latter alternative.
Then in 1929 at the International Congress of Physiology in Boston
Gasser and Erlanger demonstrated their discovery of very tiny non-
myelinated nerve fibers of very slow conduction (Class C). I
understood my failure, but I had no idea how to succeed. So I had
to turn to psychophysical experiments.

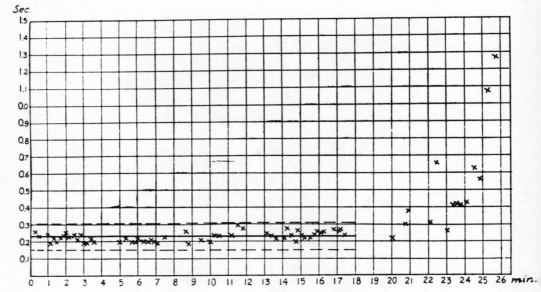

Fig. 6.   Reaction times for a needle prick on the hand while the
           blood flow to the arm was arrested. Distribution chart
           from exp. 5, see Table I. (Zotterman 1933).

     I started to record the reaction time of the first and second
pain sensation. I found that the reaction time for the second
pain-- 1 - 2 sec.-- fitted in very well with the slow conduction
rate of only 0.3 to 1.0 m/sec of these non-myelinated C-fibers
which entered the dorsal horns, while the first pain could be
attributed to A σ-fibers with conduction rates below 30 m/sec.
Further, by inflating a cuff around the upper arm, arresting the
blood flow to the lower part of the arm, I found that touch and
pressure were lost after about 18 min. while pain still could be
elicited; and this pain showed a reaction time of more than 1 sec
corresponding to the "second pain".

     On the evidence I was able to write my doctoral thesis "Studies
in the Peripheral Nervous Mechanism of Pain" in the spring of 1933.
It was a very dramatic disputation, as I had disproved Torsten
Thunberg's idea about the two pain sensations in his doctoral
thesis in Uppsala 1900. Thunberg, who had succeeded great Professor Magnus Blix at Lund was now the leading physiologist of
Sweden. I got the lowest possible points for a further university
career. Nevertheless, I found it a great turning point after
having hunted the pain fibers for six years.

     Already in 1932 I had managed to get an iron-tongue oscillo-

Table 1   Results from reaction time determinations during cuff experiment.

		1	2	3	4	5	6	7
Exp. 1	Subject B. Z.	T_{0-18} 0.223	σ 0.027	T_{18-19} 0.476		l 0.83	v_{18-19} 3.1	
Exp. 2	Subject E. H.	T_{0-17} 0.303	σ 0.061	T_{17-18} 0.618	T_{20-22} 1.75	l 0.76	v_{17-18} 2.3	v_{20-22} 0.5
Exp. 3	Subject G. D.	T_{0-18} 0.397	σ 0.077	T_{18-19} 1.1	T_{19-22} 1.62	l 0.97	v_{18-19} 1.3	v_{19-22} 0.8
Exp. 4	Subject B. L.	T_{0-20} 0.216	σ 0.057	T_{20-22} 0.381	T_{22-24} 1.69	l 0.75	v_{20-22} 4.2	v_{22-24} 0.5
Exp. 5	Subject B. L.	T_{0-18} 0.230	σ 0.026	T_{22-25} 0.467	T_{25-26} 1.17	l 0.75	v_{22-25} 3	v_{25-26} 0.8
Exp. 6	Subject B. L.	T_{0-19} 0.253	σ 0.037	T_{20-22} 0.360		l 0.75	v_{20-22} 6.1	

The interval between the moment when the needle reaches the skin and the moment when impulses inducing the reaction of the subject reach the central nervous system, can be calculated for the different periods taking a reasonable value for the afferent conduction time in the first long period of the compression experiment. The value in question can be estimated by taking the velocity of e.g. the touch fibers, v_0 = 50 m/sec, and by measuring the distance, l, between the stimulated spot on the hand and the median line at C_8. Thus we obtain

$$ T - T_8 = \frac{1}{V} - \frac{1}{V_0} ; $$

where T_0 is the mean of the observed reaction time for the first period and T the mean for the following period. The calculated conduction velocities for the afferent fibers involved are given in columns 6 and 7 (Zotterman, 1933).

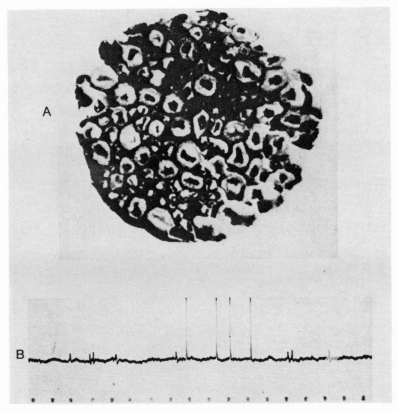

Fig. 7. A. Microphoto of lingual nerve preparation. Magnification
         940. Largest fibers measure 10 μm in diameter. Alsheimer
         Mann staining. B. Records from the same preparation
         showing the ratio between the spike heights of cold and
         touch fibers. The irregular response of small spikes is
         due to the exposure of the cat's tongue to the air. The
         four large spikes were charted by touching the tip of
         the tongue with a fine brush. (Zotterman 1936)

scope made. It was a poor copy of Bryan Matthew's very useful
oscillograph but in 1934 I could exchange it to a cathode-ray
oscilloscope designed by Manfred von Ardenne, the great German
electronic engineer, who later designed the electronics for the
V_1 and V_2, Hitler's rockets in World War II, and who later was
taken to work for the Russians. It gave excellent recordings.
One day I found a paper by Johnson and Llewellyn in the Bell
Telephone Technical Bulletin. Its title was "Signal-to-Noise

Ratio in Thermionic Valves". I shall never forget how thrilled I
was on realizing that this paper resolved the dilemma I had met
when trying to record impulses in the tiny C-fibers. I understood
that I had to make much thinner preparations than hitherto in order
to obtain a signal-to-noise ratio enabling me to record the spikes
of single C-fibers. Their spikes had previously been masked by the
noise level originating from the thermal agitation of the input
circuit. When I got a better amplifier with input valves with
lower internal noise to the cathode ray oscilloscope I was very
anxious to test whether my calculations would prove correct.
Leading off from a fine strand of the lingual nerve of the cat, I
was able to record not only from the smallest A-σ fibers mediating
cold and warmth (Fig. 7) but also from single C-fibers. These C-
spikes appeared as soon as a mechanical or thermal stimulus reached
the pain threshold (Fig. 8).

When further analyzing the response to different mechanical
stimuli, I found that a very light touch on the skin with a fine
brush elicited from the saphenous nerve of the cat volleys of very
small spikes most likely derived from small A σ- and C-fibers,
particularly when the stimulus was repeated several times. These
fibers must end very superficially. If you scratch with your nails
the skin of your palm, you can produce a tickling sensation. Only
after about 15 min can you tickle the skin again when the fiber
endings have restored their extreme mechanoreceptive property.

In 1936 my friend Olof Sjöqvist had returned from a few years
as house surgeon in the provinces to assist Herbert Olivecrona,
who pioneered brain surgery in Sweden. Sjöqvist became very interested in my pain research. One night I suggested that he should
consider how different nerve fibers run in the roots of the trigeminal nerve. Perhaps the small myelinated and the C-fibers run
in separate tracts in the brainstem as they do in the spinal cord.
He made fiber analyses of the trigeminal fibers and found that the
smaller fibers run in the bulbospinal tract (Fig. 12). Subsequently in 1937 he performed his first trigeminal tractotomies at the
level corresponding to the boundry between the caudal two-thirds
of the inferior olive. This produced a complete analgesia and
thermal anesthesia in the entire homo-lateral trigeminal area.

I had another interest in these cases. I managed to make a
sensory study of a few cases operated by Sjöqvist's tractotomy.
I asked them to shut their eyes. Then I touched the skin on the
lips and on the cheek on the operated side. They correctly reported "yes" each time I touched the skin and even when I pricked
the skin with a needle, but reported no pain nor any response to
cold or warmth in contrast to the other side of the face. But
then I touched the patient slightly on the nose with a wisp of
cotton wool, his face twitched. "It tickles", he said. I applied

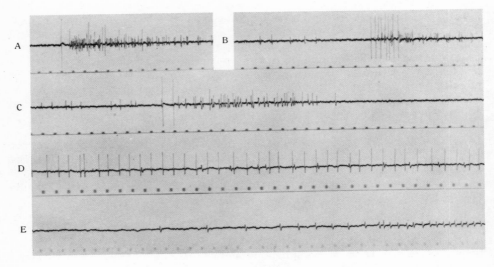

Fig. 8.   A. Record from a lingual nerve preparation approximately
          0.1 mm in diameter showing the effect of a drop of water
          of 14° C upon the tip of the tongue. The moment of the
          drop's impact is signalled by a large spike. Note the
          following massive volley of smaller spikes elicited by the
          cooling of the tip of the tongue. B. Record from the
          same preparation showing to the left a short small volley
          of low spikes elicited by a weak puff of air, which did
          not cause any deformation of the surface followed by a
          volley of large spikes due to the visible deformation of
          the surface and a subsequent volley of small cold fiber
          spikes when a strong puff of air is applied to the re-
          ceptive field. C. Same preparation. To the left is an
          irregular series of cold fiber spikes. The two large
          spikes signal the moment of impact of a drop of water of
          80°C falling upon the tongue. These are followed by a
          volley of spikes slightly diphasic. Among these warm
          fiber spikes are seen a specific type of spike of lower
          height and a configuration which indicates a much slower
          rate of conduction. Note that the cold spikes seen to the
          left disappeared. When I let a drop of 80°C fall upon my
          own tongue I experienced a sensation of warmth accompanied
          with a distinct burning sensation. D. This record shows
          the effect of applying pressure on the tongue by a wooden
          pin 1 mm in diameter. Observe how small diphasic spikes
          gradually appear among the large spikes as the pressure

is increased. E. Same preparation as in D showing the
effect of a continuous stream of water of 60°C upon the
tongue. The first small spike arrives in 0.36 sec after
the beginning of the stimulation. Note the identical
shape of these C-fiber spikes with those in D elicited by
hard, noxious stimulation. Squirting hot water like that
inhibited the response of the large myelinated mechanoreceptive fiber endings. The procedure caused a burning
sensation on my own tongue and complete numbness of the
surface of the tongue exposed. The numbness disappeared
generally in a few minutes as did the response of the
large myelinated fibers. Although the rate of conduction
of these spikes were not directly measured, there is no
doubt whatever that I recorded single C-fiber spikes.

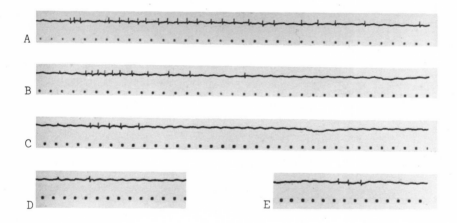

Fig. 9. Record from a single cold fiber from the lingual nerve of
the cat when applying drops of water at: A. 0°; B. 10°;
C. 20°; and D. 30°C. E. shows the effect of a very light
puff of air. (Zotterman, 1936).

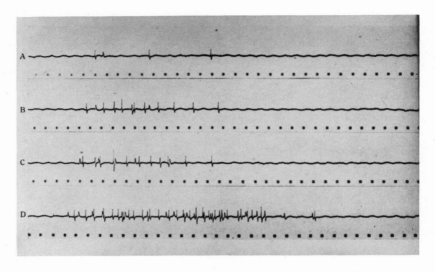

Fig. 10. Records from the same preparations as in Fig. 9 showing
          the effect of drops of water at: A. 50°; B. 60°; C. 70°;
          and D. 80°C. Repeating the same experiment on my own
          tongue. I found that a drop at 40°C was not felt as
          warm; a drop at 50°C was always felt as warm. A drop at
          70°C gave a faint burning sensation while a drop at 80°C
          always gave a distinct burning sensation. (Zotterman,
          1936)

the same stimulus to the operated side, and there was no twitching.
The patient correctly reported every touch and then said "It's
funny, I can't be tickled on this side of my face any longer." I
obtained identical results in other cases.

     It became evident for me from these studies that the sensation
generally spoken of as touch cannot be due to a simple mechanism.
This was also in good agreement with subjective experience in that
touch produces different sensations in different parts of the skin,
and that quantitative changes in the strength of a mechanical stimulus produce definite qualitative changes in sensation, indicating
different nervous mechanisms (Zotterman, 1939b). There has been
much debate ever since the days of Thunberg and Alrutz, 77 years
ago, whether tickle or itch is subserved by specific fibers separate from the "touch" and "pressure" fibers -- RA and SA fibers.
I am personally inclined to agree with Alrutz (1901) that we have

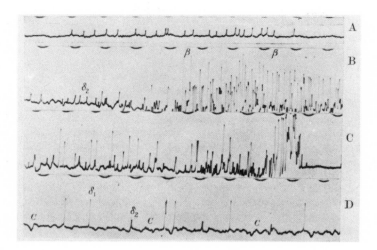

Fig. 11.   (To be read from the right). All strips from one record
           from a tiny strand of the saphenous nerve of the cat.
           A. Shows the response of two A-δ fibers alone to a light
           touch with cotton wool. B. The end of a very firm stroke.
           C. A needle prick. D. Four sec later with the needle
           still pressing on the skin with a constant pressure of
           52 g. time 1/40 sec. (Zotterman, 1939a)

specific endings for tickle in the skin.[1] In 1956 I received a
letter from Lord Adrian in which he writes that he is inclined to
accept my view "but what is the function of itching and tickling
receptors". "Well", I replied, "if you enter a cow stable you will
see how the flies touching the skin elicit a continuous reflex
activity of tails and heads. You must picture how the sensory
mechanisms of the skin have developed during millions of years while
mammals as well as humans have been living in and fighting a world
of insects".

     Finally I had reached what I had worked very hard for during 10
years. I kept on studying the behavior of cutaneous fibers but
they gave principally the same results as were described in my
paper of 1936, "Specific Impulses from the Lingual Nerve of the
Cat".

---

[1]Alrutz suggested that the "second pain" is mediated by a different neural mechanism than "first pain", a theory which was
ardently rejected by Thunberg in his chapter in the German Handbook
of Physiology, 1905. I am anxious to mention this because it shows
once again that you should trust your introspective analysis.

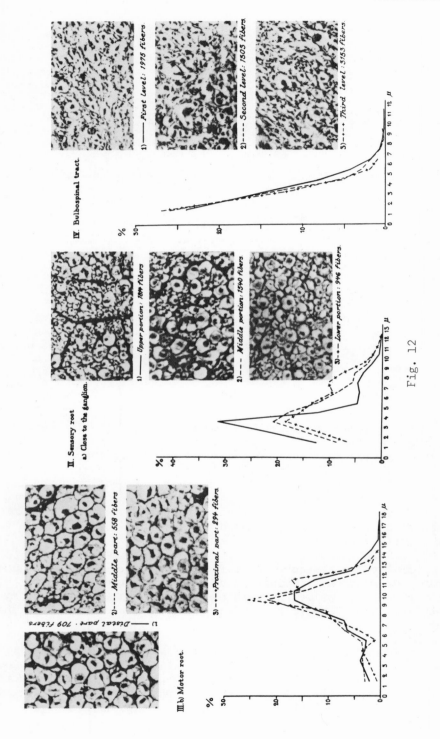

Fig. 12

Fig. 12.   A. Diagram and microphoto showing the diameter distribu-
           tion of the myelinated fibers of the trigeminal motor root.
           B. Diagram and microphoto of the fibers of the trigeminal
           sensory root near pons. C. Diagram and distribution of
           fibers in the bulbospinal trigeminal tract. (O. Sjöqvist,
           1938).

        Here I end my story on hunting pain fibers and other cutaneous
fibers. The rest of the story from the 1940s up to date which has
brought such great advances to our knowledge of the behavior of
sensory cutaneous fibers of all categories from amphibians and mammals to human beings, is largely due to the brillant contributions
of our gracious host Professor Dan Kenshalo and to many of his
guests at this symposium on "Sensory Functions of the Skin of Man".
I wish you further luck in hunting this big game.

        And now let me show the last photo I took of Edgar Douglas
Adrian in 1975 and let us honor the memory of our great master and
noble friend with a silent minute.

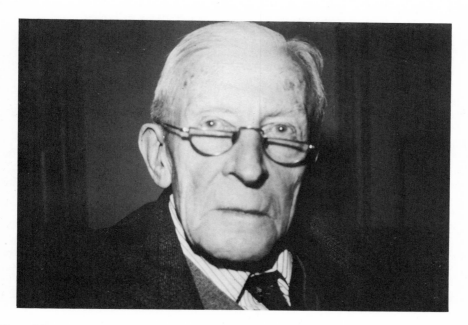

Fig. 13.   My last photo of Lord Adrian taken on March 1, 1975, in
           Cambridge. Lord Adrian was born on November 30, 1889,
           in London and died in Cambridge on August 4, 1977.

REFERENCES

Adrian, E. D. & Lucas, K. On the summation of propagated distur-
    bances in nerve and muscle. Journal of Physiology, 1912, 44,
    68-124.
Adrian, E. D. & Zotterman, Y. The impulses produced by sensory
    nerve endings. Part 2. The response of a single end-organ.
    Journal of Physiology, 1926a, 61, 151-171.
Adrian, E. D. & Zotterman, Y. The impulses produced by sensory
    nerve endings. Part 3. Impulses set up by touch and pres-
    sure. Journal of Physiology, 1926b, 61, 465-483.
Alrutz, S. Undersökningar över smärtsinnet (Studies in the sense
    of pain). Uppsala University Yearbook, 1901, 91,
Gasser, H. S., & Erlanger, J. American Journal of Physiology,
    1929, 88, 581-591.
Lucas, K. On the rate of development of the excitatory process in
    muscle and in nerve. Journal of Physiology, 1908, 37, 459-
    480.
Sjöqvist, O. Studies in pain conduction in the trigeminal nerve.
    Acta Psychiatrica and Neurologica, Suppl. XVIII, 1938, 139.
Thunberg, T. Undersökning över de köld-, värme-och smärtperci-
    pierande nervändarna. (Studies of cold, warmth and pain
    perceiving nerve-endings), Dissertation, Uppsala University,
    1900.
Zotterman, Y. Studies in the peripheral neural mechanism of pain.
    Acta Medica Scandinavica, 1933, 80, 185-242.
Zotterman, Y. Specific action potentials in the lingual nerve of
    cat. Scandinavica Archiv Physiologica, 1936, 75, 105-116.
Zotterman, Y. Touch, pain and tickling. An electrophysiological
    investigation on cutaneous sensory nerve. Journal of Phy-
    siology, 1939a, 95, 1-28.
Zotterman, Y. The nervous mechanism of touch and pain. Acta Psy-
    chiatrica and Neurologica, 1939b, 14, 91-97.

PSYCHOPHYSICAL AND NEUROPHYSIOLOGICAL METHODS TO STUDY PATIENTS

WITH SENSORY DISTURBANCES

R. G. Hallin, U. Lindblom and Z. Wiesenfeld

Departments of Clinical Neurophysiology and Neurology

Huddinge University Hospital, S-141 86 Huddinge (Sweden)

A specific diagnosis is essential for the optimal management and treatment of patients with somatosensory loss and/or dysesthesia. The diagnostic need can be met by utilizing a number of techniques from several disciplines. Recently developed methods have opened up new possibilities to study and reexamine clinical syndromes accompanied by sensory disturbances.

The aim of this paper is to focus interest on some old and new techniques which can be used in a combined approach to study sensory impairment following peripheral nerve lesions. In the investigations to be described, previously used psychophysical methods were integrated with new techniques for quantitative mechanical and thermal skin stimulation. The electrophysiological examinations included conventional neurography and electromyography. Percutaneous microelectrode recordings from the peripheral nerves (microneurography) were done in selected patients, since it was believed that such explorations would contribute to our understanding of the underlying pathophysiology.

As an introduction to each main section below, some basic findings obtained with the different technqiues will be briefly described. The latter parts of the sections concern more recent preliminary results found by using this multiple approach on patients with sutured median nerves.

SOME GENERAL METHODOLOGICAL CONSIDERATIONS

The psychophysical methods and the techniques for quantitative estimation of mechanical and thermal thresholds used have been applied repeatedly in normals and in patients with various neurological

disorders. Since these procedures are safe, relatively simple to
perform, and not very time consuming they can be applied clinically
as routine screening methods in centers with basic technical and
medical facilities.

Conventionally used electromyographic and neurographic techniques require some engineering aid and they also call for a certain skill and experience by the investigator executing the examinations.

The microneurographic technique demands much more both in
terms of technical facilities available, and in terms of personal
qualifications of the investigator. A common situation during the
exploring procedure is that the microelectrode fails to record
neural activity although the electrode appears to be situated
within the nerve. This is most probably due to positioning of the
electrode tip in epineural tissue between the nerve fascicles

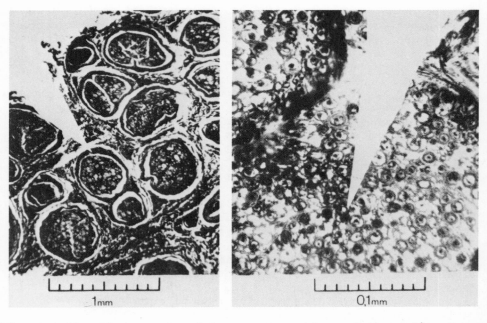

1mm   0,1mm

Fig. 1. Microphotographs of tranverse sections of the median nerve
         at the wrist level with the silhouette of a microelec-
         trode superimposed. Sections stained by eosin. Nerve
         shrinkage estimated at about 20%. The approximate length
         of the bare electrode tip is indicated schematically by
         the phantoms. (Hagbarth, Hongell, and Hallin, 1970).

as indicated in Fig. 1 (left). A thorough search for neural activities may be rewarding, however, since the electrode tip once within a fascicle (Fig. 1, right) sometimes can pick up signals from
the full nerve fiber spectrum, including the thin unmyelinated C-
fibers (Fig. 2). Since the search for nerve activity sometimes
takes more than an hour, there is a risk of nerve fiber damage involved in the explorations. Even if shown to be small (Torebjörk
and Hallin, 1978) this risk cannot be neglected. It must be considered as an ethical problem especially when recording from patients with manifest nerve lesions. The person executing these
nerve explorations should preferably have been trained in a laboratory where this technique has been in use for some time.

PSYCHOPHYSICAL METHODS FOR MEASUREMENTS OF TACTILE SENSITIVITY

There is a vast literature on psychophysical methods for studying cutaneous sensation in normal man (for references, see Marks,
1974; Stevens, S. S., 1957). Comparatively few investigators have
used quantitative measurements of mechanical stimuli to study skin
sensitivity in patients (Dyck, 1975; Verrillo and Ecker, 1977).
Recently, threshold amplitudes for passive touch were measured in
human glabrous skin using single mechanical pulses delivered to
the skin (Lindblom, 1974). Threshold functions have been investigated both in normals (Lindblom and Lindström, 1976; Vallbo
and Johansson, 1976) and in patients (Franzén and Lindblom, 1976;
Lindblom and Meyerson, 1975; Lindblom and Verrillo, 1978). The
threshold values for touch were of the order of 5 to 10 μm in the
finger tips of normals, and the finger tips were all about equally
sensitive. More proximally in the hand the thresholds were higher,
which in part might reflect anatomical differences in receptor
density, the palm being less densely innervated than the finger tips
(Johansson and Vallbo, 1976; Vallbo and Johansson, 1976). Patho-
logically low threshold values for touch have been found in patients with hyperalgesia (Lindblom, 1978).

Patients previously subjected to a complete traumatic uni-
lateral cut of the median nerve at the wrist have been studied with
different modes of mechanical stimulation. The investigations were
performed several years after nerve suture. The patients were all
somewhat handicapped by their nerve lesions and displayed a variety
of sensory disturbances. Fine motor control in the hand was impaired and routine electromyography revealed a reduced number of
motor units in some of the intrinsic muscles of the injured hand.

Conventional neurological screening methods for sensory examinations, such as light touch with cotton wool and pin pricking
(Moberg, 1958; 1962), revealed hyposensitivity in the skin of the
palm and fingers of the affected hand. Hypersensitivity in the
form of tingling and unpleasant paresthesias radiating into the
whole innervation area of the nerve was unmasked when testing with

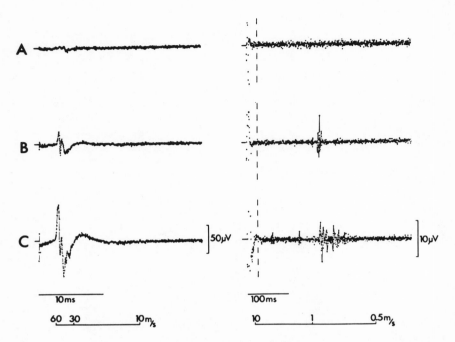

Fig. 2.   Median nerve responses induced by intradermal electrical
          shocks delivered at 0.5/sec to the volar aspect of the in-
          dex finger 15.5 cm from the recording site.   Electronic
          averaging of 50 successive sweeps.   To emphasize waves in
          the records, individual dots in the computer display have
          been joined by drawn lines.   The left row shows parts of
          the early A-fiber response, and the right row shows late
          C deflections.   The vertical interrupted line delimits
          the extension of the early waves visualized in the left
          row on displaying the response with long time base (right).
          Horizontal scales indicate the conduction velocity in
          m/sec for various components in the multifiber response.
          A.   On stimulation at the threshold for perception an
          early response was just discernible from the noise but no
          late waves appeared.   B.   When the stimulus was experi-
          enced as a prickling sensation both early A and late C
          waves were identified.   C.   On painful stimulation, addi-
          tional components were recruited to the nerve response.
          (Hallin and Torebjörk, 1973)

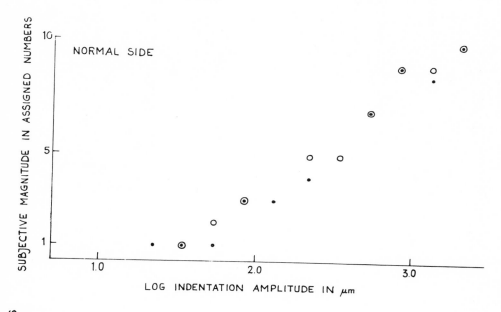

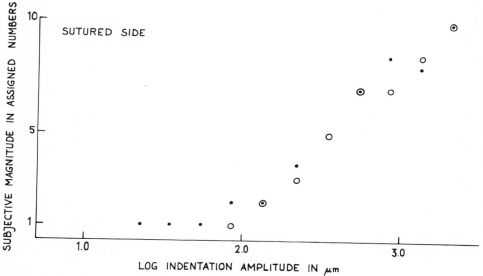

Fig. 3.   Magnitude estimation of tactile sensation by a patient with
          8 year old sutured median nerve lesion. Stimulation with
          single mechanical pulses of 50 Hz. Above and below are
          the responses to stimulation of the finger pad of the
          normal and injured hands, respectively. Abscissa: stimu-
          lus amplitude in μm of skin indentation, logarithmic
          scale. Ordinate: numberical subjective estimates, linear

scale. Filled circles indicate stimulation of index finger pad, open circles stimulation of thenar eminence.
Sensation thresholds on normal and abnormal side, respectively: finger pad, 6 and 26 μm; thenar eminence,
28 and 46 μm. Note graded intensity function on both
sides but steeper on sutured side.

strong mechanical or noxious skin stimuli. As previously shown
(Franzén and Lindblom,1976), and exemplified by the quantitative
testing visualized in Fig. 3, the threshold for single mechanical
pulses was generally raised on the affected side. The suprathreshold intensity functions were smoothly graded on both the
normal (Fig. 3-top) and the injured side (Fig. 3-bottom), the only
difference being a steeper slope in the hand with defective sensitivity.

These findings indicate that the innervation of a hand many
years after median nerve suture, although not adequate for normal
tactile sensibility, still may be sufficient for discriminating
some types of mechanical stimuli.

QUANTITATIVE ESTIMATIONS OF THERMAL THRESHOLDS

A previously used psychophysical research method to study
temperature sensitivity (Kenshalo and Scott, 1966) was recently
improved to enable relatively simple measurements of warm, cold,
cold pain and heat pain thresholds in patients (Fruhstorfer,
Lindblom, and Schmidt, 1976). The stimulator used consists of semi-
conductor junctions operating on the Peltier principle. A current
passing through the thermally buffered device produces a temperature difference between its two sides. Depending on the direction
of the current, the stimulated skin surface can be either warmed
or cooled with great accuracy. This method of testing thermal
sensibility has been applied both to normals and to patients with
various neurological disorders (Fruhstorfer, Goldberg, and Lindblom,
1976; Lindblom and Verrillo, 1978). Normally, the thermal thresholds
vary regionally and among individuals, whereas intraindividual determinations are more stable provided that the perceptive criteria of
the subjects are unchanged. A comparison of the normal data with
values obtained in patients with uremia neuropathy indicates that,
in particular, the difference in warm and cold thresholds, the
warm-cold difference limen, is a relatively sensitive parameter to
distinguish between normal and pathological thermosensitivity
(Fruhstorfer, Goldberg, and Lindblom, 1976).

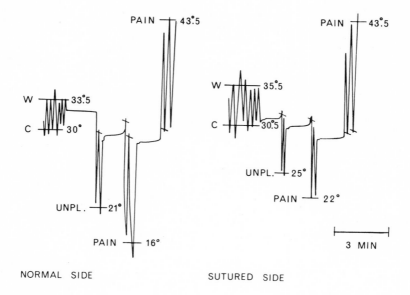

NORMAL SIDE   SUTURED SIDE

Fig. 4.   Marstock record from same patient as illustrated in Fig.
3 showing in °C, estimated warm and cold detection thresholds, levels of unpleasant and painful cold, and of heat
pain.   Note increase of warm detection threshold and higher level of cold pain (cold "hyperalgesia"), but retained
heat pain level on sutured side.

In cases of median nerve lesions, the above finding was confirmed, as illustrated in Fig. 4.   In comparison with the normal
values in the left hand the warm threshold on the sutured side, as
well as the tactile thresholds (Fig. 3), were still raised eight
years after the nerve suture.   Interestingly, this patient also had
a pathological cold pain threshold on the affected side whereas the
heat pain threshold was within the normal range.

The results of the previously discussed psychophysical testing
with mechanical stimuli agreed with the impression from the clinical
examination in indicating marked sensory disturbances in the affected hand of the patient.   The outcome of the quantitative thermal
tests added additional information in suggesting a deficit of the
thermal sensibility as well.   The results are indicative of in-
complete and abnormal regeneration of the sutured nerve.   As will
be shown below the sensory loss can be further evaluated by neurophysiological investigations of the functions of the regenerated
nerves.

CLINICAL NEUROPHYSIOLOGICAL INVESTIGATIONS

Conventional Neurography

        In studies of peripheral sensory nerve function in man,
electric skin nerve shocks are often used to elicit nerual activity,
which can be recorded as compound potentials with macroelectrodes
placed proximally near the nerve trunk (Buchthal and Rosenfalck,
1966; Dawson, 1956; Dawson and Scott, 1949; Eichler, 1937). This
method permits recording of synchronized volleys in myelinated fibers
and has been used by many investigators in clinical diagnostic work.

        In the patients with sutured nerves who had been previously
tested psychophysically, we performed conventional median nerve
neurography bilaterally to get objective measurements of the function of the various digital nerves. Ring electrodes were placed
around each individual finger for stimulating the digital nerves as
described by Buchthal and Rosenfalck (1966). The recording surface
electrode was positioned on the skin overlying the median nerve
proximal to the site of injury. As expected the potentials recorded from the digital nerves in the injured hand had lower amplitudes and longer durations than on the normal side, suggesting
a decreased number and reduced conduction velocities of myelinated
fibers. The pathological changes in the neural responses were
most pronounced in the digital nerves that supplied the skin areas
where the subjective sensory loss was greatest. In this context it
might be worth mentioning that Almqvist and Eeg-Olofsson (1970)
found no correlation between two-point discrimination (as test for
skin sensibility) and conduction velocity when examining skin sensation in patients with sutured nerves.

Microneurography

        Percutaneously inserted tungsten microelectrodes permit re-
cording of sensory impulses from intact human peripheral nerves
(Hagbarth, Hongell, and Hallin, 1970; Vallbo and Hagbarth, 1968)
either as multiunit or as single unit activity. When multiunit
activity is recorded the electrode has passed partly or completely
into a fascicle where it selectively picks up signals from intact
fibers within this particular fascicle (Fig. 1). Single unit activity
is derived from individual nerve fibers which are often damaged by
the electrode tip. In skin nerves Hallin and Torebjörk (1970; 1973)
and Torebjörk and Hallin (1970; 1973; 1974) demonstrated that this
technique permits recording of both multiunit and single unit
activity derived from the entire spectrum of nerve fibers (Fig. 2)
including the thin, unmyelinated C-fibers.

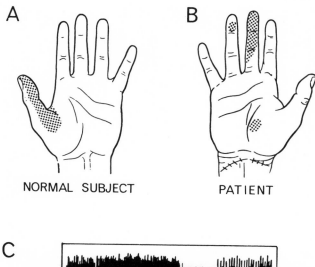

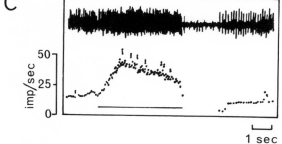

Fig. 5. Examples of receptive fields encountered in normals (A)
and in patients with sutured median nerves (B). C. Responses of a SA II afferent with a receptive field in reinnervated skin to stretching of the skin around the nail
in dorsal-volar direction. On the top is the actual response of the unit and on the bottom the instantaneous
firing frequency. The duration of the stretch is indicated with a bar under the record of the firing frequency.

Multiunit activity was recorded with microelectrodes from
the patients' median nerves proximal to the site of the injury.
Normally the fascicular median nerve receptive fields, as tested
with brief touch stimuli, are contiguous and more or less correspond to the innervation zone of one digital nerve, as shown in
Fig. 5A. By contrast, in two of the patients explored so far we
repeatedly observed patchy types of receptive fields with innervation zones distributed in 3 or 4 different areas on several

fingers and the palm (Fig. 5B). In a few cases unitary activity was recorded in the sutured nerve but so far only one afferent unit has been reliably classified. This unit showed a regular static spontaneous discharge of around 10 imp/sec in the absence of intentional stimuli. Its receptive field was located in reinnervated skin near the nail on the index finger. The unit responded in a slowly adapting manner. It showed a substantial increase in discharge frequency, up to a maximum of about 40 imp/sec, when the skin near the nail was stretched in volar-dorsal direction (Fig. 5C). Upon release of the skin stretch there was a short pause in the firing until, after a few seconds, the spontaneous unitary firing was resumed at the previous rate. The unit was identified as a slowly adapting Type II unit (Iggo, 1966) and its overall response characteristics suggested that its behavior most probably did not notably differ from that of a normal afferent of this type.

The outcome of the psychophysical tests performed on the patient group with sutured nerves are in accordance with the neurographic data described above in suggesting a deficient median nerve reinnervation after conventional nerve suture in man. The findings derived from the few microelectrode explorations done so far in sutured nerves go further and may indicate that the organization of the nerve fascicles in such nerves is pathological. In spite of this at least some cutaneous receptors in reinnervated skin appear to acquire virtually normal firing characteristics, agreeing with previous observations on regenerated cutaneous afferents in the cat (Burgess and Horch, 1973). The preliminary data described demonstrate that it is possible to study the firing characteristics of single regenerated sensory afferents in man.

COMMENTS

Conditions with sensory disturbances are common in clinical neurology. As shown here, an analysis of such syndromes with a whole battery of tests may give new detailed information concerning the underlying pathophysiology. As an example we present data from patients with sutured peripheral nerves, but the techniques can be used for investigation of other types of patients as well. This multiple approach is of interest from both the clinical and basic neurophysiological points of view and may eventually have therapeutic implications in elective cases.

ACKNOWLEDGMENTS

The study was supported by the Swedish Medical Research Council (projects no. B78-14X-04256-05C and K78-04V-5318-01), the Research Funds of Karolinska Institute, and Harald and Greta Jeansson's Foundations.

REFERENCES

Almquist, E. & Eeg-Olofsson, O. Sensory-nerve-conducting velocity and two-point discrimination in sutured nerves. Journal of Bone and Joint Surgery, 1970, 52-A, 791-796.

Buchthal, F. & Rosenfalck, A. Evoked action potentials and conduction velocity in human sensation nerves. Brain Research, 1966, 3, 1-122.

Burgess, P. R. & Horch, K. W. Specific regeneration of cutaneous fibers in the cat. Journal of Neurophysiology, 1973, 36, 101-114.

Dawson, G. D. The relative excitability and conduction velocity of sensory and motor nerve fibers in man. Journal of Physiology (London), 1956, 131, 436-451.

Dawson, G. D. & Scott, J. W. The recordings of nerve action potentials through skin in man. Journal of Neurology, Neurosurgery and Psychiatry, 1949, 12, 259-267.

Dyck, P. J. Quantitation of cutaneous sensation in man. In P. J. Dyck, P. K. Thomas and E. T. Lambert (Eds.), Peripheral neuropathy. Philadelphia: W. B. Saunders, 1975.

Eichler, W. Über die Ableitung der Aktionspotentiale vom menschlichen Nerven in situ. Zeitschrift für Biology, 1937, 98, 182-214.

Franzén. O. & Lindblom, U. Tactile intensity functions in patients with sutured peripheral nerve. In Y. Zotterman (Ed.), Sensory functions of the skin in primates. Oxford: Pergamon Press, 1976.

Fruhstorfer, H., Lindblom, U., & Schmidt, W. G. Temperature sensitivity and pain thresholds in patients with peripheral neuropathy. In Y. Zotterman (Ed.), Sensory functions of the skin of primates. Oxford: Pergamon Press, 1976.

Fruhstorfer, H., Lindblom, U., & Schmidt, W. G. Method for quantitative estimation of thermal thresholds in patients. Journal of Neurology, Neurosurgery, and Psychiatry, 1976, 39,1071-1076.

Hagbarth, K.-E., Hongell, A., Hallin, R. G., & Torebjörk, H. E. Afferent impulses in median nerve fascicles evoked by tactile stimuli of the human hand. Brain Research, 1970, 24, 423-442.

Hallin, R. G. & Torebjörk, H. E. C-fibre components in electrically evoked compound potentials recorded from human median nerve fascicles in situ. Acta Societatis Medicorum Upsaliensis, 1970, 73, 77-80.

Hallin, R. G. & Torebjörk, H. E. Electrically induced A and C fibre responses in intact human skin nerves. Experimental Brain Research, 1973, 16, 309-320.

Iggo, A. Cutaneous receptors with a high sensitivity mechanical
    displacement. In A. V. S. DeRueck and J. Knight (Eds.),
    Ciba foundation symposium, touch, heat and pain. Boston:
    Little, Brown and Co., 1966.
Johansson, R. & Vallbo, Å. B. Skin mechanoreceptors in the human
    hand: an inference of some population properties. In Y.
    Zotterman (Ed.), Sensory functions of the skin of primates,
    Oxford and New York: Pergamon Press, 1976.
Kenshalo, D. R. & Scott, H. S. Temporal course of thermal adapta-
    tion. Science, 1966, 151, 1095-1096.
Lindblom, U. Touch perception threshold in human glabrous skin in
    terms of displacement amplitude on stimulation with single
    mechanical pulses. Brain Research, 1974, 82, 205-210.
Lindblom, U. Sensory abnormalities in neuralgia. In J. Bonica,
    J. Liebeskind and D. Albe-Fessard (Eds.),Advances in pain
    research and therapy (Vol. 3). 1978. In press.
Lindblom, U. & Lindström, B. Tactile thresholds of normal and
    blind subjects on stimulation of finger pads with short
    mechanical pulses of variable amplitude. In Y. Zotterman
    (Ed.), Sensory functions of the skin of primates. Oxford and
    New York: Pergamon Press, 1976.
Lindblom, U. & Meyerson, B.A. Influence on touch, vibration and
    cutaneous pain of dorsal column stimulation in man. Pain,
    1975, 1, 257-270.
Lindblom, U. & Verrillo, R. T. Sensory functions in chronic
    neuralgia. Journal of Neurology, Neurosurgery and Psychiatry,
    1978. In press.
Marks, L. E. Sensory processes. New York: Academic Press, 1974.
Moberg, E. Objective methods in determining the functional value
    of sensibility in the hand. Journal of Bone and Joint Surgery,
    1958, 40-B, 454-476.
Moberg, E. Criticism and study of methods for examining sensibility
    in the hand. Neurology, 1962, 12, 8-19.
Stevens, S. S. On the psychophysical law. Psychological Review,
    1957, 64, 153-181.
Torebjörk, H. E. & Hallin, R. G. C-fibre units recorded from hu-
    man sensory nerve fascicles in situ. Acta Societatis Medi-
    corum Upsaliensis, 1970, 75, 81-84.
Torebjörk, H. E. & Hallin, R. G. Perceptual changes accompanying
    controlled preferential blocking of A and C fibre responses
    in intact human nerves. Experimental Brain Research, 1973,
    16, 321-332.
Torebjörk, H. E. & Hallin, R. G. Identifcation of afferent C
    units in intact human skin nerves. Brain Research, 1974, 67,
    387-403.
Torebjörk, H. E. & Hallin, R. G. Microneurographic studies of peri-
    pheral pain mechanisms in man. In J. Bonica, J. Liebeskind
    & D. Albe-Fessard (Eds.), Advances in pain research and thera-
    py (Vol. 3). 1978, In press.

Vallbo, Å. B. & Hagbarth, K.-E. Activity from skin mechano-re-
    ceptors recorded percutaneously in awake human subjects.
    Experimental Neurology, 1968, 21, 270-289.
Vallbo, Å. B. & Johansson, R. Skin mechanoreceptors in the human
    hand: neural and psychophysical thresholds. In Y. Zotterman
    (Ed.), Sensory functions of the skin in primates. Oxford
    and New York: Pergamon Press, 1976.
Verrillo, R. T. & Ecker, A. D. Effects of root or nerve des-
    truction on vibrotactile sensitivity in trigeminal neuralgia.
    Pain, 1977, 3, 239-255.

DISCUSSION

DR. TOREBJÖRK: Your Fig. 5C illustrates some of the drawbacks with the microneurographic technique in clinical studies. It has the obvious advantage that one can record activity from the entire nerve fiber spectrum including the thinnest fibers which, for example, you cannot do with the Buchthal method (Buchthal & Rosenfalck, 1966). But it has the drawback that it is perhaps too selective. A single unit can dominate the recording, as in this case which is taken from the median nerve (Hallin & Torebjörk, 1974), and you may see that a single fiber, with conduction velocity of 17 m/sec, is actually dominating the recording at the threshold for perception. One can see it all the time when one increases the stimulus intensity. It is very difficult, then, to use this method in order to estimate the absolute numbers of fibers from which a record is made. All that can be said is that there are fibers of different types, but it cannot be used to count the number of fibers.

DR. LINDBLOM: I quite agree. That is an important point that one cannot conclude too much from single unit studies. The whole fiber spectrum can only be studied with biopsy. This is done sometimes, but in the median nerve patients biopsies are not possible for ethical reasons.

DR. HENSEL: You have shown a picture of the response of an SA II fiber and I would like to know if you have done any experiments with thermal stimulation as well.

DR. LINDBLOM: No, we have not.

DR. ZOTTERMAN: Does anyone know the reason why the C fibers regenerate so much quicker than the myelinated fibers?

DR. LINDBLOM: No, it is very difficult to explain. It is an old observation that C fiber functions recover much quicker then the coarse fiber functions.

DR. FRANZEN: Just a short comment to our previous study (Franzén & Lindblom, 1976). I think the reason we got a good fit the last time was that we had a shorter stimulus range. Here, however, when one gets close to threshold the function deviates from a straight line in a log-log plot, and is what we found also, because some of the functions can be corrected by an additive constant.

DR. VERRILLO: I have a question about this figure (Fig. 3). This is for one subject?

DR. LINDBLOM: Yes, this is one subject. Two samples of data were obtained, the filled points are from the finger pad and the open circles are from the thenar. It shows that the finger tips and the thenar behave similarly, although the threshold is a bit higher on the thenar.

DR. VERRILLO: I am a little surprised that you got the same slope from the finger pad and the thenar eminence with your conditions.

DR. LINDBLOM: So am I, but, nevertheless, with our conditions we got it. It is possible that one would get a separation between the functions for the thenar eminence and the finger tip, if one were to make a very careful study in normal subjects where one had plenty of time and could make several trials.

DR. VERRILLO: Because our studies on the finger pad and the thenar eminence show the steeper slope for the latter, we said it was because of the denser innervation of the finger tip. Do you agree with that?

DR. STEVENS: As you said, Dr. Lindblom, hypoesthesias usually appear in measurements of threshold and hyperesthesias at suprathreshold levels. I thought you might be interested in one apparent exception to that rule. A colleague of mine at the Pierce Foundation, Dr. Linda Bartoshuk, has studied thresholds and suprathresholds responses to taste in patients who are undergoing radiation therapy. What typically happened was that after radiation, suprathreshold responses remain greatly depressed long after the thresholds had recovered. That may be the only example in the entire nervous system of a phenomenon like that, but it is interesting to know that it can occur, and I think that it underscores your own apparent conviction that it is important to look at suprathreshold magnitudes as well as at the threshold.

DR. LINDBLOM: It is very interesting to hear.

REFERENCES

Buchthal, F., & Rosenfalck, A. Evoked action and conduction velocity in human sensory nerves. Brain Research, 1966, 3, 1-122.
Franzén, O., & Lindblom, U. Tactile intensity functions in patients with sutured peripheral nerve. In Y. Zotterman (Ed.), Sensory functions of the skin in primates. Oxford: Pergamon, 1976.
Hallin, R. G. & Torebjörk, H. E. Activity in unmyelinated nerve fibers in man. In J. J. Bonica (Ed.), Advances in neurology (Vol. 4). New York: Raven Press, 1974.

PRECISION AND AMBIGUITY IN CODING VIBROTACTILE INFORMATION

Ove Franzén
Department of Psychology, University of Uppsala

Erik Torebjörk, Department of Clinical Neurophysiology,
University Hospital, Uppsala, Sweden

In diagnosing a disease palpation and percussion carried out by the hand depends among other things, on its great vibrotactile sensibility (pallaethesia). Helen Keller has also witnessed about the importance of somesthesis:..." I perceive countless vibrations. By placing my hand on a person's lips and throat, I gain an idea of many specific vibrations...".

Mechanoreception through the skin can be described as touch, pressure and vibration. As stimuli, touch is transient, pressure static and vibration intermittent deformation of the integument. Tickling elicited by light mechanical stimuli as e.g., a stroke with a piece of cotton-wool is considered a separate sub-sense as we have learned from Zotterman's pioneering work (1939).

The receptor apparatus for touch, pressure and vibration is assumed to be partly separate, partly shared. Velocity-sensitive receptors that respond to tactile stimuli are located both in glabrous and hairy skin as well as in subcutaneous and deeper tissue (Montagna, 1960; Quilliam, 1966). Certain receptors are rapidly adapting (RA) whereas others are slow in that respect. The latter may contribute to the sensation of pressure.

Input-output characteristics of the RA receptors have been studied under pulse stimulation or linear deformation in combination with psychophysical measurements (Franzén and Lindblom, 1976) and the PC receptors under sinusoidal stimulation (Sato, 1961; Lindblom and Lund, 1966; Talbot, Darian-Smith, Kornhuber, and Mountcastle, 1968). The steady discharge from slowly adapting endings has been explored by means of static deformation of variable force and amplitude (Knibestöl, 1975; Werner and Mountcastle, 1965).

39

In the middle of the sixties there was still much debate about the process underlying the perception of mechanical vibration because some psychophysical results seemed to be in conflict with the neurophysiological finding (Lindblom, 1966, pp. 158-163). However, Franzén (1965) pointed out that vibratory stimulation produces a U-shaped threshold curve as a function of frequency with a minimum in the neighborhood of 250 Hz and that isolated Pacinian corpuscles also have best tuning frequencies at about 250 Hz (Sato, 1961). The two sets of data show striking similarities. It was also noted that the behavior of the Pacinian corpuscles cannot singly explain the characteristics of the whole threshold curve. The same comments were made by Verrillo (1966) in his discussion of a duplex mechanism of vibrotaction.

An important contribution to this issue was made by Talbot et al. (1968) in their psychophysical threshold studies on humans and electrophysiological recordings from mechanoreceptive afferents in primates. The dual mechanism of vibrotaction of the hand is so far best understood in terms of the intracutaneously located Meissner receptors and the subcutaneously located Pacinian receptors.

The purpose of the present study is to fill a gap between receptor function and perception at liminal and supraliminal levels of stimulation by a combined use of psychophysical methods and a single unit recording technique in humans and, specifically, to understand the mechanisms by which the two fundamental dimensions of intensity and frequency are coded in an unambiguous fashion.

CODING OF INTENSITY

Psychophysics

Procedures of modern psychophysics to establish scales of subjective magnitude fall mainly into two classes: indirect and direct methods (Torgerson, 1958; Marks, 1974). In our experiments the direct method of magnitude estimation developed by S. S. Stevens (1957) was employed to determine the form of the psychophysical functions for vibratory sinusoidal stimuli applied to the finger tip. The signals varied in both intensity and frequency. The task of the observer was to assign numbers to each stimulus in such a way that the numbers corresponded to his impressions. The method is of course based on the possibly strong assumption that the number continuum is proportional to sensory experience. With a standard stimulus prescribed by the experimenter a sensory ratio between subjective magnitudes can be assessed. For further details see Franzén (1969).

The average estimates for a group of six subjects were computed and plotted in logarithmic coordinates (Fig. 1). For these ranges

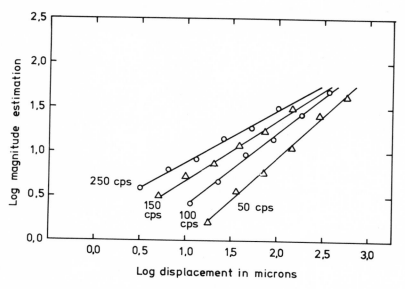

Fig. 1.   Intensity functions for vibratory stimulation of different
           frequencies. (Franzén, 1969)

of displacement amplitudes the data approximate straight lines indicating that the scales are well described by power functions of
the form $R=cA^n$ where R is the subjective magnitude, c is the multiplicative constant (related to the unit of measurement), A is the
displacement amplitude and n is the exponent. For the four frequencies examined - 50, 100, 150 and 250 Hz - the best fitting
power functions describing the relationship between the subjective
and physical intensity were as follows:

$$R_{50} = 0.11 \cdot A^{0.95}$$

$$R_{100} = 0.35 \cdot A^{0.81}$$

$$R^{150} = 1.12 \cdot A^{0.70}$$

$$R_{250} = 2.04 \cdot A^{0.58}$$

Growth rate is clearly a linear function of the stimulus raised to
a power. The psychophysical exponent and the multiplicative constant depend on stimulation frequency i.e. the higher the frequency
the flatter is the log-log function. The parameters of this family
of functions are plotted in semi-logarithmic coordinates (Fig. 2)

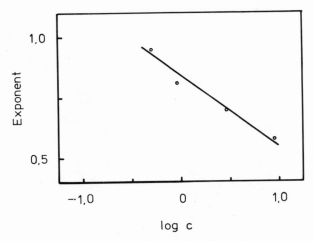

Fig. 2.   The constants of the psychophysical power function, R = cA^n, in Fig. 1 plotted in semi-logarithmic coordinates.

where the inverse relation between the constants of the power functions is best summarized by a function of the form, $n = a - 0.28 \log c$. Similar relationships can be derived for other sense modalities (e.g. Stevens and Stevens, 1963; Franzén and Berkley, 1975).

   Detection threshold examined for frequencies above the flutter range (> 40 Hz) (Talbot et al., 1968) exhibited its well-established dependency on frequency (Fig. 3). The average tuning curve for a sample of Pacinian afferents innervating the glabrous skin of the monkey hand (Talbot et al., 1968) is displayed in the same graph. As was noted above the multiplicative constant of the psychophysical power functions that is related to the unit of measurement covered quite one log as do the threshold data. A most interesting relationship is therefore observed in Fig. 3 namely, that the reciprocal of this constant runs almost parallel to the perceptual and neurophysiological thresholds. Thus, the subjective magnitude estimation function for frequencies between 50 to 250 Hz is directly reflected in the response characteristics of Pacinian afferents, in all likelihood subserving the vibratory sensation.

   If we slice horizontally the magnitude functions in Fig. 1 a family of equal-vibness curves could be mapped as shown in Fig. 4.

   These curves are very similar to two curves obtained by Goff (1959) and confirmed in an extended matching study carried out by

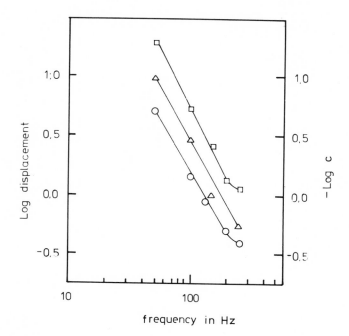

Fig. 3. Comparison of neural and perceptual threshold functions and
         the reciprocal of the multiplicative constant of the psy-
         chophysical power functions for four different frequencies.
         a) squares represent the average tuning curve for primate
         Pacinian afferents (replotted from Talbot et al., 1968).
         b) triangles represent the inverse of the multiplicative
         constant (c) of the power functions in Fig. 1.
         c) circles represent detection threshold as a function of
         frequency for the same subjects as in Fig. 1.
         The displacement amplitude is specified in microns RMS.

Ross and reported by Stevens (1968). All these data taken together
indicate that we are dealing with genuine perceptual phenomena.

     The vibrotactile functions bear also a resemblance to analogous
curves in audition (Kingsbury, 1927; Fletcher and Munson, 1933)
suggesting that similar underlying mechanisms may be operative in
the two senses.

Single Unit Activity in Pacinian Afferents

     Because of the good agreement between the psychophysical and
electrophysiological observations presented in Fig. 3 we will

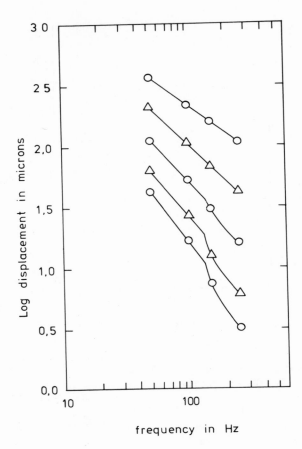

Fig. 4.   Equal-vibness contours derived from the magnitude func-
          tions in Fig. 1.   (Franzen, 1969).

concentrate our interest on Pacinian receptors in what follows.

        Single fiber recordings were made from median nerve fascicles
10 cm proximal to the elbow. Tungsten electrodes with a shaft
diameter of 0.2 mm and a tip of 1-5 microns were used (Hagbarth and
Vallbo, 1967; Vallbo and Hagbarth, 1968). The signals were amplified by an AC preamplifier and recorded on magnetic tape for later
analysis of the experimental data. Half-wave rectified sinusoids
from a waveform generator energized a vibrator mounted on a stand
that allowed the delivery of pulses to almost any area of the palm
of the hand. The waveform and duration of the pulses can be seen
in Fig. 5 and 7. The stimulator probe had a diameter of 2 mm.

During our search for Pacinian afferents we could confirm the existence of the four different types of mechanoreceptive afferents that were first shown by Knibestöl and Vallbo (1970). The Pacinian receptors which are rarely found are recognized by their receptive field characteristics: large field with indistinct borders and one single sensitivity maximum and absence of steady discharge at constant skin indentation. The discharge of Pacinian fibers was entrained by the stimulus up to 250 pps for a stimulus duration of at least one second which was the longest duration in the psychophysical experiments. The conduction velocity for these fibers ranged between 25-45 m/sec. In these measurements a' step skin indentation was used to determine the latency. This way of measuring conduction velocity presumably leads to an underestimation of the real velocity since transduction time is not known and consequently cannot be subtracted.

In Fig. 5 it is seen that the fiber discharges on all-or-nothing spike per cycle and that no change in the synchronous impulse pattern takes place with increasing intensity although this increment in amplitude was accompanied by a clear change in subjective intensity. Double discharges were occasionally observed for this particular frequency (50 Hz). At higher rates (200 Hz) this observation was never made.

Since the transducer mechanism transmits effectively the stimulus frequency but saturates at low intensity levels, the magnitude of the vibratory stimulus (50 - 250 Hz) is signalled to the brain by progressive recruitment of PC receptors. Thus, the subjective impression is based on the integrated peripheral activity. A direct comparison between the integrated receptor potential recorded from the human olfactory mucosa and sensory experience has

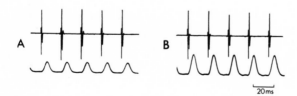

Fig. 5. Single unit activity from a PC fiber innervating the glabrous skin of the hand. Stimulation frequency 50 Hz. Indentation amplitude: A,50μm; B,100μm. Lower trace shows the waveform of the stimulus.

been made by Franzén, Osterhammel, Terkildsen, and Zilstorff,
(1970) who found a close correspondence between the two sets of
measurements. The sensitivity of the Pacinian system seems to determine the rate at which the neural elements are recruited and
consequently the form of the supraliminal functions for the frequencies investigated. This mechanism is suggestive of recent observations on the intensity functions in patients with peripheral
nerve lesions (Franzén and Lindblom,1976). Furthermore, the point
of convergence of the subjective magnitude functions is thus interpreted as that intensity level at which the same number of receptors are excited independently of the carrier frequency of the
vibratory stimulus.

CODING OF FREQUENCY

     What precision has the perceptual pathway in a frequency dis-
crimination task and what constitutes the code for vibratory pitch?

Psychophysics

     Half-wave rectified sinusoids of 2 msec duration were applied
to the finger-tip. By using trains of short mechanical pulses instead of sinusoids and thus removing any ambiguity as to the time
of application of the stimulus, measurements of frequency discrimination could be extended down to 1 Hz. An added advantage to short
pulses in preference to sinusoids was to eliminate a possible source
of variation in the presentation of the vibratory stimulus. The
subject was asked to match pairs of pulse frequency between 1 and
256 Hz. The standard frequency set by the experimenter was separated by a silent interval of 0.4 msec from that under the subject's control. Thus, the subject had to adjust the frequency of
the comparison stimulus to produce a subjective match with the
standard. Each of the six subjects made 20 settings per frequency.
A timer determined the interval between the two pulses of the pulse
train corresponding to the setting. For further details see
Franzén and Nordmark (1975).

     The estimation of frequency for mechanical pulses delivered
at rates of 1 to 4 per second is obviously based on time interval
measurements. We assume, however, that the same time mechanism
is operative over the whole frequency range. It seems therefore
logical to represent the standard and comparison stimuli in the
time domain as is done in Fig. 6. Although the percept changes as
frequency is changed from the lowest pulse rates to that range in
which the pulse trains elicit a sensation of vibratory pitch, the
match between the input and output data is excellent as indicated
by the nice fit of a straight line of unit slope. (Pulse frequency
of 1 to 256 Hz correspond to 1000 to 3.91 msec in the time domain).
The central detector appears to reproduce faithfully the stimulus

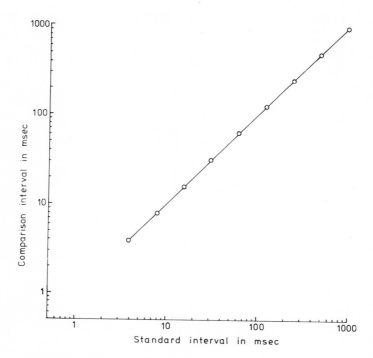

Fig. 6.   Standard intervals plotted against comparison intervals
           corresponding to 1 to 256 Hz.

event.   Also, an almost perfect neural replica of the input must be
stored in the sensory register for at least 1 sec in order to attain
the precision suggested by the matchings.

Electrophysiological Recordings from Paciniform Receptors.

     Two Paciniform receptors were held long enough to study the
impulse pattern for several frequencies between 1 to 250 pps covering a nearly identical range as used in the matching experiments.
A sample of records is presented in Fig. 7.   It is evident from
Fig. 8 that the average impulse interval of the primary afferents
is proportional to the cycle length of the stimulus.   Inspection
of Fig. 6 and Fig. 8 leads to the simple conclusion that the central detector works with a precision that almost mirrors the input
from the peripheral mechanoreceptive fibers.

     Within the projection area of the hand represented in S I,
Mountcastle, Talbot, Sakata, and Hyvärinen (1969) recorded from

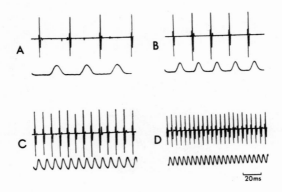

Fig. 7. Unitary responses evoked by vibratory stimuli at A 30 Hz,
         B 50 Hz, C 100 Hz, D 200 Hz. Indentation amplitude 50 µm.

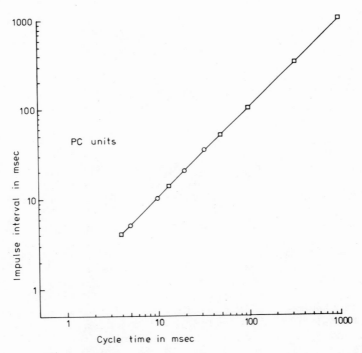

Fig. 8. Cycle time (corresponding to 1 to 250 Hz) plotted against
         average impulse interval for two PC afferents.

individual neurones in unanaesthetized monkeys. Periodic signals
elicited in Pacinian fibers did not appear in the discharge pattern
of "Pacinian" cortical neurones in response to cutaneous vibrations
above 100 Hz. The lack of periodicity in the cortical discharges
following high-frequency stimulation is obviously at variance with
the precision by which subjects can discriminate frequencies over
100 Hz as has already been shown. These observations could be interpreted as though frequency discriminations are mediated by subcortical mechanisms (Franzén and Nordmark, 1975).

Uncertainty in the Estimates of Stimulus Period.

       In equating the frequency of the standard and comparison pulse
trains a method of adjustment was employed. The arithmetic mean of
the subject's settings provided a measure of the point of subjective equality (PSE). If a temporal mechanism is at work, we
would except the standard deviation of the time distribution of the
PSE values for each frequency to decrease as a function of frequency. Differential sensitivity (difference limen) conforms
approximately to the simplest form of Weber's law since the majority of the points fall on a straight line with a slope of about
-1.0 (Fig. 9). The standard deviations decrease from 22.5 msec
at 1 pps to 0.1 msec at 256 pps.

Analysis of Peripheral Jitter

       To what extent can the uncertainty in the subject's estimates
of the pulse intervals be understood in terms of peripheral jitter?
By using short mechanical pulses presumably all mechanoreceptive
elements are activated at the lower stimulus rates which could be
a contributory cause to the large DL's for that range of frequencies.
Differences in conduction velocity among afferents (25 - 50 m/sec)
could also explain part of the scatter in the psychophysical settings. A difference limen of 22.5 msec at e.g. a rate of 1 pps,
however, has no counterpart in the way Pacinian afferents transmit
the time interval.

       At higher rates, only Pacinian fibers may be excited. We have
made a preliminary analysis of the jitter in the discharge pattern
of the Paciniform afferents (see Fig. 10). The spikes are not
locked to a particular phase of the stimulus but do vary relative
to the stimulus cycle with time. At supraliminal stimulation amplitudes at 100 Hz we estimated the jitter to be about 0.2 msec for
the first second of the mechanical vibration which is relevant for
our psychophysical measurements. This estimate is rather close to
a DL of 0.3 msec (see Fig. 9).

Ambiguity in the Sensory Input

       Earlier it has been suggested that vibratory perception was
the result of successive stimulation of "pressure receptors"

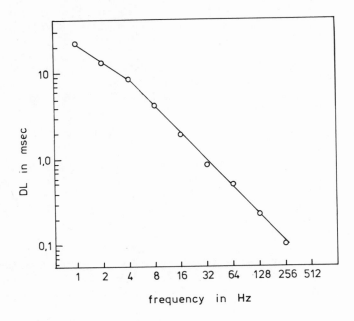

Fig. 9.   Difference limen (DL) for short mechanical pulse as a
          function of frequency in Hz. (Franzén and Nordmark, 1975)

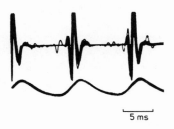

5 ms

Fig. 10. The amount of jitter in a PC fiber relative to the stimu-
          lus cycle during the first sec of the stimulation at 100
          Hz. The spikes are photographically superimposed. The
          interquartile range was calculated to be 0.18 msec. The
          lower trace shows the movement of the stimulator probe
          at 50 μm.

(Geldard, 1940). We may say that this idea is partly revived in a paper by Järvilehto, Hämäläinen, and Laurinen (1976) who suggested that a SA receptor could tell the difference between constant pressure and vibration on the basis of the variability in the discharge pattern. By the regular static discharge of the fiber shown in Fig. 11 is classified as a slowly adapting type II receptor. At a sustained pressure of 2 mm amplitude the unit fires at a rate of 50 i/s (Fig. 11). A response of a SA fiber to a vibratory stimulus of 50 Hz is presented in Fig. 12 (Järvilehto et al., 1976, Fig. 8, p. 54). This unit also transmits 50 i/s to the CNS. Since vibration is easily discriminated from a pressure stimulus, could variability in the discharge provide the CNS with a reliable cue as to what physical event is impinging upon the peripheral transducer?

First, how well does the impulse interval reproduce the cycle time of the vibratory stimulus? As seen in Fig. 13 this kind of receptor fails to do the job and the result is just the opposite of what we have presented for psychophysical matchings in Fig. 6 and for the PC afferents in Fig. 8. Now, what about the uncertainty in the impulse pattern as a function of frequency? In fact, the standard deviation in the discharge increases with increasing frequency (Fig. 14) which is contrary to what has been reported for the psychophysical settings (Fig. 9). All this evidence appears to rule out any possible significance of the SA receptors in perception of vibratory stimuli. (See also Talbot et al., 1968; Konietzny and Hensel, 1977). A receptor can presumably give rise to only one percept although the same unit can be driven by more than one kind of mechanical stimulus. This notion is also supported by the swiftness and accuracy static and vibratory stimuli are differentiated from one another.

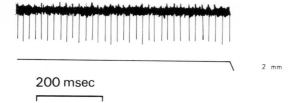

2 mm

200 msec

Fig. 11.   Unitary discharges in a slowly adapting (SA) Type II
            afferent innervating the hand. Mean discharge frequency
            50 i/s. Skin indentation 2 mm.

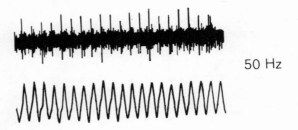

50 Hz

Fig. 12.   Response of SA fiber to each cycle of a vibration of 50
Hz.   (From Fig. 8 in Järvilehto et al., 1976)

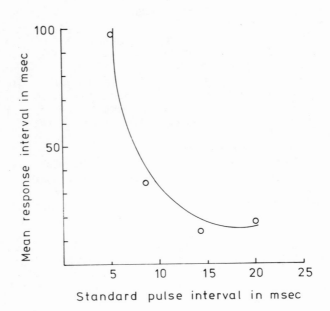

Fig. 13.   Interval analysis of the same fiber as in Fig. 12.   Response interval as a function of stimulus corresponding
to 50 to 200 Hz vibration.   (From Fig. 9 in Järvilehto,
et al., 1976).   Compare this graph with Fig. 8 of the
present paper.

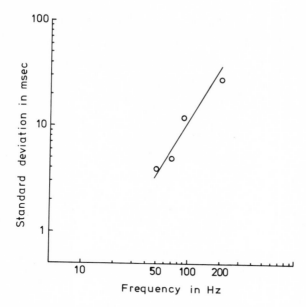

Fig. 14. Standard deviation of the impulse distribution as a function of frequency for the same unit as in Figs. 12 and 13. (From Fig. 9 in Järvilehto, et al., 1976). Compare this graph with Fig. 9 of the present paper.

SUMMARY

The present study aims at linking receptor function to perception using a combined approach of psychophysics and single unit recording technique in humans. The response characteristics of Pacinian afferents, in all likelihood subserving the vibratory sensation, were examined.

There are two basic modes of furnishing the central nervous system with unambiguous information about vibrotactile signals: intensity discrimination is based on an increment in the number of receptors excited and frequency discrimination is based on a change in the temporal pattern of the neural discharges.

ACKNOWLEDGEMENTS

This study was partly supported by a grant from the Swedish Council for Research in the Humanities and Social Sciences.

REFERENCES

Fletcher, H., & Munson, W. A.   Loudness, its definition, measurement
    and calculation. Journal of the Acoustical Society of America,
    1933, 5, 82-108.
Franzén, O.   On summation: a psychophysical study of the tactual
    sense. STL-QPSR 4/65, 1965, 14-25. Royal Institute of Tech-
    nology, Stockholm.
Franzén, O.   The dependence of vibrotactile threshold and magnitude
    functions on stimulation frequency and signal level. A percep-
    tual and neural comparison. Scandinavian Journal of Psycho-
    logy, 1969, 10, 289-298.
Franzén, O., Osterhammel, P., Terkildsen, K., & Zilstorff, K.
    What man's nose tells man's mind. A comparison between sen-
    sory scales of odor intensity and the electro-olfactogram in
    man. In G. Ohloff, G. & A. F. Thomas (Eds.), Gustation and
    olfaction. New York: Academic Press, 1970.
Franzén, O., & Berkley, M.   Apparent contrast as a function of modu-
    lation depth and spatial frequency. A comparison between per-
    ceptual and electrophysiological measures. Vision Research,
    1975, 15, 655-660.
Franzén, O., & Nordmark, J.   Vibrotactile frequency discrimination.
    Perception and Psychophysics, 1975, 17, 480-484.
Franzén, O., & Lindblom, U.   Coding of velocity of skin indentation
    in man and monkey. In Y. Zotterman (Ed.), Sensory functions
    of the skin in primates. New York: Pergamon Press, 1976.
Franzén, O., & Lindblom, U.   Tactile intensity functions in patients
    with sutured peripheral nerve. In Y. Zotterman (Ed.), Sensory
    functions of the skin in primates. New York: Pergamon Press,
    1976.
Geldard, F. A.   The perception of mechanical vibration III. The
    frequency function. Journal of General Psychology, 1940, 22,
    281-289.
Goff, G. D.   Differential discrimination of frequency of cutaneous
    mechanical vibration. Doctoral dissertation, University of
    Virginia, Charlottesville, 1959.
Hagbarth, E., & Vallbo, Å. G.   Mechanoreceptor activity recorded
    percutaneously with semimicroelectrodes in human peripheral
    nerves. Acta Physiologica Scandinavica, 1967, 69, 121-122.
Järvilehto, T., Hämäläinen, H., & Laurinen, P.   Characteristics of
    single mechanoreceptive fibers innervating hairy skin of the
    human hand. Experimental Brain Research, 1976, 25, 45-61.
Kingsbury, B. A.   A direct comparison of the loudness of pure tones.
    Physical Review, 1927, 29, 588-600.
Knibestöl, M.   Stimulus-response functions of slowly adapting mech-
    anoreceptors in the human glabrous skin area. Journal of Phy-
    siology (London), 1975, 245, 63-80.

Knibestöl, M., & Vallbo, Å. B.   Single unit analysis of mechano-
    receptor activity from the human glabrous skin.   Acta Physio-
    logica Scandinavica, 1970, 80, 178-195.
Konietzny, F., & Hensel, H.   Response of rapidly and slowly adapting
    mechanoreceptors and vibratory sensitivity in human hairy skin.
    Pflügers Archiv, 1977, 368, 39-44.
Lindblom, U.   Basic mechanisms: biophysics of supporting tissues
    and receptors.   In A.V.S. deReuck and J. Knight (Eds.), Touch,
    heat and pain.   London: Churchill, 1966.
Lindblom, U., & Lund, L.   The discharge from vibration-sensitive re-
    ceptors in the monkey foot.   Experimental Neurology, 1966, 15,
    401-417.
Marks, L. E.   Sensory processes: the new psychophysics.   New York:
    Academic Press, 1974.
Montagna, W.   Cutaneous innervation.   New York: Pergamon Press, 1960.
Mountcastle, V.B., Talbot, W. H., Sakata, H., & Hyvärinen, J.
    Cortical neuronal mechanisms in flutter vibration studied in
    unanesthetized monkeys.   Journal of Neurophysiology, 1969, 32
    452-484.
Sato, M.   Response of Pacinian corpuscles to sinusoidal vibration.
    Journal of Physiology (London), 1961, 159, 391-409.
Stevens, J. C., & Stevens, S. S.   Brightness function: Effects of
    adaptation.   Journal of Optical Society of America, 1963, 53,
    375-385.
Stevens, S. S.   On the psychophysical law.   Psychological Review,
    1957, 64, 153-181.
Stevens, S. S.   Tactile vibration: change of exponent with fre-
    quency.   Perception and Psychophysics, 1968, 3, 223-228.
Talbot, W. H., Darian-Smith, I., Kornhuber, H. H., & Mountcastle,
    V.B.   The sense of flutter-vibration: Comparison of the human
    capacity with response patterns of mechanoreceptive afferents
    from the monkey hand.   Journal of Neurophysiology, 1968, 31,
    301-334.
Torgerson, W. S.   Theory and methods of scaling.   New York: Wiley,
    1958.
Vallbo, Å. B., & Hagbarth, K. E.   Activity from skin mechanorecep-
    tors recorded percutaneously in awake human subjects.   Experi-
    mental Neurology, 1968, 21, 270-289.
Verrillo, R. T.   Vibrotactile sensitivity and the frequency response
    of the Pacinian corpuscle.   Psychonomic Science, 1966, 4, 135-
    136.
Werner, G., & Mountcastle, V. B.   Neural activity in mechanorecep-
    tive cutaneous afferents: stimulus-response relations, Weber's
    functions, and information transmission.   Journal of Neuro-
    physiology, 1965, 28, 359-397.
Zotterman, Y.   Touch, pain and tickling: an electrophysiological
    investigation on cutaneous sensory nerves. Journal of Physio-
    logy (London), 1939, 95, 1-28.

DISCUSSION

DR. GESCHEIDER: You plot the standard deviation as a function of frequency for the frequency matching?

DR. FRANZÉN: That is correct.

DR. GESCHEIDER: Figure 9 indicates a remarkable frequency discrimination when compared with the earlier data of, say, Goff or more recent data of Verrillo. Do you have any explanation for why frequency discrimination is so good in your experiment?

DR. FRANZÉN: Yes, I think so. Our interest is to study the precision of the system. We want to push the system to its limit. There can be discrepancies in the results because different methods were used. The task of the subject was to match the standard with the variable frequency so that the pulse trains were identical. This method minimizes the dispersion of the data. One gets larger difference limen with a method in which the subject is asked to report when a difference in frequency is experienced.

DR. IGGO: There is another aspect that is perhaps worth commenting on. When you are using the different frequencies are you applying similar pulses at different frequencies or are you applying a sinusoidally varying stimulus?

DR. FRANZÉN: The point is that we used pulses with exactly the same shape and of 2 msec duration presented from 1 Hz up to 256 Hz.

DR. IGGO: So the actual stimulus delivered to the Pacinian corpulse is the same at different frequencies and the Pacinian corpuscles may be responding to stimuli 1 sec apart or 100 msec apart and so on. It is not as in the older work where sinusoidal stimuli were used.

DR. FRANZÉN: Yes, that is one of the points of the paper, and also there is no ambiguity at low frequencies. The experience is of a sharply defined tactile pulse.

DR. JÄRVILEHTO: Your results appear to fit quite well with ours. We have said that SA fibers might mediate vibratory information in low frequency range with, perhaps, RA fibers serving at somewhat higher frequencies as Talbot et al (1968) suggested. We have further suggested (Järvilehto, Hämäläinen, and Laurinen, 1976), that information transmission could be based on the variability in the interspike interval. When there is a steady pressure on an SA receptor then the intervals are dispersed more than with vibration. In Fig. 4 of that paper we have applied two von Frey hairs, one of

1.7 g and the other 7.15 g. We carried out an interval analysis during the time from stimulus onset to its offset. In Fig. 5 are shown
the interval histograms. There is quite a lot of scatter with
the smaller stimulus but, with increased stimulus intensity, the
intervals become shorter. If you look at the standard deviation
there is still a considerable variability. In Fig. 9 is shown
the interval analysis of an SA fiber response to a static pressure
and there is again a dispersion of the interstimulus intervals.
This is actually the response to steady pressure by the vibrator
tip. When we start vibrating the intervals correspond very well
to the stimulating frequency. When we increased the frequency
then the response failed to follow the probe frequency above 70 Hz.
The intervals were no longer scattered around the stimulus
frequency but the fiber may follow at half frequency. I would
predict that the threshold of the fiber increased in this range
but it seems quite clear that the fiber is able to transmit the
information up to these frequencies, then it is actually not so
ambiguous.

DR. FRANZÉN: Well, yes, at least your figure is not ambiguous
but, I think the information is ambiguous for the central nervous
system. I prefer to take the simple minded view, that if we
consider receptors, like the SA II receptors that also react to
temperature change, the percept is not a change in temperature, it
is a change in the tactile sensation. Dr. Hensel may comment
on that. He has given a presentation (Hensel, 1978) in which he
talked about Weber's illusion that was mentioned in Weber's (1834)
paper.

DR. IGGO: Could I interrupt here to make one point we should be
quite clear about at the very beginning of the meeting. It has to
do with the stimulus conditions. Dr. Franzén has been talking
about applying a stimulus at different frequencies. He has been
applying the same envelope of mechanical displacement at different
frequencies, whereas a lot of the analytical work done on the
primary afferent fibers has involved changing frequency of a
sinusoid. This has quite a different effect, especially on the
kind of afferent fiber that is excited. If, for example, you try
to excite a Pacinian corpuscle, a sinusoidally varying stimulus
at 1 Hz will not excite it, whereas, if you apply a rapid pulse
envelope to the Pacinian corpuscle at 1 Hz in which the frequency
components of that stimulus are quite high, then it will be excited.
This, I think, is an important distinction. I recollect when we
had the 1966 meeting here, there was the question of adaptation
being discussed and the point made then was that some experimental
workers were applying what they called a square wave stimulus, but
in fact it was a stimulus lasting 0.5 sec, but not just a constant
displacement as the receptor workers would use, but an envelope

of a vibrating stimulus. It would be worthwhile at the very onset
of this meeting to be quite clear when we are talking about different stimulus conditions, that we really are talking about the same
thing.

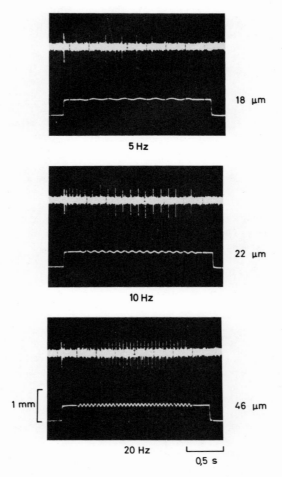

Fig. 1.   Response of a Type I slowly adapting mechanoreceptor (SA
          I) from hairy skin of the human hand to stimulation with
          stepwise indentations (500 /um) of the skin at ampli-
          tudes of the superimposed sine wave required to evoke a
          one - to - one following of the fiber at stimulation
          frequencies of 5, 10, and 20 Hz.

DR. HENSEL: Another point that has to be considered when talking about ambiguity is the possibility of synchronization of several receptors. When applying a constant pressure to the slowly adapting receptors, you will get an asynchronous discharge of the population, whereas with vibration you will get a synchronized discharge. This will give, perhaps, the information necessary to discriminate in steady pressure and vibration.

DR. KONIETZNY: I am not sure from our experiments that the SA I mechanoreceptors will transmit information about vibration in the very low frequency range. We have stimulated human SA I receptors at 5, 10, and 20 Hz, and you see in Fig. 1 a one to one following of the fiber to the superimposed sine waves. In Fig. 2, you can see the average sensation threshold in 10 subjects and the average threshold of the SA I mechanoreceptor. This curve, in the frequency range from 5 to 20 Hz, lies very low so that in this frequency range this type of receptor, in my opinion, could not transmit enough information to be detected as a vibration. I think the frequency range between 50 to about 100 Hz, as Dr. Järvilehto has investigated this receptor, might transmit enough information on vibration.

DR. STEVENS: Your plot (text, Fig. 1) of the various psychophysical functions for various vibration frequencies looks to me like they are going, on extrapolation, to meet at a common point corresponding to a single point on the abscissa. And indeed if the constant n is linearly related to the constant log c, it follows mathematically that these functions must intersect at a common point. I have found that to be true of many families of psychophysical functions and very often that point has empirical meaning. For example, in the case of warmth functions for various areal extents of stimulation, the functions always meet at the threshold for thermal pain.

DR. FRANZEN: I agree with you Dr. Stevens, completely. We know that at very high intensities the equal vibratory curve is almost flat, and that is an indication that these curves, in fact, converge (unpublished observations).

If there are no further comments, I would like to stress the point of why we used the kind of stimulus that we did. The point is that when you use very short tactile pulses, you can go down to 1 Hz. You would not be able to do that if you used sinusoidal stimuli. But since we support the idea that there is a temporal analysis carried out by the tactile system, and at very low frequencies, as I have already pointed out, there was no indication of vibration, there was just the task of determining the time interval. Although the quality of the sensation changed, over frequency, the function was a straight line, indicating that the same underlying mechanism is at work. That was the idea behind it.

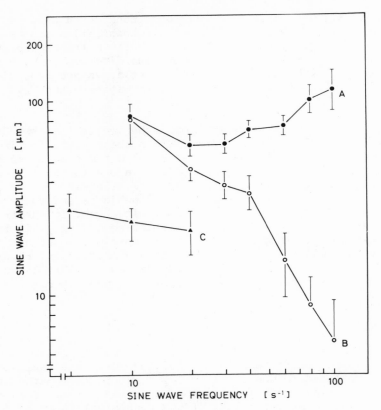

Fig. 2. Mean tuning curves of RA fibers (A) and SA I fibers (C)
from the superficial branch of the radial nerve in human
subjects and the human threshold function for the perceptions of sine wave oscillation applied to the hairy
skin of the hand (B).

REFERENCES

Buchthal, F., & Rosenfalck, A. Evoked potentials and conduction
velocity in human sensory nerves. Brain Research, 1966, 3,
1-122.
Franzén, O. & Lindblom, U. Tactile intensity functions in patients
with sutured peripheral nerve. In Y. Zotterman (Ed.), Sensory functions of the skin in primates. Oxford: Pergamon,
1976.

Goff, G. D. Differential discrimination of frequency of cutaneous
    mechanical vibration. Journal of Experimental Psychology,
    1967, 74, 294-299.

Hallin, R. G. & Torebjörk, H. E. Activity in unmyelinated nerve
    fibers in man. In J. J. Bonica (Ed.), Advances in neurology,
    (Vol. 4). New York: Raven, 1974.

Hensel, H. Phenomenal and neural structures of touch. In Workshop
    on sensory and perceptual processes. 20. Tagung experimentell
    arbeitender Psychologen, Markurg 20-22 März 1978.

Järvilehto, T., Hämäläinen, H., & Laurinen, P. Characteristics
    of single mechanoreceptor fibers innervating hairy skin of
    the hand. Experimental Brain Research, 1976, 25, 46-61.

Quilliam, T. A. Unit design and array patterns in receptor organs.
    In A.V.S.de Reuck and J. Knight (Eds.), Touch, heat and pain.
    London: Churchill, 1966.

Rothenberg, M., Verrillo, R. T., Azhorian, S. A., Brachman, M. L.,
    & Bolanowski, S. J., Jr. Vibrotactile frequency for encoding
    a speech parameter. Journal of Acoustical Society of America,
    1977, 62, 1003-1012.

Talbot, W. H., Darian-Smith, I., Kornhuber, H. H., & Mountcastle,
    V. B. The sense of flutter-vibration: Comparison of the human
    capacity with response patterns of mechanoreceptive afferents
    from the monkey hand. Journal of Neurophysiology, 1968, 31,
    301-334.

Weber, E. H. De pulsu, resorptione, auditu et tactu: annotationes
    anatomicae et physiologiae, 1834.

CUES SUPPORTING RECOGNITION OF THE ORIENTATION OR DIRECTION OF

MOVEMENT OF TACTILE STIMULI

William R. Gould, Charles J. Vierck, Jr. and Mary
Margaret Luck
Department of Neuroscience and Center for Neurobiological
Sciences
University of Florida College of Medicine, Gainesville,
Florida, U.S.A., 32610

In a previous investigation of human subjects with stimulation
of the volar surface of the forearm (Jones and Vierck, 1973), it was
shown that discrimination of line lengths is quite good, relative
to traditional measures of spatial resolution, such as the two-
point or compass test. Whereas two-point thresholds of 30 to 40 mm
are reported for the forearm (Weinstein, 1968), line-length thresholds ranged from 4.8 mm to 9.6 mm, depending on the length of the
standard, the orientation of the stimuli and the method of presentation (i.e. whether the standard and comparison stimuli were
presented separately or in sequence on a given trial). Considering
the large receptive fields that have been observed for CNS neurons
receiving tactile input from the forearm (Powell and Mountcastle,
1959), these results support the contention that certain spatial
attributes can be coded effectively by systems of neurons with
large, overlapping receptive fields (Erickson, 1968; McIlwain,
1976); and it is pertinent to inquire as to the variety of spatial
discriminations that are mediated with reasonable acuity on the
basis of input from the skin of the forearm.

The previous experiment on line-length discrimination and the
first studies to be reported here involved the use of stimuli that
were presented manually. Clearly, this method of stimulus presentation sacrificed precise control of a number of features of
skin deformations. By using hand-held stimuli, the experimenter
effectively randomized the depth, pressure and rate of each skin
identation and asked the subjects to attend to certain spatial
features of the stimulus. Similarly, an animal in its natural environment may well recognize certain tactile stimuli on the basis
of spatial cues, despite wide fluctuations of indentation rate,
pressure and depth. In principle the variability of tactile

impressions can be attenuated greatly by active touch, but the forearm skin is seldom used directly in the process of haptic exploration. Much of the stimulation received by forearm skin occurs in passage, as the animal moves about with attention directed away from that skin region. Thus, we are interested in knowing what spatial cues are most salient in a noisy environment of varying pressures, depths, durations, and velocities of indentation. Also, the clinical examination of neurological patients would benefit from a greater appreciation of the variety of spatio-tactile features that can be evaluated reliably and conveniently (without the technology that is required for sophisticated stimulus control). The traditional two-point measure of spatio-tactile resolution is not sensitive to lesion of the dorsal columns, the spinal somato-sensory pathway containing the most precise somatopic map of the skin (Cook and Browder, 1965; Levitt and Schwartzman, 1966), and therefore it should be supplemented or replaced by other tests that are representative of "lemniscal" functions (Vierck, 1974; Azulay and Schwartz, 1975; Wall and Noordenbos, 1977).

     Given evidence that forearm skin supports reasonably good discrimination of the length of a line impressed on the skin, we were interested in gaining an appreciation of the resolution of the skin for specifying the orientation of such an edge contour. As a first exploration of this question, we determined the length of a line that was just sufficient to support discrimination of the easiest orientation problem (i.e., a 90° alignment of the standard and comparison orientations). Fourteen college students (8 males and 6 females) received sets of 25 trials in which one edge of a 3 mm thick plexiglas rectangle was placed on the antero-medial aspect of one forearm. The line stimulus was presented in either a longitudinal or a transverse orientation, and the subjects were instructed to report the orientation. Trials were presented in sets of 25, with approximately 1 sec contact and a 5 sec intertrial interval. Thresholds for line orientation were tracked by choosing the length of line (in 3 mm increments) used on each set of trials on the basis of whether performance on the preceding set exceeded or fell short of 75 percent correct responses. The reported threshold value for each subject was bracketed by at least 100 trials on each side and was calculated by linear interpolation.

     The average threshold line length for discriminating proximal-distal vs. medial-lateral orientations was 16.8 mm. Although it may be the case that relative orientations of much less than 90° are discriminated quite accurately once the minimum contour length (of approximately 17 mm) is exceeded, this result suggests either: (a) that contour orientation is not a particularly useful cue for object recognition (on the forearm) or (b) that shapes which can be discriminated when applied to this patch of skin must be quite large. It seems reasonable, both in terms of the organization of the neural system supplying forearm skin (e.g., large receptive fields) and the reliance of the organism on the distal extremities for tactile exploration, that proximal appendicular regions of skin can support reasonably good recognition of the location and size of tactile stimuli but poor specification of shape. However, returning to the question of orientation detection, proximal appendicular skin is frequently subjected to stimuli that move across the skin surface, and it could be that orientation detection is greatly enhanced when sequential cues are present. Accordingly, the first set of studies included stimuli that progressed from point to point along a given orientation.

In the most impoverished conditions, the separation of two points that was required to discriminate proximal-distal vs. medial-lateral orientations was compared when the points were applied simultaneously or sequentially. Sequential application did improve orientation discrimination somewhat, generating thresholds of 8.7 mm as opposed to 13.1 mm when the points were delivered simultaneously. Similarly, plastic arcs were cut from a 19 mm diameter disc of 1.6 mm thick plastic, and these arcs were "rolled" over the skin, providing stimuli that progressed continuously over the surface, for comparision with the uninterrupted lines. Again, the threshold length of the moving stimulus for orientation detection was less (10.5 mm circumference of the arc) than that required for the lines (16.8 mm). However, by far the most dramatic improvement in orientation discrimination was observed when the stimulus was a simple stroke of the skin with a probe having a tip diameter of 1 mm. All subjects performed well above chance, with a group average of 89.4 percent correct responses, at the minimum stroke length that could be generated with the hand-held probe (approximately 3 mm).

In a previous experiment with monkey subjects that had sustained interruption of the dorsal spinal columns, a substantial and enduring deficit was observed on a behavioral task requiring tactile direction sensitivity (Vierck, 1974). This deficit stood in contrast to other measures of spatio-tactile resolution that had been shown to be minimally affected by dorsal column lesions (Cook and Browder, 1965; Schwartz, Eidelberg, Marchok, and Azulay, 1972; Schwartzman and Bogdonoff, 1969; Wall, 1970), suggesting that the dorsal columns are particularly adapted to the coding of spatio-temporal stimulus sequences. The small receptive fields, fast conduction, fast adaptation, secure synaptic transmission and precise afferent inhibition of the dorsal column pathway (see Mountcastle, 1961) could well constitute essential input characteristics for the directionally sensitive cells that have been observed in somatosensory cortex (Whitsel, Roppolo, and Werner, 1972). However, this logic assumes that directional sensitivity arises from the generation of discrete spatio-temporal patterns of activity in populations of central cells that converge selectively on the

feature detector cells (e.g., see Whitsel et al., 1972), and such
a mechanism presupposes the sequential crossing of a reasonable
number of receptive field boundaries by the stimulus as it moves
across the skin surface. Thus, we were surprised to observe that
minimal movement of a punctate probe generated excellent discrimination of orientation. However, it is important to note that while
the probe moved over a very small extent of skin, the elasticity of
the skin could have permitted selective excitation of different
populations of stretch sensitive receptors with movements in different directions. Accordingly, the following experiments sought
to measure orientation and direction sensitivity under stimulation
conditions that varied the relative contributions of skin stretch
and movement across the skin surface.

Ten college students (8 females, 2 males) were seated at a
table with the right forearm supinated and resting on a foam pad
with sandbags placed over the arm at several locations to secure
and stabilize the arm comfortably. Hair was removed with a depila-
tory in the area to be stimulated on the volar forearm. In one
testing condition, a "floating" steel probe weighing 5 grams was
fitted into a plastic sleeve, which was attached to a rack and
pinion manipulator with adjustable stops that permitted accurate
movement of the probe for set excursions over the skin surface.
Observations of skin movement were made with a dissecting microscope, and it was determined that, at a point 5 mm in the wake of
the moving probe, up to 50 μm of movement could occur for each mm
of probe excursion. On a given trial, the probe was moved medially,
laterally, proximally or distally from a start point on the volar
forearm surface; the subjects reported the orientation and direction
of the perceived movement; and then the probe was returned to the
start point. Sets of 25 trials were delivered at a given excursion,
and thresholds were tracked by sets of trials as before. Under
these conditions, the average excursion at threshold for identification of the orientation of the movement was 4.3 mm. At the excursion value just above orientation threshold for each subject
(in 0.5 mm steps), the direction of probe movement was correctly
identified on 89.3 percent of the medial-lateral trials and on 73.6
percent of the proximal-distal trials. Thus, the direction of probe
movement was specified at approximately the excursion length sufficient to reveal the orientation of the stimulus.

In order to appreciate the significance of skin stretch as a
cue for discriminating the direction of movement of an object across
the skin surface, the 10 subjects that were tested with the floating probe also received trials on which a 2 mm diameter, rubber-
tipped probe was glued, with contact cement, to the skin. Once firmly
affixed to the skin, the probe was adjusted in height so that there
was no observable indentation of the skin, and then 4 sets of 25
trials were delivered with 1 mm excursions in the medial, lateral,

proximal or distal directions (as dictated by a quasi-random
schedule). All subjects performed above chance for discrimination
of medial vs. lateral movement (mean of 96.7 percent correct responses) and for discrimination of proximal vs. distal movement
(94.9 percent correct responses). This suggests strongly that skin
stretch ordinarily provides the most salient cue for discrimination
of the direction of movement of objects across the skin surface.

To evaluate further the contribution of skin stretch to directional sensitivity, we wished to utilize a stimulus that produced
an indentation that could be moved along the skin without a component of friction that would stretch the skin. Accordingly, a
group of 4 male subjects was tested with a stream of air that was
forced, at 20 lb/sq in. through a 24 gauge needle. The squared-off
tip of the needle was positioned as close to the skin as possible
without touching the skin at any point in its excursion. The overall force of the air stream was approximately 0.7g, and the elicited
sensation was a very light and well localized touch. The tubing
from the air tank was coiled in a hot water bath to bring the
temperature of the air within the thermoneutral zone for the subjects. Hair was removed from the tested area of forearm skin. At
the beginning of each trial, the air stream was turned on and then
moved medially or laterally a set distance; after the subject responded, the air flow was terminated and the needle returned to the
start position. Sets of 25 trials were run at each excursion, and
thresholds were determined as in the other experiments. The mean
excursion required to discriminate the direction of movement of the
air stream across the skin surface was 11.3 mm. These 4 subjects
were also tested with a 0.7g "floating" probe (with a 1 mm diameter
spherical tip), and the mean threshold for direction sensitivity
with this light stimulus was 14.0 mm. Finally, these subjects were
tested with the probe glued to the skin, and they all responded
above chance with a 2 mm excursion. Thus, in the various conditions
in which stretch of the skin was not a significant factor in speci-
fying the orientation or direction of stimuli placed on the skin or
moved across the skin surface (i.e. lines, 2-points, rolling an arc,
stroking with a 0.7g probe or moving a stream of air) orientation or
direction thresholds for the length of the stimulus or its excursion
ranged from 8.7 mm to 16.8 mm (see Table 1). In contrast, stretching
the skin less than 1 mm appears to be sufficient to specify the
direction of the skin distortion, representing approximately an
order of magnitude greater sensitivity for stretch than for utiliza-
tion of the spatial pattern of normal indentation(s).

The final experiment in this series was designed to accurately
determine the length of excursion sufficient to specify the direction
of skin stretch. Stimulation was produced by a Ling vibrator which
was serve-controlled to produce ramp excursions either at 1 cm/sec
or at 1 mm/sec. Three subjects (2 female) were tested with medial

Table 1   Thresholds for the extent of different stimulations re-
          quired to specify the orientation or direction of the
          tactile stimulus.

Stimulus	Discrimination Task	No. of Subjects	Threshold	S.E.
Line	90° orientation	14	16.8 mm	1.4
Arc (rolled)	90° orientation	14	10.5 mm	1.1
2-pts. simul- taneous	90° orientation	14	13.1 mm	1.0
2-pts. se- quential	90° orientation	14	8.7 mm	0.9
5 g stroke	90° orientation	10	4.3 mm	0.4
stretch	M-L or P-D direction	10	< 1 mm	---
0.7g stroke	M-L direction	4	14.0 mm	1.9
0.7g air stream	M-L direction	4	11.3 mm	2.5
stretch	M-L direction	4	< 2 mm	---

vs. lateral movement of a 2 mm diameter probe that was glued to de-
pilated skin of the right volar forearm. The Ling vibrator was
mounted to a stereotaxic manipulator which permitted adjustment of
the height of the probe so that there was no observable indentation
or elevation of the skin underneath the probe at the start position.
On each set of 50 trials, medial and lateral excursions of a set
length were randomly interchanged, and thresholds were bracketed by
at least 500 trials (10 sets) in steps of 0.1 mm (at 1 cm/sec) or
0.5 mm (at 1 mm/sec). On each trial, the ramp stimulus was produced, the probe was held at the end position until the subject responded, and then the probe was reset to the start position. The
output of a displacement transducer, mounted on the shaft of the vibrator, was monitored on a memory oscilloscope to insure reliability
of the individual stimuli. When the probe moved at 1 cm/sec, the
mean threshold was 0.6 mm, but performance was impaired at the
slow excursion velocity (see Table 2). At 1 mm/sec, the mean
threshold for stretch direction was greater than 2 mm (one subject could not discriminate at the maximum excursion of 3.0).
Two of the subjects received further testing sessions in which
they were instructed to report when they felt movement of the probe
(at 1 cm/sec), regardless of the direction of movement. Their
thresholds for simple detection of skin stretch were less (mean of
0.15 mm) than those for discrimination of the direction of stretch
at the same velocity.

Table 2   Individual thresholds for the extent of skin stretch
           sufficient to detect the movement of the probe or to
           discriminate the direction of stretch.

Subject	Stretch Detection (1 cm/sec)	Stretch Direction (1 cm/sec)	Stretch Direction (1 mm/sec)
J K	0.1 mm	0.5 mm	>3.9 mm
P N	0.2 mm	0.3 mm	0.6 mm
R C	-----	1.0 mm	2.5 mm

The major implication of the observations reported here is that skin stretch must be considered as an important source of information for the somatosensory system. In terms of tactile capacities such as those emphasized here (sensing the direction of movement of an object across the skin surface), the advantage of stretch sensitivity is that a tangential perturbation at one skin locus will involve stretch receptors over a considerable area with a distinctive spatial pattern. For example, considering one of the tactile receptors that is exquisitely sensitive to skin stretch (the slowly adapting, type II or Ruffini Corpuscle; Chambers, Andres, Duering, and Iggo, 1972) and plentiful in human skin (Järvilehto, Hämäläinen, and Laurinen, 1976), a medial stretch of the skin should activate a portion of the type II receptors lateral to the probe (i.e., those with a mediolateral polar orientation) and unload a similar proportion of receptors medial to the probe. This would provide a sharp border of excitation near the probe and a trailing area of lateral receptor activity (Fig. 1). Microscopic observations on a single subject indicated that medial or lateral excursions of 1 mm produced 0.5 mm movements of skin 4 cm from the probe, suggesting that the area of receptor involvement from a 0.6 mm stretch at threshold for discrimination of the direction of movement could well match or exceed the spatial extent of receptors activated by a 17 mm line at threshold for orientation discrimination.

Another implication of the present findings relates to the contribution of the dorsal column-medial lemniscal system to spatio tactile discrimination capacities. The relevant bits of information are as follows: (a) tactile direction sensitivity of the hindlimb is one of the few discriminations that has been shown to be impaired for months following dorsal column lesions (Vierck, 1974); (b) tactile direction sensitivity is determined primarily by cues

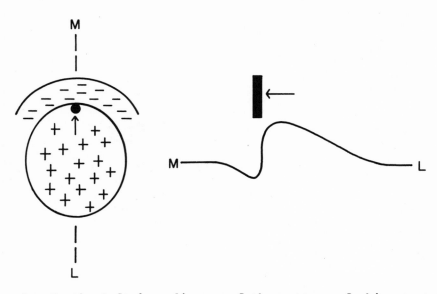

Fig. 1.   On the left is a diagram of the pattern of skin stretch
          and relaxation that is produced by medial (M) movement of
          a probe (small black circle) that is glued to the skin.
          Lateral (L) to the probe is an area of stretched skin
          (marked by + symbols), and medial to the probe is an area
          of elevated or relaxed skin (marked by - symbols). On the
          right is a hypothetical representation of the amount of
          activity that should be observed if recording in sequence
          from skin stretch receptors located along a medial to
          lateral line that passes underneath the probe. Assuming
          a level of ongoing discharge in receptors outside the in-
          fluence of the moving probe (resulting from normal skin
          tension), receptors medial to the probe would be relatively
          silent, while the activity of receptors lateral to the
          probe would increase in proportion to their proximity to
          the probe.

provided by stretching the skin (present report); and (c) the receptors that are most likely to be responsible for tactile stretch
sensitivity are the slowly adapting (SA) type II receptors (Chambers,
et al., 1972). Similarly, difference limens for tactile pressure
sensitivity are temporarily elevated by dorsal column lesions
(Vierck, 1977), and slowly adapting receptors appear to be the only
tactile receptors capable of differential responding to a wide
range of identation pressures (Harrington and Merzenich, 1970;
Werner and Mountcastle, 1965). However, these behavioral results

are in conflict with physiological evidence that afferent fibers from SA receptors (including type II) exit the fasciculus gracilis and synapse on cells of the dorsal horn (Whitsel, Petrucelli, and Sapiro, 1969). Thus, the behavioral results suggest that the ascending projection pattern of slowly adapting afferents should be reevaluated in primates. This need is reinforced by the lack of clear evidence that the slowly adapting tactile afferents project onto dorsal horn cells of origin of any of the major ascending routes to the thalamus and cerebral cortex (i.e. the spinothalamic or spinocervicothalamic tracts or secondary fibers that ascend the dorsal or dorsolateral columns to synapse in the nucleus gracilis; Angaut-Petit, 1975; Bryan, Coulter, and Willis, 1975). If one of the pathways outside the dorsal columns does receive a substantial input from SA type II afferents, then it is likely that stretch sensitivity is not mediated primarily by SA type II receptors, and the possibility should be considered that quickly adapting field receptors contribute the most salient input related to skin stretch (Burgess and Perl, 1973). Alternatively, the primary condition for tactile direction sensitivity may not be stretch of the skin per se but could be related to shear forces generated by movement of superficial layers of the skin relative to underlying tissues.

Looking more generally at somatosensory functions that might be served by receptors that respond to stretch of the skin, it seems worth noting that different joint movements produce quite distinct patterns of stretch and relaxation of extensive skin regions. The reader is encouraged to observe these patterns with extension, flexion, pronation and supination of a forearm. Thus, while muscle and joint receptors have been emphasized as the major contributors to the sense of limb movement and position, a contributing role for tactile receptors has not been ruled out (Cross and McCloskey, 1973), and the present results provide evidence that skin stretch sensitivity of human subjects is sufficient to merit consideration of a tactile contribution to some aspects of proprioception. For example, determination of the direction of movement at a joint would appear to be coded effectively by the associated pattern of skin regions that are stretched and relaxed. The finding that stretch sensitivity deteriorated at the slower rate (1 mm/sec) indicates that skin stretch would contribute most significantly to proprioceptive sensations accompanying relatively fast limb movements.

ACKNOWLEDGEMENTS

Supported by Grant NS-07261 from the National Institute of Neurological and Communicative Disorders and Stroke.
Present address of W. R. Gould: Department of Physical Therapy, School of Community and Allied Health Resources, The University of Alabama at Birmingham Medical Center, Birmingham, Alabama 35294.
College of Health Related Professions, University of Florida, Gainesville, Florida, U.S.A., 32610

REFERENCES

Angaut-Petit, D. The dorsal column system. II. Functional pro-
    perties and bulbar relay of the postsynaptic fibers of the
    cat's fasciculus gracilis. Experimental Brain Research,
    1975, 22, 471-493.
Azulay, A. & Schwartz, A. S. The role of the dorsal funiculus cf
    the primate in tactual discrimination. Experimental Neurology,
    1975, 46, 315-332.
Bryan, R. N., Coulter, J. D., & Willis, W. D. Cells of origin of
    the spinocervical tract in the monkey. Experimental Neuro-
    logy, 1974, 42, 574-586.
Burgess, P. R., & Perl, E. R. Cutaneous mechanoreceptors and no-
    ciceptors. In A. Iggo (Ed.), Handbook of sensory physiology
    (Vol. 2). Berlin: Springer-Verlag, 1973.
Chambers, M. F., Andres, K. H., Duering, M. V., & Iggo, A. The
    structure and function of the slowly adaptive type II re-
    ceptor in hairy skin. Quarterly Journal of Experimental Phy-
    siology, 1972, 57, 417-445.
Cook, A. W. & Browder, E. J. Function of posterior columns in man.
    Archives of Neurology (Chicago), 1965, 12, 72-79.
Cross, M. J. & McCloskey, D. I. Position sense following surgical
    removal of joints in man. Brain Research, 1973, 55, 443-445.
Dart, A. M. & Gordon, G. Some properties of spinal connections of
    the cat's dorsal column nuclei which do not involve the dor-
    sal columns. Brain Research, 1973, 58, 61-68.
Erickson, R. P. Stimulus coding in topographic and non-topographic
    modalities: on the significance of the activity of individual
    sensory neurons. Psychological Review, 1968, 75, 447-465.
Harrington, T. & Merzenich, M. M. Neural coding in the sense of
    touch: human sensations of skin identation compared with
    the responses of slowly adapting mechanoreceptive afferents
    innervating the hairy skin of monkeys. Experimental Brain
    Research, 1970, 10, 251-264.
Järvilehto, T., Hämäläinen, H., & Laurinen, P. Characteristics of
    single mechanoreceptive fibers innervating hairy skin of the
    human hand. Experimental Brain Research, 1976, 25, 45-61.
Jones, M. B. & Vierck, C. J., Jr. Length discrimination on the
    skin. American Journal of Psychology, 1973, 86, 49-60.
Levitt, M. & Schwartzman, R. J. Spinal sensory tracts and two-
    point tactile sensitivity. Anatomical Record, 1966, 154, 377.
McIlwain, J. T. Large receptive fields and spatial transformation
    in the visual system. In R. Porter (Ed.), International re-
    view of physiology, neurophysiology, 1976, 10, 223-248.
Mountcastle, V. B. Some functional properties of the somatic af-
    ferent system. In W. A. Rosenblith (Ed.), Sensory communic-
    ation. New York: John Wiley, 1961.

Powell, T. P. S. & Mountcastle, V.B. Some aspects of the functional organization of the cortex of the postcentral gyrus of the monkey: a correlation of findings obtained in a single unit analysis with cytoarchitecture. Johns Hopkins Medical Journal, 1959, 105, 133-162.

Rustioni, A. Spinal neurons project to the dorsal column nuclei of Rhesus monkeys. Science, 1977, 196, 656-658.

Schwartz, A. S., Eidelberg, E., Marchok, P., & Azulay, A. Tactile discrimination in the monkey after section of the dorsal funiculus and lateral lemniscus. Experimental Neurology, 1972, 37, 582-596.

Schwartzman, R. J. & Bogdonoff, M. D. Proprioception and vibration sensibility discriminations in the absence of the posterior columns. Archives of Neurology, 1969, 20, 349-353.

Vierck, C. J., Jr. Tactile movement detection and discrimination following dorsal column lesions in monkeys. Experimental Brain Research, 1974, 20, 331-346.

Vierck, C. J., Jr. Absolute and differential sensitivities to touch stimuli after spinal cord lesions in monkeys. Brain Research, 1977, 134, 529-539.

Wall, P. D. The sensory and motor role of impulses traveling in the dorsal columns toward cerebral cortex. Brain, 1970, 30, 159-193.

Wall, P. D. & Noordenbos, W. Sensory functions which remain in man after complete transection of dorsal columns. Brain, 1977, 100, 641-658.

Weinstein, S. Intensive and extensive aspects of tactile sensitivity as a function of body part, sex and laterality. In D. R. Kenshalo (Ed.), The skin senses. Springfield, Ill: Thomas, 1968.

Werner, G. and Mountcastle, V. B. Neural activity in mechanoreceptive cutaneous afferents: stimulus-response relations, Weber functions and information transmission. Journal of Neurophysiology, 1965, 28, 359-397.

Whitsel, B. L., Petrucelli, L. M., & Sapiro, G. Modality representation in the lumbar and cervical fasciculus gracilis of squirrel monkeys. Brain Research, 1969, 15, 67-78.

Whitsel, B. L., Roppolo, J. R., & Werner, G. Cortical information processing of stimulus motion on primate skin. Journal of Neurophysiology, 1972, 35, 691-717.

Willis, W. D., Maunz, R. A., Foreman, R. D., & Coulter, J. D. Static and dynamic responses of spinothalamic tract neurons to mechanical stimuli. Journal of Neurophysiology, 1975, 38, 587-600.

DISCUSSION

DR. IGGO: This is a very interesting attempt to try to extend the analysis that has been going on, into the input characteristics of another kind of receptor. Earlier we heard about Pacinian corpuscles and now we have moved to the SA II receptors.

DR. VIERCK: I have a question to ask of the audience. My impression, from the few peripheral nerve recordings that I have made, is that the SA II receptors are selective for orientation but not for direction. The ones I saw would respond very well, let us say, to a medial or a lateral stretch but not a proximal or distal stretch. As near as I could tell they did not give a differetial response to, say, one quadrant of the circle. So, I tend to think in terms, not of the receptors themselves as being selectively responsive to direction, but more in terms of a population of fibers.

DR. JÄRVILEHTO: I have some information that is relevant to this question. We have found, actually one unit, in the hairy skin of the hand which I think was not an SA II receptor. It was however, spontaneously active. When we moved the pin over the hand, distally quite gently, it increased firing and when we moved the pin proximally it was inhibited. I do not know what the receptor was because we did not find a receptive field for it.

DR. IGGO: In terms of the behavior of the receptors, these SA II receptors are Ruffini endings. They are spindle shaped and attached to the connective tissue at both ends. So, one would not expect them to show a differential effect of pulling in one direction and then in the opposite direction. They respond, at least when the stimulus is applied, even though the receptor is lying somewhere in the skin underneath, it is going to be stretched you pull to one side or the other.

DR. VIERCK: My expectation of what happens when you stretch in one direction is that you are involving a number of SA II units in the wake of the stimulus, when you stretch in the opposite direction, you would then stimulate a different population of receptors and the discrimination may well be made in terms of the location of receptors driven rather than by activation of a set of cells precisley tuned to the direction of movement.

DR. JOHANSSON: Our studies on SA II units in the glabrous skin area of the human hand have revealed some new data which may be of interest in this context. We found two basically different types of such units, one type responded, to skin stretch in principally two opposite directions from the zone of maximum sensitivity to indentation. The zone of maximum sensitivity probably reflects the location of the receptor in the skin. The other type of SA II unit responds when the skin is stretched in only one direction from its zone of maximum sensitivity. When stretched in the opposite direction any activity present is decreased. The frequency of occurrence of these two types is about equal (for further details see Johansson, 1978).

DR. VERRILLO: You mentioned in the beginning that you used hand-held stimuli because these may be of value in clinical practice. I think it is very important when you report data, because you have decreased the precision of your measuring instrument, that you report something about the variability of your means because you may see differences that may or may not be real. It would be a good idea, I think, to report some statistical tests on how much faith you have in the differences that you report.

DR. VIERCK: I agree with you; the statistics will be presented in the publication. The major point to be emphasigned in this presentation is the advantage of skin stretch over indentation for orientation or direction sensitivity, and that comparison does not require statistics to appreciate the differences in discriminability.

DR. LINDBLOM: I would like to ask you if the rate of application on the hand-held lines was important. One criticism which you can have with all of these manual methods is that you have no control of the rate of indentation and of the depth. With the von Frey hairs you, at least, have some measure of the pressure. But with the compass test you do as you feel practical for the moment. The indentation velocity and depth may vary from one time to the next and from one investigator to the other. That, to my mind, is one serious criticism of these easy methods. How do you view that, with orientation and with the line length discriminations?

DR. VIERCK: We have not looked at those parameters of stimulus application. That certainly needs to be done to appreciate the limits of discriminability under different conditions. Rate might be important as it was for stretch sensitivity.

DR. STEVENS: There is another measure of spatial discrimination, often called the V test or gap detection, that is kind of analogous to two-point limen except that you are discriminating two lines. I do not recall whether that gave better discrimination than the two-point limen. Do you?

DR. VIERCK: No, I do not remember. We have used a different kind of gap discrimination that gives thresholds comparable to the two-point limen. Of course, one of the problems with the two-point measure is that when you compare two against one, if those two points define a line, you vary the external dimensions as well as the gap size when you change the distance between the two points. We used stimuli that were cut out of lines so that the gaps were of different dimensions and the outside length of the line remained constant. These stimuli gave essentially the same thresholds as the two-point threshold.

DR. VERRILLO: You have another problem when you are using two points, I assume the same thing is true for the line, and that is the person could be making an intensity discrimination rather than a spatial discrimination because two could feel greater than one.

DR. VIERCK: The two points have the additional problem of the temporal discrimination that might be made if you do not apply the two stimuli exactly simultaneously. There is much less of a problem with the gaps in the lines in terms of intensity or temporal discriminations, but certainly these cues could be present for the two-point method.

DR. STARR: I am not a cutaneous individual, I work in the auditory system but I can see one of the problems that you are talking about is the coupling between some environmental event and the response of the skin and then the nervous system. Has anybody looked at, for instance, how young skin differs from old skin or what is the turgor of the skin? Is there any way that one can define whether some of these are the differences you are talking about? Are they really neural events or are they skin elastic quality events?

DR. VIERCK: Probably other people are better equipped to answer that than I. I am only aware of the extensive literature on vibratory sensitivity that shows changes with old age. Would someone else like to speak on the point of young versus old skin?

DR. LINDBLOM: I can only say that the type of skin, the glabrous skin versus the hairy skin, is important and that the thickness of the corneal layer of the glabrous skin is very important as far as the threshold measurements are concerned, for instance of the Meissner corpuscles. That has been studied in human skin and in the cat's pad but I do not know about the suprathreshold functions. The type of skin will also influence the discrimination. If you have a stiff corneal layer the indentation will spread in a wider circle and make the neural excitation less precise.

DR. IGGO: It is also true that the responses of the primary afferent fibers can be affected by the condition of the skin. During the course of an experiment, but under general anesthesia, the sweat in the monkey's glabrous skin more or less stops and

gradually the skin becomes much stiffer. In those conditions the
thresholds of rapidly adapting receptors, for example, will increase quite a lot, and if the skin is then moistened the threshold
decreases again. It is clear that the condition surrounding the
skin is quite important. If you cut away some of the stratum
corneum in glabrous skin in the cat you can alter considerably the
threshold of the receptors lying beneath. I do not know, however,
of any systematic study of the problem.

DR. VERRILLO: I have systematic studies on the psychophysics of
vibratory sensitivity with age (Verrillo, in press) and I can
quickly show you the results. If you plot the threshold as a
function of frequency with very young children you get the standard
duplex threshold curve as shown in Fig. 1. With older people, up
to 70 or so years old, the non-Pacinian portion remains unchanged
but the minimum at about 250 Hz, the Pacinian portion, increases.
You can see that there is a very systematic change in the Pacinian
portion of the curve and this correlates very well with Cauna's
findings that the Pacinian corpuscle keeps adding lamellae with
age. They get large and distorted and become more efficient as a
filter. The non-Pacinian portion of the curve does not change with
age.

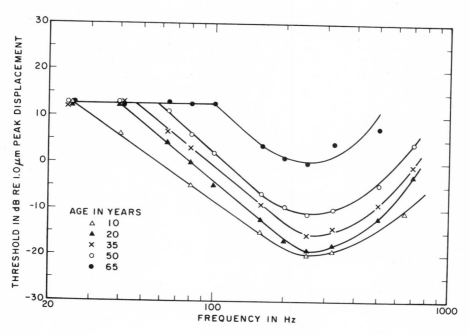

Fig. 1

DR. IGGO: Could I perhaps comment on the effect that you (Vierck) had when you were using a moving rather than a static displacement. The RA receptors in the hairy skin occupy quite large receptive fields. If the stimulus probe were placed directly on the field there will be a response as the stimulus is applied and then nothing. But if, for the same afferent unit, you then moved a stimulus across the field the total number of impulses and the duration of the discharge would be very much greater. This may account for the alteration of thresholds that you report when you use a moving rather than a static stimulus, at least a stimulus applied immediately over its whole length. This, however, then invokes the RA receptors in the exercise and does not leave it restricted to a consideration of only the RA receptors.

DR. VIERCK: Yes, I think that it is likely a very significant contributor to directional sensitivity of the skin and I think Barry (Whitsel) is going to speak on that point in a minute, when he shows directional sensitivity under conditions that should minimize skin stretch.

DR. FRANZEN: You talked about the motion of the stimulus and you move it quite fast. Does the subject ever over estimate the length of the excursion of the probe? There is an analagous situation in the visual system. If you have a line and move it very quickly, then ask the subject to point how far it has moved he will always over-estimate the distance it has moved away (Franzén, 1976). This is called "motion track enlargement," and if you use a monocular presentation the motion track enlargement is smaller than in the binocular situation, so you not only have the motion track enlargement you also have binocular summation. I wonder if you can see anything of this nature in your skin studies.

DR. VIERCK: No, I have not, but, this type of thing is being addressed much more by Barry Whitsel and he can probably interact with you on that.

REFERENCES

Franzén, O. On binocular vision. Scandinavian Journal of Psychology, 1976, 19, 223-229.
Johansson. R. S. Tactile sensitivity in the human hand: Receptive field characteristics of mechanoreceptive units in the glabrous skin area. Journal of Physiology (London), 1978, 281, 101-123.
Verrillo, R. T. Age-related changes in the sensitivity to vibration. Journal of Gerontology, in press.

THE CODING OF DIRECTION OF TACTILE STIMULUS MOVEMENT: CORRELATIVE PSYCHOPHYSICAL AND ELECTROPHYSIOLOGICAL DATA

B. L. Whitsel, D. A. Dreyer, M. Hollins, & M. G. Young

Departments of Physiology and Psychology,
Dental Research Center, and Neurobiology Program
University of North Carolina
Chapel Hill, North Carolina 27514

Recently published psychophysical studies have shown that the capacity of human subjects to identify direction of tactile stimuli that move in a linear path across the thenar eminence and the upper arm is a function of velocity, of the distance traversed by the moving stimulus ("traverse length") and of the cutaneous inner-vation density (Dreyer, Hollins, and Whitsel, 1976; Dreyer, Duncan, and Wong, 1978a; Dreyer, Hollins, and Whitsel, 1978b). Moreover, a subject's capacity to identify direction of linear movement on either the hairy or glabrous skin is independent of the orienta-tion of the stimulus path (Whitsel and Dreyer, unpublished obser-vations).

The primary objective of the present study was to identify an experimental approach that could provide quantitative estimates of the influence of stimulus parameters and of centrally acting drugs on the capacity of individual neurons in the postcentral gyrus of the cerebral cortex (area SI) to signal the direction of linear stimulus motion on the skin. Of specific interest were the stimu-lus parameters shown to exert prominent effects in our human psy-chophysical studies (e.g., velocity, traverse length, and stimulus location), and the general anesthetic drugs that are commonly em-ployed in studies of information processing by the somatic sen-sory nervous system. A secondary objective was to obtain additional psychophysical data bearing on the proposal that the well-known topographic variations in the density of cutaneous innervation are paralleled by topographic variations in cutaneous directional sensitivity (Dreyer, et al., 1976, 1978a,b).

The neurophysiological results to be presented demonstrate that directionally selective SI neurons of unanesthetized macaque

79

monkeys exhibit a prominent dependency on stimulus velocity and
traverse length. Moreover, comparison of the psychophysical and
neurophysiological data reveals that the capacities of SI neurons
to signal stimulus direction and of human subjects to discriminate
stimulus direction exhibit a similar dependence on stimulus velocity
and traverse length. All of the general anesthetics employed were
found to interfere dramatically, at subanesthetic dose levels,
with the information transmitting capacity of a population of SI
neurons which, in the absence of general anesthesia, reliably responded differentially to opposite directions of stimulus motion
on the skin. The psychophysical results provide further support
for the suggestion that the minimal distance a stimulus must move
in order for its direction to be accurately detected ("the critical
traverse length") is least for body regions that receive a dense
cutaneous innervation. The psychophysical data are also consistent
with the finding that SI neurons with receptive fields on the distal portions of the limbs continue to respond differentially to
stimuli moving in opposite directions at traverse lengths less
than the minimal traverse length required to demonstrate the directionally selectivity of neurons with receptive fields on more
proximal body regions.

METHODS

Neurophysiological Experiments

     Single unit recording. Extracellular recordings were obtained
with glass-insulated tungsten microelectrodes: their preparation
and characteristics have been described previously, as have our
methods for determining receptive-field location, submodality
class, and response properties of individual cerebral cortical
neurons (Werner and Whitsel, 1968). The impulses discharged by
individual neurons were amplified and displayed in the conventional
manner.

     At the end of the experiment, the animal was deeply anes-
thesized and then perfused with 0.9 percent saline and 10 percent
neutral buffered formalin. The brain was embedded in celloidin,
sectioned at 30 μm, and the sections were stained with cresyl fast
violet and/or Mahon's stain. Each microelectrode penetration was
reconstructured, and the cytoarchitectonic areas encountered by the
electrode were identified according to the criteria of Powell and
Mountcastle (1959). Electrolytic lesions (created by passing DC
currents of 2.5 to 5 sec through the recording electrode) were made
in order to identify the sites at which single neurons were studied
quantitatively.

     Stimulus control, data collection and analysis. The mechanical
stimulator employed consisted of a servomotor and controlling

electronic circuitry enabling the delivery of constant-velocity
tactile stimuli that traversed a selected region of skin at a
predetermined orientation and direction (for details see Schreiner
and Whitsel, 1978). Stimuli consisted of movements of a camel's
hair brush (Fig. 1) across the skin at constant velocity. The
handle of the brush was connected to the shaft of the servomotor
so that as the shaft rotated through 360°, the brush described a
large circle. None of the brushes used in the present study ex-
erted a force greater than 10 gm, nor did they produce significant
distortion of the skin at any of the velocities employed. Stimuli
were delivered at velocities between 0.25 and 400 cm/sec: the
stimuli were controlled by a PDP-11/20 computer (for details of
stimulus control see Schreiner and Whitsel, 1978).

At least eight different stimulus velocities were applied in
the course of study of an SI neuron; in addition, stimuli differing in velocity were applied in opposite directions, at several
orientations, and over several traverse lengths whenever possible
(see next section for method of controlling traverse length).
Stimuli differing in velocity were randomized for each neuron
studied and successive stimulus presentations were separated by an
interval of at least 3.5 sec during which the stimulator did not
contact the skin.

For the characterization of the discharge activity evoked by
tactile stimuli moving at constant velocity, we plotted the data
as post stimulus time histograms (PST histograms). Each PST histogram was constructed from the responses to $\underline{n}$ replications of a
stimulus having velocity $\underline{v}$, traverse length $\underline{TL}$ and direction $\underline{d}$.

Psychophysical Experiments

The subject was comfortably seated in a dental chair, and the
region of the forelimb to be studied was immobilized using a suction-
evacuated plastic bag containing polystyrene beads (Nuclear Associates, Inc.). A plate of 0.6 cm thick plexiglas was positioned
gently on the skin and then clamped in place. In the center of
the plate was an aperture 0.5 cm in width and 0.25, 0.5, 1, 2, or
4 cm in length. The servomotor stimulator was positioned so that
with each 360° rotation of its drive shaft (both clockwise and
counterclockwise rotations were possible) the brush moved over the
aperture plate that had been placed on the skin. The plate was
machined to allow the brush to move smoothly onto and off the skin.
Since the brush was slightly wider than the aperture, the width
of the skin field stimulated was defined by the aperture width
(0.5 cm) and the length of the stimulated field (traverse
length) by aperture length. The motor and the plate were always

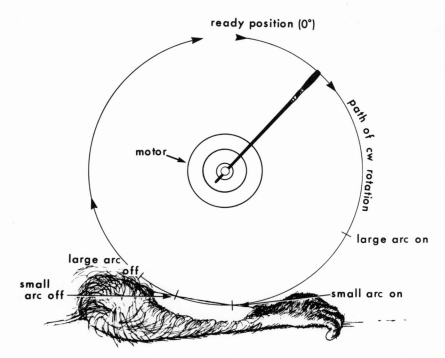

Fig. 1.   The mechanical stimulator used to deliver constant velocity
          moving stimuli to the skin. The motor is connected to a
          position encoder that indicates the position of the brush
          with an accuracy of ½°. On command, either manually or by
          program control, brush movement (either CW or CCW) begins
          at the 0° (ready) position and moves at high velocity
          (slew) to a preset position called "large arc on." This
          position and the other three preset positions are set by
          thumb wheel switches on the motor controller. At large
          arc on, the motor slows to the test velocity which has
          been set either manually or by the program control via a
          D/A converter. The brush moves to the "small arc on" pre-
          set position (always inside large arc on) at which time
          an interupt is generated so that the computer can obtain
          a clock reading. Similarly, at the "small arc off"
          position another interrupt is generated. The small arc
          positions are usually employed to mark the point of initial
          brush contact and the point at which the brush leaves the
          skin. As movement continues, the brush finally reaches
          the "large arc off" position where it slews to the ready
          position and stops. A third interrupt is generated when
          the ready position is reached and, at this time, the
          stimulus cycle can be repeated.

oriented so that when the servomotor shaft rotated in the counter-clockwise direction the brush swept from proximal to distal (P→D) over the skin; a clockwise rotation moved the brush in the opposite (D→P) direction. The opposite directions of brush motion and the different stimulus velocities were delivered and monitored by the PDP-11/20 computer and were randomized within each block of trials.

Surgical towels were draped across adjacent skin regions to prevent air currents from serving as cues. The subject's view of the apparatus was blocked by a curtain, and headphones were used to eliminate auditory cues.

A green panel light mounted in front of the subject informed him that a stimulus presentation (a single sweep of the brush) was about to begin; after each presentation, the green light was turned off and a blue light came on indicating that a response was required. A two-option forced choice procedure was used. The subject operated a toggle switch to indicate whether he thought the brush moved in a proximal to distal direction, or the reverse. No feedback was given during a run. The computer stored the response to each stimulus. Following each block, the actual direction and velocity of each stimulus as well as the subject's response to that stimulus were printed out in tabular format and the subject's performance (in terms of per cent correct responses at each velocity) was plotted automatically.

RESULTS

Neurophysiological Experiments

Determinants of design. Prior work (Whitsel, Roppolo, and Werner, 1972; Whitsel, Dreyer, and Hollins, 1978; Hyvärinen, Poranen, Jokinen, Näätänen, and Linnankoski, 1973; Hyvärinen, Poranen, and Jokinen, 1974) has shown that stimulus motion across the cutaneous receptive field (RF) of an SI neuron usually evokes a higher rate of discharge than that produced by a stimulus moving perpendicular to the skin surface (i.e., by skin indentation). Although most SI cutaneous neurons do not respond differentially to stimuli that move across their RFs in different directions (non-directional neurons), for a certain population of SI neurons one particular direction is particularly effective (Whitsel, et al., 1972; Hyvärinen, et al., 1973, 1974). These directionally selective neurons are differentially distributed within SI of primates, i.e., they are found most frequently in cortical laminae located superficial and deep to lamina IV of cytoarchitectural area 1 (Whitsel, et al., 1972).

Figure 2 shows the spike trains obtained from a directionally selective SI neuron whose RF was located on the glabrous skin of the contralateral hand. This figure illustrates that the two PST

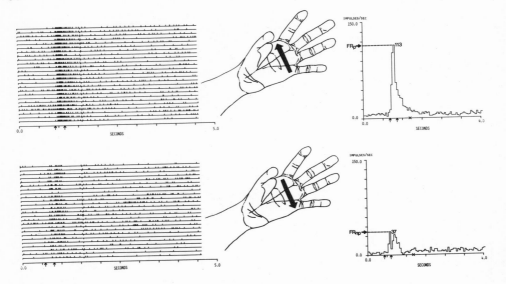

Fig. 2. The response of a directionally selective SI neuron
(18-5-A) to stimuli moving at constant velocity (15 cm/sec
in opposite directions across the receptive field. On the
left: spike trains evoked by stimulus movements from
lateral to medial (the preferred direction: at the top)
and in the opposite direction (the non-preferred direction;
at the botton) across a 3.0 x 0.5 cm path on the palmar
surface of the contralateral hand. On the right: PST
histograms computed for the spike trains shown on the left.
FR_p = peak mean firing rate (bin width 50 msec) in preferred direction: FR_{np} = peak mean firing rate in non-
preferred direction. See text for details.

histograms computed for the spike trains evoked by the opposite
directions of stimulus motion can be used to obtain an estimate of
the capacity of the neuron to distinguish, using a mean rate code,
between stimuli moving at identical velocities but in opposite
directions across the RF. This estimate (hereafter referred to as
"D") is the difference between the peak mean firing rates evoked
by the opposite directions of stimulus motion. Mean firing rate
was selected as the measure of neuronal response since it is independent of changes in stimulus and, as a consequence, it can be
used to assess the effects of stimulus velocity on SI neuron responses. Figure 3 illustrates this point of view with representative trains of discharge activity obtained from an SI neuron at
different velocities as well as with a plot of stimulus velocity

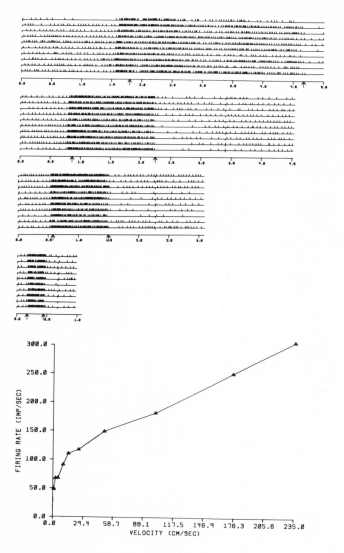

Fig. 3. Effects of velocity on SI neuron responses to moving tactile stimuli. At the top: 4 sets of spike trains (10
stimulus replicates/set) obtained for an SI neuron (12-4-
C) during the application of stimuli moving from caudal to
rostal across the skin of the dorsal trunk. The different sets of spike trains were evoked by brushing stimuli
that moved the same distance (13.6 cm) across the receptive field at 4 different velocities: i.e., 5, 10, 15
and 50 cm/sec, respectively. At the bottom: the velocity-
response (peak mean firing rate) relationship between
1.0 and 235 cm/sec.

versus peak mean firing rate for the same neuron. Inspection of
these spike train data clearly reveals that, due to changes in
stimulus duration, the mean number of spikes evoked per stimulus
is a decreasing function of stimulus velocity. On the other hand,
the velocity-response plot demonstrates that for this SI neuron
increments in peak mean firing rate accompanied increases in

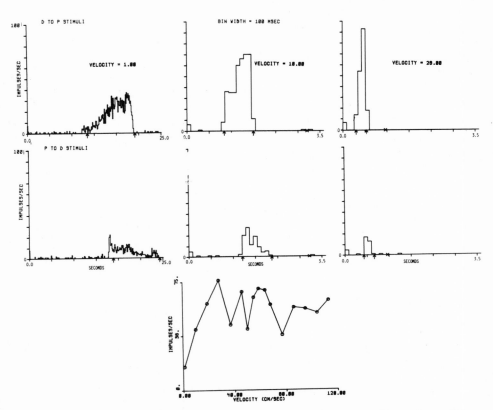

Fig. 4.   Effects of stimulus velocity on the capacity of an SI
           neurons (7-2-A) to respond differentially to opposite
           directions of stimulus motion. At the top: three PST
           histograms computed for the responses to stimulus move-
           ment from distal-to-proximal (D→P) at 1.0 (left), 10
           (middle), and 28 (right) cm/sec over 7.5 cm of the dorsal
           preaxial thigh. Middle: PST histograms for the responses
           to stimulus movement from proximal-to-distal (P→D) at the
           same distance and velocities employed in the opposite
           direction. Each histogram was computed from the response
           of 25 identical stimulus replications. Botton: plot of
           the difference in peak mean firing rates (D) evoked by
           the opposite directions of stimulus motion. Bin width
           of all histograms 100 msec.

stimulus velocity over the range of 1 to 250 cm/sec.

The PST histograms of Fig. 4 show that the magnitude of the difference in peak mean firing rate (D) evoked from a directional SI neuron by opposite directions of stimulus motion is prominently and systematically influenced by stimulus velocity. In the experiments of this study and in earlier investigations (Whitsel, et al., 1972, 1978), it was also demonstrated that the directionally selective response of SI neurons (as estimated by D) could be prominently inlfuenced by the orientation of the linear stimulus path. On the basis of the available data, it appears that the population of directionally selective SI neurons that represent a given cutaneous field consists of individuals each of which is rather narrowly tuned to detect stimulus movement in a particular direction, and that for a given cutaneous field there are SI neurons tuned to movement across the RF in all of the available directions. It also seems clear that our failure in previous studies to utilize a sufficiently wide range of stimulus velocities and orientation led us to underestimate grossly the number of directionally selective neurons present in SI (Whitsel, et al., 1972).

Figure 5 shows the effect of a rapidly acting barbiturate (Methohexital 4 mg/kg, administered intravenously) on the directional response of the same neuron illustrated in Fig. 2. Similar effects were obtained with Ketamine, Pentobarbital, and halothane.

In view of the observations described above, we adpoted the following approach to the quantitative analysis of the effects of stimulus velocity and traverse length on the representation of stimulus direction by SI neurons. In the first place, the experiments were conducted in the absence of general anesthesia.[1]

---

[1]The effects of the neuromuscular blocking drugs on SI discharge activity are not easy to assess experimentally. There are grounds, however, to believe that use of non-depolarizing neuromuscular blocking agents (e.g., gallamine) does not lead to intense pain and discomfort and in fact, after several hours of adaptation, does not lead to a situation appreciably more disorienting or stressful than that experienced by restrained animals subjected to similar neurophysiological recording and stimulus procedures. For instance, the demonstration that unambiguous representation of stimulus direction by some SI neurons requires the behaving animal to be selectively attending to his stimulus environment (Werner, 1978; see also Hyvärinen, et al., 1974) suggests that under our conditions the animal is attending to the cutaneous stimuli and makes it seem quite unlikely that the condition of neuromuscular block (provided it is produced with non-depolarizing drugs, that no pain producing

Second, at the initial stage of our study of a neuron, moving
stimuli were applied (using the servo-controlled stimulator in the
"manual" mode) in opposite directions at each of several orientations in order to determine the orientation at which the maximal
differential response was evoked by linear motion in opposite
directions. Once the optimal orientation had been determined,
the remainder of the experiment was conducted with the stimulator
under computer control. At each stimulus traverse length (most
frequently determined by use of an aperture) brushing stimuli
moving at different velocities were presented. Whenever possible,
at least eight stimulus velocities ranging between 1 and 250

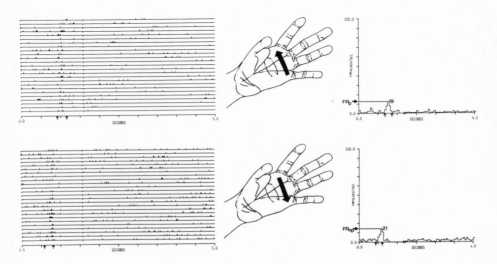

Fig. 5.   The response of a directionally selective SI neuron
          (18-5-A) to stimuli moving at a constant velocity (15
          cm/sec) in opposite directions across 3 cm of its re-
          ceptive field 20 minutes after the intravenous adminis-
          tration of Methohexital (4 mg/kg). Format is the same
          as that of Fig. 2.

mechanical stimuli are delivered, and that ventilation is adequate)
is, in itself, pain producing. On the other hand, the depolarizing
neuromuscular blocking drugs (e.g., succinylcholine, decamethonium)
must be avoided in the absence of general anesthesia, for the intense activation of peripheral mechanoreceptors and chemoreceptors
they produce would be certain to evoke painful and distressful
sensations.

cm/sec were employed, each velocity was replicated at least 10 times and, in all cases, the velocities were presented in random order. For a given traverse length, a complete set of velocities was delivered in one direction and then in the other. Successive stimulus presentations were separated by 3.5 seconds.

Effects of velocity at different traverse lengths. Figures 6. 7 and 8 show the PST histograms computed from the activity evoked from a directionally selective SI neuron (18-5-A) at three different velocities (1.0, 25 and 175 cm/sec). At each velocity, the stimuli were applied in opposite directions at each of three different traverse lengths: 3.0 cm (Fig. 6), 1.0 cm (Fig. 7), and 0.5 cm (Fig. 8). It can be seen that at a traverse length of 3.0 cm (Fig. 6) the neuron responds differentially to stimuli moving in opposite directions at all three velocities, and that the differential response is maximal at 25 cm/sec. As traverse length is reduced, however, (to 1.0 cm in Fig. 7, and to 0.5 cm in Fig. 8) the response evoked by the moving stimuli applied in the preferred direction falls off to a much greater extent than that evoked by movement in the non-preferred direction. When traverse length was reduced to 0.5 cm or less, the neuron continued to respond to stimulus movement with a clear-cut elevation in firing rate, but opposite directions of movement no longer evoked significantly different peak mean firing rates.

Figure 9 summarizes an extensive set of observations obtained from SI neuron 18-5-A. The velocity-response relations for the preferred (0-0) and non-preferred (Δ-Δ) directions of movement at the three traverse lengths are shown on the left: on the right the difference in the peak mean firing rates evoked by the opposite directions of stimulus movement (D) is plotted as a function of velocity for each of the three traverse lengths.

Effects of velocity at a given traverse length are dependent on receptive field location. Figure 10 compares the effects of stimulus velocity on the capacity of SI neurons representing different body regions to respond differentially to stimuli moving in opposite directions. Traverse length was held constant at 13.6 cm for 12-4-C and at 15.0 cm for neuron 12-5-A. For both neurons, D increased progressively as velocity was increased from 1.0 to 15 cm/sec. Further increases in velocity revealed substantial differences between the neurons. For neuron 12-5-A (RF on dorsal trunk), D decreased sharply as velocity was increased above 15 cm/sec, whereas for neuron 12-4-C (RF on distal forelimb) there was little, if any, significant decrease of D at the higher velocities. These data are representative of those obtained from neurons with RFs positioned on either proximal or distal body regions when large traverse lengths are employed. Fig. 11 shows the effects of reductions in traverse length on the velocity

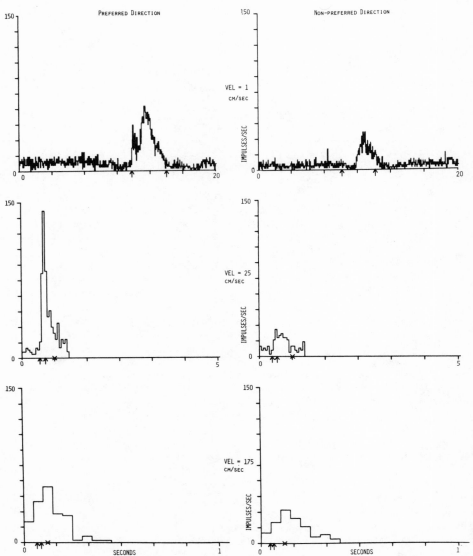

Fig. 6. PST histograms illustrating the responses of an SI neuron
(18-5-A) to stimuli moving in opposite directions, i.e.,
preferred (on the left) and non-preferred (on the right).
For all histograms in Figs. 6,7 and 8 intertrial interval-
3.5 sec and bin width = 50 msec. Time at which the brush
made contact and at which it left the skin are indicated
by arrows below the ordinate. Traverse length = 3.0 cm
and brush velocities were 1 cm/sec (top), 25 cm/sec
(middle) and 175 cm/sec (bottom).

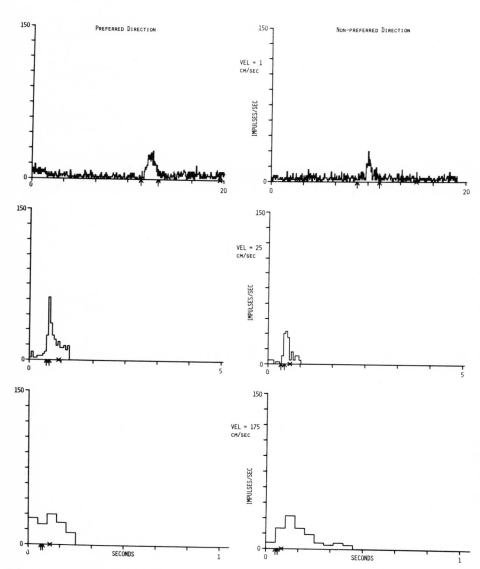

Fig. 7. PST histograms illustrating the responses of SI neuron (18-5-A) to stimuli moving in opposite directions. Traverse length = 1.0 cm. See legend to Fig. 6 for other parameters and details.

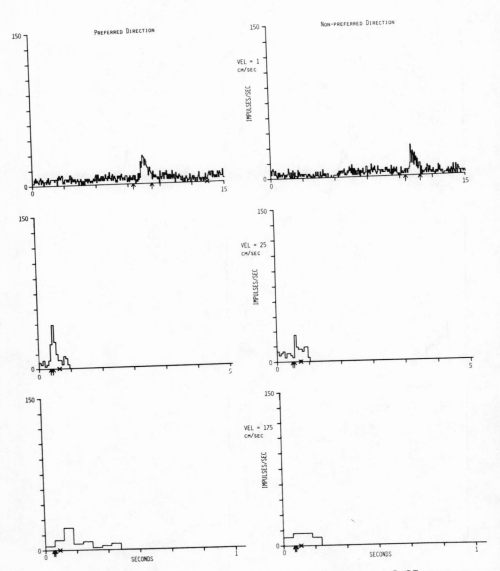

Fig. 8.   PST histograms illustrating the response of SI neuron
          (18-5-A) to stimuli moving in opposite directions. Tra-
          verse length = 0.5 cm. See legend to Fig. 6 for other
          parameters and details.

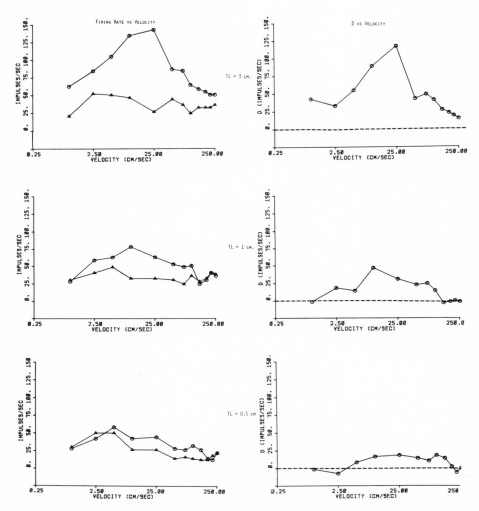

Fig. 9. Summary of the effects of velocity and traverse length on
the capacity of SI neuron 18-5-A to respond differentially
to stimuli moving in opposite directions over its receptive field. Circles represent preferred and triangles
non-preferred direction. See text for details. When
D ≃ 0, there is no difference in the peak mean firing rate
evoked by stimulus movement in opposite directions.

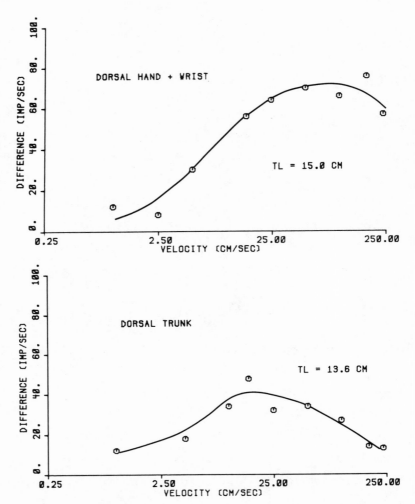

Fig. 10.   The effects of stimulus velocity on the capacity of two
           SI neurons with different receptive fields to respond
           differentially to stimuli moving in opposite directions.
           For both neurons, traverse length was held constant
           (13.6 cm for neuron 12-4-C, 15.0 cm for neuron 12-5-A;
           it is extremely unlikely that this difference in the
           traverse lengths could account for the substantial differ-
           ence in the effects of velocity on the directional selec-
           tivity of the two neurons).   The substantial differences
           in the effect of velocity are particularly evident at
           velocities above 25 cm/sec.

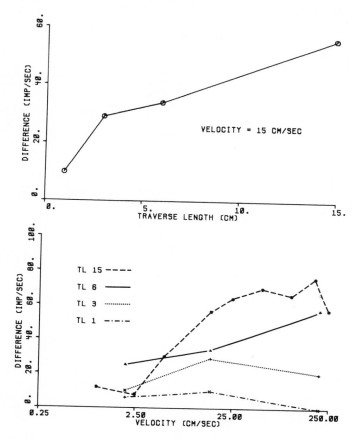

Fig. 11.   Effects of different traverse lengths on the capacity of
SI neuron 12-5-A to respond differentially to stimuli
moving in opposite directions across the receptive field.
The top graph is a plot of D as a function of traverse
length at a single velocity (15 cm/sec). Similar relationships would be obtained at other velocities over
the range of 5 to 200 cm/sec. The bottom graph shows
the effects of four different traverse lengths on the
difference in peak mean firing rate evoked by opposite
directions of stimulus movement.

dependent directional selectivity of neuron 12-5-A (RF on distal
forelimb). It can be seen (a) that at traverse lengths as small
as 3 cm, this neuron continued to respond differentially (in terms
of peak mean firing rate) to stimuli moving in opposite directions:
and (b) that at this near minimum traverse length, opposite directions of movement are signalled best at intermediate velocities
(velocities in the vicinity of 15 cm/sec) and poorly at either the
high (200 cm/sec) or low (1 cm/sec) extremes of the velocity range

employed. It should also be noted that although D approaches zero
(when D=0 there is no difference in the mean firing rate evoked by
opposite directions of movement) for all stimulus velocities when
traverse length was 1 cm, the moving stimuli were still quite
effective in evoking a response whose peak mean firing rate significantly exceeded the firing rate of the neuron in the absence
of stimulation. Figure 11 (top) plots, for neuron 12-5-A, D as a
function of traverse length at a single velocity. It is apparent
that a similar relationship would obtain at most velocities within the range of 5 to 200 cm/sec.

In general, we interpret the available data to indicate (a)
that for directionally selective SI neurons representing different
body regions a reproducible and systematic relationship exists
among traverse length, velocity, and the neuron's capacity to respond differentially to opposite directions of stimulus motion,
and (b) that a major difference between neurons with proximal and
distal receptive fields is that the former require larger traverse
lengths to manifest significant directionality.

Psychophysical Experiments

Figure 12 illustrates the performance of two subjects when
moving stimuli were applied to the most distal region of the volar
surface of digit 2 on the left hand. Subject performance (expressed
in terms of the per cent of correct responses) is plotted as a
function of brush velocity. Each point is based on 40 trials and
different symbols are used to represent the different traverse
lenghts employed. The data obtained from subject B.L.W. are shown
in Fig. 12 (top). When the stimuli moved a distance of 4 cm, this
subject's performance exceeded the 75 per cent criterion level at
all velocities tested. Progressive reductions in traverse length
led to a decrease in performance at both the higher (100-250 cm/
sec) and lower (0.75-1.0 cm/sec) velocities until, at a traverse
length of 0.5 cm, the subject exceeded the criterion level only at
velocities between 3 and 10 cm/sec. Criterion performance was
never attained by subject B.L.W. when the stimulus traverse length
was 0.25 cm.

Figure 12 (bottom) plots the data obtained from subject D.A.D.
Since this subject exceeded the 75 per cent criterion at all velocities when the stimulus moved 2 cm across the volar surface of
digit 2, the 4 cm aperture was not tested. Similar to the data
shown for B.L.W., this subject's performance fell below the 75 per
cent criterion at velocities of 100 cm/sec and higher when a traverse length of 1 cm aperture was used. With the 0.5 cm aperture,
criterion was reached or exceeded only at velocities of 1, 3 and
10 cm/sec. Once again, criterion performance was not attained at
any velocity when the traverse length was 0.25 cm.

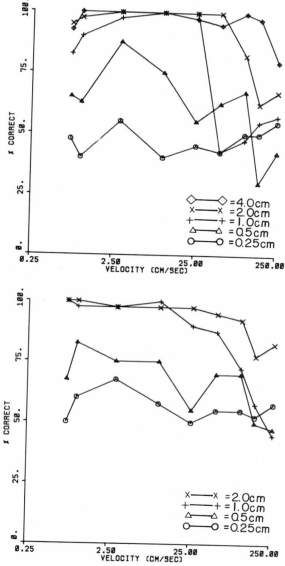

Fig. 12.   Performance (percent correct) as a function of velocity
for B.L.W. (top) and D.A.D. (bottom) when stimuli were
delivered to the volar surface of digit 2 of the left
hand. Stimulus velocities applied were 0.75, 1, 3, 10,
25, 50, 100, 150 and 250 cm/sec. Five traverse lengths
were used for B.L.W.: 4, 2, 1, 0.5 and 0.25 cm. The 4
cm plate was not used with D.A.D. Each points represents 40 trials.

Two general trends can be observed in the psychophysical data plotted in Fig. 12: (i) a subject correctly distinguishes stimulus direction of the skin at the longer traverse lengths and (ii) at a given traverse length, a subject generally performed better at velocities between 3 and 10 cm/sec than he did at the lower or higher velocities. This tendency is most evident at intermediate traverse lengths since performance versus velocity functions of the longest and shortest traverse lengths are necessarily flattened as they reach the ceiling (100 percent) and floor (50 percent) of the range over which performance varies.

Figure 13 replots the performance of a single subject (B.L.W.) as a function of traverse length for stimuli moving at 1.0 cm/sec. Since similar relationships were found at nearly all the other velocities used in this study, we have characterized performance at each velocity by a single number which we call the "critical length" (CL) for that velocity. As indicated in Fig. 13, the critical length for a given velocity is that traverse length,

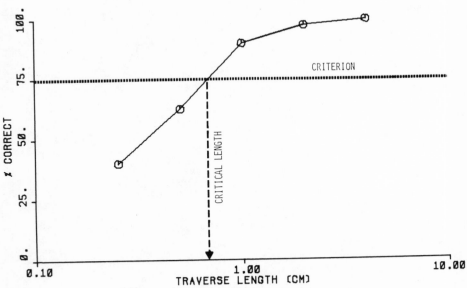

Fig. 13.   Data from one subject (B.L.W.) for one velocity (1.0 cm/sec) are plotted from Fig. 12 to illustrate the method for determining critical length: i.e. that traverse length, determined by interpolation, at which 75 percent of the responses would be correct.

determined by interpolation, at which the subject would respond correctly on 75 per cent of the trials.

Critical length data for digit 2 are shown in Fig. 14 along with previously described data (Dreyer et al., 1978a,b) for other body regions. The more accurately a subject can identify direction of brush movement at a particular velocity, the lower will be the computed critical length and, as predicted by the data in Fig. 12, critical length is minimal (directional sensitivity is maximal) at intermediate stimulus velocities. Figure 14 illustrates that CL

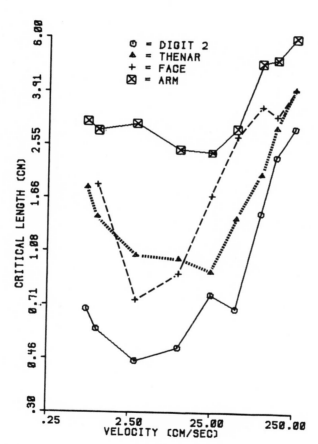

Fig. 14. Critical length as a function of velocity for four different body regions. Data points for digit 2 are averages of individual data from two subjects: data points for all other body regions are averages from three subjects.

for digit 2 is minimal (i.e., directional sensitivity is maximal) at velocities between 3 and 10 cm/sec and declines at lower and particularly at the higher velocities. Figure 14 also illustrates (a) that all regions tested, velocity exerts similar effects on the capacity to distinguish stimulus direction, and (b) that the relative sensitivity to tactile stimulus direction exhibits systematic topographic variations that are highly reproducible from one subject to the next. When ranked according to directional sensitivity the sequence is as follows: volar digit 2 > face > thenar eminence > arm.

DISCUSSION

The neural data available at this time are still too meager to be compared quantitatively with the data obtained in the psychophysical studies of human subjects. Nevertheless, for all SI neurons examined the data indicate (a) that the velocity range required for maximal differential response to cutaneous stimuli moving in opposite directions corresponds closely to that required for optimal cutaneous direction discrimination by human subjects, and (b) that the dependency of the directional response on traverse length is qualitatively similar to that of the human subjects. In addition, the finding that the minimal traverse length necessary for an SI neuron to respond differentially to opposite directions of stimulus movement is smaller for distal than it is for proximal body regions corresponds nicely with the psychophysical evidence that the minimal traverse length required for direction discrimination (the "critical length") is greater for body regions lacking a dense cutaneous innervation (e.g., the upper arm) than it is for densely innervated regions (the thenar eminence, the face, and the digits).

The above observations, taken together with (a) the evidence that the postcentral gyrus is the earliest stage of the somatosensory nervous system to contain neurons with directional selectivity (Whitsel, et al., 1972) and (b) that the capacity of macaque monkeys to discriminate direction of stimulus motion is permanently lost following interruption of the spinal afferent input to this cortical region (Vierck, 1974; Dreyer, et al., 1974) leads us to suggest that the population of directionally selective neurons in SI contributes in a fundamental way to the capacity of primates to evaluate and respond appropriately to natural stimuli that move across the skin.

ACKNOWLEDGEMENTS

The technical assistance of Ann Cooper, Pat Whitaker and Calvin Wong is gratefully acknowledged. The authors wish to express their appreciation to Robert Schreiner for developing the computer programs for collection and off-line analysis of the neurophysiological data as well as for program control of the stimulator in both the neurophysiological and psychophysical experiments.

Principal support for this project was provided by PHS Grant NS10865 awarded by the NINCDS. Additional support was provided through grants RR05333 and DE02668. General facilities support was provided, in part, by Grant NS11132. D. A. Dreyer is the recipient of NIH Career Development Award DE00011.

REFERENCES

Dreyer, D. A., Hollins, M. & Whitsel, B. L. Behavioral measures of cutaneous sensitivity. Neuroscience Abstracts, 1976, 2, 933.

Dreyer, D. A., Duncan, G., Wong, C. & Whitsel, B. L. Factors influencing capacity to judge direction of tactile stimulus movement on the face. Submitted to Archives of Oral Biology, 1978a.

Dreyer, D. A., Hollins, M. & Whitsel, B. L. Factors influencing cutaneous directional sensitivity. Sensory Processes, 1978b, 2, 71-79.

Dreyer, D. A., Schneider, R. J., Metz, C. B. & Whitsel, B. L. Differential contributions of spinal pathways to body representation in postcentral cyrus of Macaca mulatta. Journal of Neurophysiology, 1974, 37, 119-145.

Hyvärinen, J., Poranen, A., Jokinen, Y., Näätänen, R. & Linnankoski, I. Observations on unit activity in the primary somesthetic cortex of behaving monkeys. In H. H. Kornhuber (Ed.), The somatosensory system. Stuttgart: Georg Thieme Variag, 1973.

Hyvärinen, J., Poranen, A. & Jokinen, Y. Central sensory activities between sensory input and motor output. In F. O. Schmitt & F. G. Worden (Eds.), The neurosciences, third study program. Cambridge: The MIT Press, 1974.

Powell, T. P. S. & Mountcastle, V. B. Some aspects of the functional organization of the cortex of the postcentral gyrus of the monkey: a correlation of findings obtained in a single unit analysis with cytoarchitecture. John Hopkins Medical Journal, 1959, 105, 133-162.

Schreiner, R. G. & Whitsel, B. L. A computer system for neurophysiological data acquisition and experiment control. Submitted to Computers and Biomedical Research, 1978.

Vierck, C. J. Tactile movement detection and discrimination following dorsal column lesions in monkeys. Experimental Brain Research, 1974, 20, 331-346.

Werner, G.   Static and dynamic components of object representations
     in the central nervous system.   In M. A. B. Brazier & H.
     Petsche (Eds.), In Architectonics of the cerebral cortex.
     New York: Raven Press, 1978.

Werner, G. & Whitsel, B. L.   Topology of the body representation
     in somatosensory area I of primates. Journal of Neurophy-
     siology, 1968, 31, 856-869.

Whitsel, B. L., Roppolo, J. R. & Werner, G.   Cortical information
     processing of stimulus motion on primate skin. Journal of
     Neurophysiology, 1972, 35, 691-717.

Whitsel, B. L., Dreyer, D. A. & Hollins, M.   Representation of
     moving stimuli by somatosensory neurons. Federation Proceed-
     ings, 1978, 37, 9-13.

DISCUSSION

DR. FRANZÉN: A short question as to anesthesia. When you plot
velocity and the magnitude of the response, I understand, of course,
that anesthesia affects the magnitude of the response but could it
be that the relationship is invariant? I mean you could get the
family of functions if you used different levels of anesthesia. In
that way coding would still be precise although the overall
amplitude would change.

DR. WHITSEL: For certain SI neurons that exhibit directional
selectivity we have observed that although the magnitude of response
evoked by stimuli moving in one direction is reduced by general
anesthetics, the form of the velocity-response function is
essentially unchanged. On the other hand, a total loss of directional
selectivity, but not of sensitivity to moving stimuli, has been
seen for other SI neurons. The latter effect could only occur, of
course, if the velocity-response functions for the two directions
of motion were altered differentially.

DR. POULOS: I was wondering, with the type of arc that you have,
how you control intensity, especially at the longer lengths. It
would seem that for a certain length, intensity would be more
constant than at others. One aside, perhaps you know the group
at Pittsburgh who have been working with awake animals. They show
slides very similar to your Fig. 5, i.e., a reduction in the
overall activity following injection of very small amounts of
nembutal. However, behaviorally, the animals performed better than
normals.

DR. WHITSEL: Yes, I have seen prominent reductions in overall
activity and in receptive field dimensions after nembutal injection,
but I have not performed concurrent measures of directional
sensitivity under the same conditions. To me, at least, such
increases in the capacity to identify stimulus direction would not
appear to go along with the neurons' loss of their capacity to
signal stimulus direction. Perhaps different effects appear with
different dosage levels? As to your first question regarding
stimulus control, the radius of the arc and the brush length were
maintained constant across all experiments. With the range of
velocities we studied, our apparatus permitted us to deliver all
the velocities at one brush length.

DR. FRANZÉN: What Dr. Poulos mentioned reminds me of what
happened at the last olympic games. In shooting, they found that
people who took one or two cans of beer before the game performed
better.

DR. WHITSEL: I would comment on the actions of another class of drugs on SI neurons. Since my graduate training was in pharmacology I, of course, have had more than a passing interest in the actions of centrally acting drugs and of the hallucinogens in particular on the capacity of sensory neurons to encode stimulus features. Hallucinogens do have quite prominent actions on somatosensory cortical neurons: for example, after low doses of phencyclidine certain neurons exhibit an enhanced capacity to encode stimulus direction. That is not a recommendation.

DR. VIERCK: It seems to me that by delivering the stimulus in the window that you are minimizing the effect of stretch, and also the traverse length functions that you show, indicate that stretch is probably not an important factor here. But I wonder if you have seen slowly adapting units in the cortex that are directionally sensitive. If so, how does stretch relate to that directional sensitivity?

DR. WHITSEL: The particular type of stimulus mode we are using is rather different than that conventionally used to classify the adaptation characteristics of first-order somatosensory afferents. While SI neurons could be classified on the basis of the length of time they maintain a response during stimulus movement across their receptive fields, I don't think this information would tell one which first-order afferents were projecting onto the neuron. To illustrate, since the great majority of SI neurons continue to fire as the stimulus moves through the receptive field one might tend to classify them as slowly adapting. This would lead to confusion, however, and our approach to the problem has been to use punctate stimuli with the hope of achieving a match between groups of cortical neurons and first-order afferents. With punctate stimuli (maintained skin indentation with a 1 mm stimulus probe) the great majority of cortical neurons with cutaneous receptive fields respond only weakly, if at all, and only at stimulus onset. Another approach we have taken was to study first-order afferents with moving stimulus identical to those described in today's presentation. In addition to the hair follicle afferents, the SA I and II afferents respond very well to such stimuli. True directional preferences were not seen, at least not in the relatively small sample studied to date.

DR. VIERCK: Stretch is not effective, directionally, for these units?

DR. WHITSEL: One does see, as the stimulus crosses the receptive field, an apparent unloading of the receptors that is reflected by a depression of the ongoing spontaneous activity, and when the stimulus crosses the bleeb (excitatory focus) there is a large increase in mean firing rate. After crossing the focus, there may or may not be a second unloading of the receptor organ. Such differences in the response to tactile stimuli moving in opposite directions over the focus are very subtle compared to those seen for directionally selective cortical neurons and, furthermore, the differences in the response to opposite directions of brush movement seen for first-order afferents exhibit little velocity dependency.

DR. IGGO: Do you think that the different effects that you get with direction, and so on, can be simply accounted for in terms of the number of impulses coming in from the periphery? For example, the sensitivity of thresholds vary whether you have the stimulus applied to the periphery or the upper arm and, of course, there are more afferent fibers per unit area in the periphery. When you increase the velocity, or when you change direction you may also change the number of impulses being discharged in any particular afferent fiber. Or, do you think that there is some other process at work?

DR. WHITSEL: I would be very interested in the correct answer to that question. Although I cannot give an answer, it strikes me as important to note in this context that the receptive fields of these neurons are very large compared to those recorded at first-order levels. There are, therefore, plenty of opportunities for convergence and integration. The mechanisms that could produce the directional preferences exhibited by these neurons are completely unknown. It may be that drugs can be quite useful tools for studying the mechanisms underlying somatosensory cortical neuron direction selectivity.

DR. IGGO: In cases where you used the same amount of window aperture distally on the limb and then proximally in the limb, one would certainly expect to have many more afferents engaged by the distal than proximal stimulus. This would fit with the results that you get, not the directional effects.

DR. WHITSEL: Yes, the similarly shaped functions relating critical length with velocity that we got for the four different body parts (Text Fig. 12) indicate that considerations about cutaneous innervation density do not really contribute to the form of the function.

DR. IGGO: No, not necessarily to the form of the function, but to the relative sensitivity.

DR. WHITSEL: Yes, you're right. The directional sensitivity seems to correlate very well with peripheral cutaneous innervation density.

DR. LINDBLOM: Would your stimuli be rapid enough to excite the Pacinian afferents and would simultaneously applied vibration in the receptive field interfere with the directional sensitivity?

DR. WHITSEL: I do not know the answer to either question. I suspect that at least at the intermediate and higher velocities such stimuli are adequate to activate the Pacinian afferents. I doubt very much they are sufficient at the lowest velocities. Five grams is the amount of pressure we have monitored by placing a transducer under the aperture in place of the skin. The stimulator delivers a fairly decent looking step of force when it encounters the leading edge of the transducer; and the force is well maintained as the brush proceeds across the transducer surface (a 1.0 by 3.0 cm plate). However, if the aperture is removed prominent fluctuations in force occur. The latter observation is difficult to interpret, but we suggest that since such fluctuations are not seen with the aperture, the skin "sees" a step-like and smooth force-profile when the stimulator is used with the aperture plate.

DR. IGGO: What effects do you note when you compare hairy and glabrous skin? Do you notice any difference in the hairy skin? I should think it is just brushing one way with, and the other way against the hair, but in the glabrous skin the bristles will bounce from one ridge to another.

DR. WHITSEL: With several exceptions, we have excluded from our sample most neurons whose receptive fields only involved the convoluted surfaces of the glabrous skin. In order to sample SI neurons with glabrous skin receptive fields we have preferentially sought those neurons with receptive fields that extend along the edges of the hand or foot. For these neurons the aperture plate was positioned so that the stimuli crossed only the glabrous skin on the edge of the foot or hand. The directional selectivity of such neurons does not differ fundamentally from that exhibited by neurons with receptive fields on the hairy skin.

DR. FRANZÉN: We know that there are similarities between skin and vision with respect to the cortical columnar organization. Did I understand you correctly to say that the receptive fields of these directional sensitive neurons were larger than those, for instance, that respond to common tactile stimuli?

DR. WHITSEL: No, I said that they were larger than those found at first-order levels of the somatosensory nervous system. SI neurons exhibiting direction selectivity are located only within restricted levels of the cortical cell column. Neurons in layer IV tend not to exhibit this property, but significant numbers of

neurons in the laminae located superficial and deep to layer IV
do so. For all neurons studied so far, direction selectivity is
best developed between 5 to 50 cm/sec and, in many cases, it is
exhibited only within a narrow range of orientations and at
traverse lengths equal or greater than the "critical length" for
that body part.

SOMATOSENSORY POTENTIALS IN HUMANS EVOKED BY BOTH MECHANICAL
STIMULATION OF THE SKIN AND ELECTRICAL STIMULATION OF THE NERVE

H. Pratt, R. N. Amlie and A. Starr

University of California, Irvine Medical Center

Irvine, California 92717

Somatosensory potentials evoked by electrical stimulation of peripheral nerves can be recorded by surface electrodes at various locations along the somatosensory pathway. The potentials correspond to activity in peripheral nerves (Dawson and Scott, 1949; Gilliatt and Sears, 1958; Buchthal and Rosenfalck, 1966), spinal cord (Cracco, 1973; Matthews, Beauchamp, and Small, 1974; Jones, 1977), brainstem and midbrain (Cracco and Cracco, 1976; Jones, 1977), and somatosensory cortex (Dawson, 1947; Goff, Rosner, and Allison, 1962; Cracco and Cracco, 1976). The neural generators of these potentials in humans have been proposed from comparable experiments in animals using the correlation between potentials recorded from brain structures comprising the sensory pathway and the surface derived potentials (Iragui-Madoz and Wiederholt, 1977).

While electrical stimulation of the peripheral nerve ensures their synchronous activation, its disadvantages are: (a) a lack of specificity with regard to the types of fibers activated, (b) a failure to activate nerve endings resulting in functional changes confined to them going undetected, and (c) a sensation of discomfort, and even pain that subjects may experience.

Reports on the potentials evoked by mechanical cutaneous stimuli (e.g., tapping on body surfaces) have been limited to the peripheral nerves (Sears, 1959; Bannister and Sears, 1962; McLeod, 1966) and to components whose peak latencies and scalp topography indicate their origin to be in the cerebral cortex (Kjellman, Larsson, and Prevec, 1967; Franzén and Offenloch, 1969; Larsson and Prevec, 1970; Nakanishi, Takita, and Toyokura, 1973). The potentials evoked by mechanical stimuli which originate in the spinal, brainstem, and midbrain levels have not yet been described in humans.

The purpose of this study was to examine in humans the potentials evoked by mechanical cutaneous stimulation at several levels of the somatosensory pathway, and to compare them with the potentials evoked by the customarily employed electrical stimulation of nerves.

METHODS

The subjects were 23 adults ranging in age from 18 to 68, without neurological complaints or symptoms suggestive of abnormalities of somatosensory function. They rested on a bed in a sound-attenuating chamber, with their left hand supported on a warmed plastic mold and their left index finger strapped to its surface. The skin temperature of the index finger was monitored continuously, and maintained between 33° and 36°C. The evoked potentials from each subject were collected in a single session in responses to: (a) electrical stimulation of digital nerves of the index finger, (b) electrical stimulation of the trunk of the median nerve at the wrist, and (c) mechanical stimulation on the fingernail. All stimuli were delivered at a rate of 4/sec.

The electrical stimuli were 0.2 msec square wave pulses of constant current, delivered to the digital nerves through ring electrodes around the middle and proximal phalanges of the index finger, or to the median nerve through silver cup electrodes, separated by 3 to 4 cm, placed at the wrist parallel to the nerve. The proximal electrode of each pair was the cathode. The current was adjusted to a level just below that producing discomfort or a twitch of the thenar muscles, whichever was lower.

The mechanical stimulation was produced by activating a moving coil vibrator with a 50 msec duration electric pulse. The sound produced by the vibrator's movement was masked by white noise from a speaker placed near the subject. The vibrator's spindle was attached to a rod with a hemispheric tip, 7 mm in diameter, and adjusted to be perpendicular to and just in contact with the center of the nail of the index finger. Activation of the vibrator resulted in a downward movement of the rod. In two of the subjects the displacement of the fingernail was recorded with a Linear Variable Differential Transformer (LVDT), with its core connected to a thin rod glued to the fingernail. Figure 1 shows the electrical input to the vibrator, and the resulting displacement of the fingernail. The latency of movement was 1.8 msec and peak displacement occured by 4.8 msec.

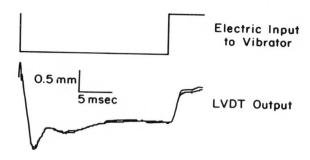

Fig. 1.   The electrical signal transduced by the vibrator and the
          resulting fingernail displacement as measured by a Linear
          Variable Differential Transformer (LVDT).

The digital nerve potentials were recorded from the ring electrodes on the index finger. The other recording electrodes were
10 mm diameter silver cups attached to the skin by collodion glue.
Electrode resistances were kept below 3k Ohm by abrading the outer
layer of the skin and applying conducting jelly. Subjects were
grounded by a metal plate attached to the dorsum of the left hand.
Median nerve potentials at the wrist were recorded from the same
electrode pair used to stimulate the nerve. Proximal median nerve
potentials were recorded by an electrode located over the brachial
artery near the axilla. Brachial plexus activity was recorded from
an electrode at Erb's point. Both of these electrodes were referenced to an electrode placed over the insertion of the deltoid muscle. Spinal cord activity was recorded from an electrode placed
over the second cervical vertebra (CII) referenced to the middle
of the forehead, or from an electrode placed over the inion (Oz)
referenced to CII. Somatosensory cortical activity was recorded
from an electrode at the scalp at C4 (according to the 10-20 system) referenced to the forehead electrode. A summary of the electrode placements and the recording configurations used in this study
is included in Figure 2.

The potentials were amplified with a gain of 200,000 using a
band pass of 30 to 3,000 c/sec (3dB down points). The digital
nerve potentials evoked by mechanical stimuli were recorded with
a gain of 50,000. The potentials evoked in response to 1,000
stimuli were averaged over a 51 msec time period by a four-channel
averager using a dwell time of 200 μsec and 256 addresses per channel. A duplicate of each average was made to assess reproducibility.
The averaged potentials were recorded by an x-y plotter (positivity
at the positive electrode of the differential configuration plotted

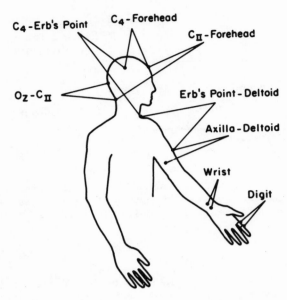

Fig. 2.   Electrode locations and recording configurations used
           in this study.

in an upward direction), and stored on magnetic tape for further
analysis. Amplitudes and latencies of various components of the
recorded potentials were determined from the computer CRT screen
with a cursor. Latencies were measured from the onset of the electrical pulse delivered to the peripheral nerves or to the mechanical vibrator. Amplitudes were measured between positive peaks and
the following negative troughs. Nerve conduction velocities between
electrode placements along the median nerve were determined by measuring the distance between the initial electrode at each placement
that recorded the propagated volley, and then dividing this distance
by the latency difference between the negative trough of the potentials recorded at the two placements.

     In one subject we determined the effects of ischemia and digi-
tal nerve block on the peripheral nerve potentials evoked by mechanical stimulation of the finger. Ischemia was produced by inflating a blood-pressure cuff around the upper arm above the systolic
pressure for 12 min. The nerve blockade was produced by injecting
2 cc of 1 percent lidocaine around the distal phalange of the index finger.

RESULTS

Figure 3 shows the potentials recorded from a subject with potentials of average amplitudes in response to the three types of stimuli at each of the electrode configurations used in this study. The results will be described in terms of the potential's presumed site of origin along the somatosensory pathway.

Median Nerve

The digital ring electrodes recorded potentials in response to both mechanical stimulation of the fingernail and to electrical stimulation of the trunk of the median nerve at the wrist. The mechanically evoked potentials were overwhelmed by an artifact of the movement interfering with the definition of neural events. This was indicated by: (a) the potentials recorded from the digital electrodes corresponded in both waveform and latency to the movement of the finger itself (Fig. 4a), and (b) the mechanically evoked potentials recorded from the digit persisted, and were paradoxically even larger following both anesthetic blockade of the digital nerve (Fig. 4b) and ischemia (Fig. 4c). If these potentials were of biological origin they should have diminished with ischemia. The increased amplitude probably represents change in tissue impedance as a result of the technique used to produce ischemia and nerve blockade. Thus, the afferent activity evoked in the digital nerves by mechanical stimulation could not be distinguished by our recording techniques. In contrast, the potentials from the digital nerves evoked by electrical stimulation of the trunk of the median nerve at the wrist were detectable and consisted of a biphasic, short duration and high amplitude component (latency: 3.2 msec) followed by a lower amplitude broad monophasic wave (latency: 9.4 msec). The monophasic component only accompanied high-intensity electrical stimulation that produced muscle twitches. An electromyogram recorded by surface electrodes over the thenar muscle had a latency comparable to that of the monophasic component recorded simultaneously from the digital ring electrodes and appeared with the same threshold of stimulus intensity. In contrast, the initial, biphasic component occurred prior to any muscle activity, assuring its neural origin.

The electrodes overlying the median nerve at the wrist recorded biphasic activity in response to both mechanical and electrical stimulation of the digit. The potentials evoked by the mechanical stimulus was not an artifact, as they diminished when the digital nerve was blocked (Fig. 4b). The relative amplitude of the positive and negative components of the whole-nerve action potential were dependent of the relative proximity of the proximal and distal recording elements to the nerve trunk, making the measure of absolute amplitudes very variable. However, in such subjects, the

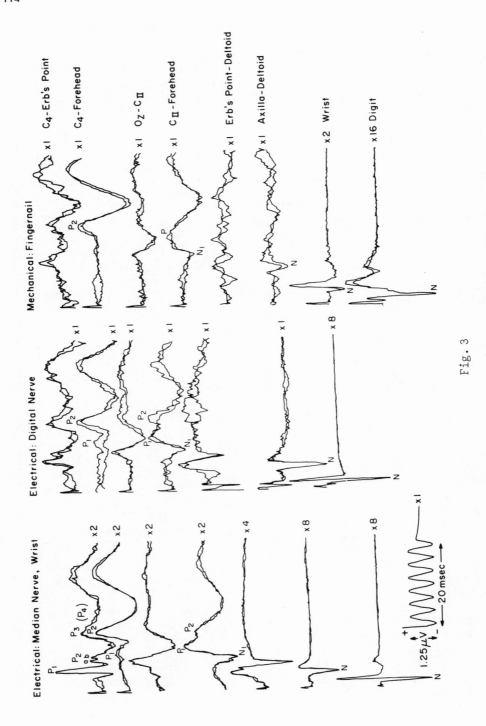

Fig. 3

Fig. 3. Potentials recorded from the same subject at each electrode
configuration in response to the three methods of stimulation used in this study. Note the different display gains
of some of the traces. The numbers next to each trace
have to be multiplied by the calibration signal's amplitude in order to read the actual amplitude from that trace.

potentials evoked by electrical stimulation of the digital nerve
can be compared to the potentials evoked by mechanical stimulation. These ratios show that the nerve potentials evoked by electrical stimulation were both of higher amplitude (10/1) and shorter
duration (2/3) than those evoked by mechanical stimulation (Fig. 3).

The electrodes overlying the proximal portion of the median
nerve at the axilla recorded activity evoked by the three stimuli
that was similar in shape, and consisted of a major negative trough
preceded and followed by smaller positive peaks. The negative
trough evoked by electrical stimulation was considerably larger
than the mechanically evoked potentials (14/1 for electrical stimulation of the median nerve at the wrist and 3/1 for electrical
stimulation of digital nerves) but were of comparable duration
(approximately 4 msec). Because the median nerve potentials evoked at the wrist by electrical stimulation of digital nerves had
shorter duration than those evoked by mechanical stimulation, the
finding of comparable durations at the axilla indicates that mechanically evoked potentials had considerably less temporal dispersion in propagating from the wrist to the axilla compared to
the electrically evoked potentials.

Brachial Plexus

The electrode overlying the brachial plexus at Erb's point
referenced to an electrode over the deltoid insertion recorded
clear potentials in response to the electrical stimuli, consisting of a major negative trough, preceded by a dual positive peak.
In contrast, the potential evoked by mechanical stimulation could
not be identified in the majority of the subjects until the number of trials comprising the average was increased five-fold from
1,000 to 5,000 (Fig. 5b).

Spinal Cord

The potentials recorded over the spinal cord at the second
cervical vertebra referenced to the forehead had a similar shape
and duration in response to the three methods of stimulation and
consisted of an initial negative trough followed by a positive

peak. This potential originated from the upper spinal cord, cere-
bellum and medulla because it reversed in polarity when the electrode at Oz was referenced to the second cervical vertebra. The
positive component of the potentials evoked by electrical stimulation had a notch, whereas this component was smooth when evoked by
mechanical stimulation. In approximately half of the subjects, the
potentials evoked by nerve truck stimulation and recorded between
cervical vertebra II and the forehead exhibited an additional later
positive component (not shown in the figures or tables) with a latency of 28.2 ± 1.4 msec. This component was not evident in Oz-
CII recordings, suggesting its origin in structures remote from the

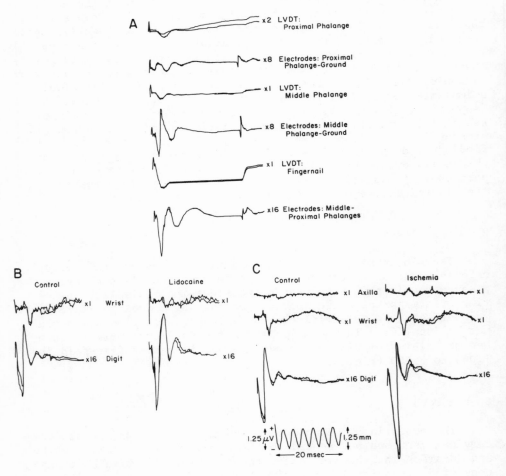

Fig. 4.

Fig. 4. Control experiments to assess the mechanically evoked
         potentials recorded by the digital electrodes. (a)
         Simultaneous recordings from electrodes and from an
         LVDT along the finger. Stimulus duration was 40 msec,
         producing an offset artifact in the electrode recordings.
         Note the identical onset and offset latencies, as well
         as the comparable waveforms of the mechanical displace-
         ments and the respective electric potentials recorded
         by the electrodes. (b) Recordings before (Control) and
         following (Lidocaine) nerve block at the distal phalange
         of the wrist finger. Note that although the potentials
         at the wrist were practically absent following the in-
         jection, the potentials recorded at the digit were ac-
         tually increased in amplitude. (c) Recordings before
         (Control) and following 12 minutes of ischemia. Note
         that the latency of the wrist potential increased as a
         result of ischemia, as did the latency difference be-
         tween the axillary and wrist potentials. In contrast,
         the latency of the potentials recorded from the digit
         remained unchanged, and their amplitude actually in-
         creased.

upper cervical region. The potential is recorded from the upper cervical region in response to electrical stimulation of the nerve were
larger than the mechanically evoked potentials (3.5/1 for electrical
stimulation of the median nerve at the wrist and 1.8/1 for electrical stimulation of digital nerves) but of comparable duration.

Cortex

     The cortical potentials recorded from the C4 electrode refer-
enced to the forehead were essentially similar in shape and duration for the three types of stimuli used in this study and consisted of an initial component followed by two prominent positive
peaks. In approximately half of the subjects, the first prominent
positivity evoked by stimulation of the nerve truck at the wrist
(P2) was notched with its later peak corresponding in latency
(28 msec) to the positive component recorded in CII-forehead recordings in some of the subjects. In distribution to the potentials recorded at all other sites, the cortical potentials evoked
by the three methods of stimulation were of comparable amplitudes.

Far-Field

     The electrode configuration of C4 referenced to Erb's point
has been recommended for use in clinical tests because of its

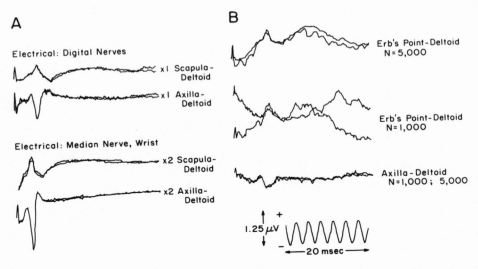

Fig. 5. (a) Potentials recorded from the same subject using electrical stimulation of the median nerve at the wrist and of digital nerves. In both recording configurations, the electrode over the deltoid insertion was negative in the differential recording. The positive electrode was over the scapula or the axilla. Note that the initial positivity of the scapula-deltoid configuration was of similar latency to the axillary-deltoid negativity. (b) Potentials recorded over Erb's point and at the axilla in response to mechanical stimulation (averaging 1,000, compared with 5,000 trials). In the axillary recording, an average of 1,000 trials was superimposed on an average of 5,000 trials. Note the marked improvement of the definition of the Erb's point recording when more trials were averaged. No such improvement was observed in the axillary recordings. The potential recorded at Erb's point was later than that recorded at the axilla or that at the scapula-deltoid configuration.

ability to define a series of components originating in structures from brachial plexus to cortex (Cracco and Cracco, 1976). The potentials evoked by electrical stimulation of the nerves has a prominent initial peak (approximately 10 msec following stimulation at the wrist and 12 msec following stimulation of the digital nerve) corresponding in latency to the potential evoked at the brachial plexus, but of reversed polarity as a result of the recording configuration (see Erb's point-deltoid recordings in Fig. 3).

Table 1. Average values of amplitude and latency (with standard deviations) of some of the components recorded at various locations in response to the three stimuli used in this study. The components listed are marked on the recordings in Fig. 3.

		NERVE-TRUNK		ELECTRICAL DIGIT		MECHANICAL DIGIT	
		Latency	Amplitude	Latency	Amplitude	Latency	Amplitude
DIGIT	N	3.2 ± 0.2	15.5 ± 11.4	-------	-------	3.8 ± 0.7	39.2 ± 24.8
WRIST	N	-------	-------	2.6 ± 0.3	14.9 ± 7.0	6.2 ± 0.8	1.5 ± 0.7
AXILLA-DELTOID	N	6.8 ± 0.6	9.9 ± 4.0	9.6 ± 0.8	1.8 ± 0.9	13.8 ± 1.4	0.7 ± 0.3
C_{II}-FOREHEAD	N_1	13.2 ± 0.8	1.4 ± 0.7	16.2 ± 1.4	0.7 ± 0.3	20.4 ± 2.0	0.4 ± 0.2
	P_1	16.8 ± 1.0	1.4 ± 0.5	20.2 ± 1.6	0.7 ± 0.4	25.4 ± 2.0	1.1 ± 0.3
	P_2	22.2 ± 2.2	2.7 ± 1.1	25.6 ± 2.4	1.0 ± 0.5		
FOREHEAD	P_1			18.8 ± 1.4	0.5 ± 0.3		
	P_2			26.4 ± 2.4	1.5 ± 0.9	30.6 ± 3.4	1.3 ± 0.6
C_4-ERB'S POINT	P_1	10.0 ± 0.6	3.8 ± 2.2				
	P_{2a}	13.2 ± 1.0	0.4 ± 0.5				
	P_{2b}	14.2 ± 0.8	2.5 ± 0.8				
	P_3	22.0 ± 1.8	0.9 ± 1.0				
	P_4	27.2 ± 2.4	1.2 ± 0.8				

This component was followed after 3 to 4 msec by a positive-negative complex corresponding in its latencies to the potentials recorded over the spinal cord (see Oz-CII recordings in Fig. 3). There was a final set of positive-negative-positive components (occurring 9 to 13 msec later) corresponding in latency to the cortical events (see C4-forehead recordings in Fig. 3). In contrast, the potentials evoked by mechanical stimulation began with the positive-negative component which occurred at the same latencies as the potentials recorded over the second cervical vertebra (see recordings from Oz-CII in Fig.,3). The subsequent components were identical to the potentials recorded at C4 referenced to the forehead. With mechanical stimulation when only 1,000 trials were averaged, no reproducible potentials corresponding in latency to the volley at Erb's point were detected.

The average values for amplitude and latency of the various components designated in Fig. 3 are listed in Table 1. In general, the potentials evoked by electrical stimulation of the nerve trunk had the largest amplitudes and the greatest number of components; potentials with intermediate amplitudes and number of components were evoked by stimulation of the digital nerve; and the lowest amplitudes and simplest waveforms were evoked by mechanical stimulation of the finger.

The average values for the conduction velocity along two portions of the median nerves of the 23 subjects are listed in Table 2. The effect of age on decreasing nerve conduction velocities is demonstrated in scatter diagrams in Fig. 6 which also contain their regression constants and correlation coefficients.

Table 2.   Nerve conduction velocities (in m/sec $\pm$ 1 SD) for two portions of the median nerve in response to the three stimuli used in this study.

| | ELECTRICAL | | MECHANICAL |
	NERVE-TRUNK	DIGIT	DIGIT
DIGIT TO WRIST	51.33 $\pm$ 3.75	48.62 $\pm$ 5.34	54.37 $\pm$ 5.72
WRIST TO AXILLA	58.35 $\pm$ 4.09	59.90 $\pm$ 4.20	56.55 $\pm$ 5.99

DISCUSSION

The results of this study show that comparable potentials can be recorded along the somatosensory pathway in response to either mechanical stimulation of the finger or electrical stimulation of

the nerves innervating the hand. In general, the mechanically
evoked potentials were of relatively low amplitude and simple waveform, and showed little temporal dispersion after propagation along
the arm, suggesting that they were recorded from a small number
of fibers of a uniform diameter. The electrically evoked potentials had relatively high amplitude and complex waveform and showed
appreciable temporal dispersion after propagation along the arm.
These findings suggest that there were many fibers activated
synchronously by electrical stimulation but the comprised a di-
verse population with regard to conduction velocity.

It is unfortunate that the potentials recorded from the electrodes overlying the digital nerve in response to mechanical stimulation of the fingernail were primarily an artifact of movement.
This measure could have provided objective evidence of the activity
of receptors and the terminal portions of the nerves. The failure
of both ischemia and nerve blockade to attenuate these potentials
coupled with their morphology being identical to that of the finger
displacement are strong evidence of their artifactual origin. Sears
(1959) and McLeod (1966) probably attributed these mechanically

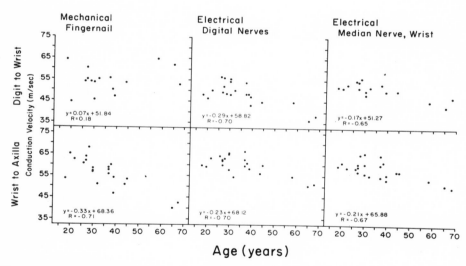

Fig. 6. Scatter diagrams of nerve conduction velocity as a func-
         tion of a subject's age, for two portions of the median
         nerve in response to the three stimuli used in this study.
         Regression constants and correlation coefficients are
         given for each scatter diagram. Note in the mechanically
         evoked nerve conduction, the.steep slope for the conduction
         in the proximal portion of the nerve, and its absence for
         the digital portion of the nerve.

evoked potentials to neural events because they did not have the benefit of transducers that recorded displacement of the finger adjacent to the electrodes and because of different interpretations of the control experiments. Nevertheless, we believe that the combination of evoked potentials recorded at the wrist in response to electrical stimulation of the digital nerves and mechanical stimulation of the finger could provide the information necessary for defining receptor and nerve-ending impairments in peripheral neuropathies.

The similarities between the mechanically and the electrically evoked potentials were both in waveform and conduction velocity. The biphasic morphology of the potentials at the digit and at the wrist is consistent with their being recorded in turn under each electrode of a differential recording pair. When the potentials recorded by each electrode of the pair were subtracted from each other by the differential recording, the biphasic shape of the response was produced (Woodbury, 1960). The triphasic morphology of the potentials recorded at the axilla is consistent with a monopolar derivation of the activity over a nerve trunk (Lorente de Nó, 1947), suggesting that the contribution from the electrode over the deltoid was minor. The complex morphology of the potentials recorded at Erb's point referenced to the deltoid insertion (Fig. 3) was due to the overlap of a high-amplitude triphasic potential recorded by the differential amplifier (Fig. 5a). The failure to clearly define potentials at Erb's point in response to mechanical stimulation was due to a poor signal-to-noise ratio as a result of the low amplitude of the neural signal evoked by mechanical stimulation coupled with high-amplitude myogenic noise from the neck. This explanation is supported by the definition of mechanically evoked potentials recorded from Erb's point when the number of trials comprising the average was increased (Fig. 5b).

The inversion of polarity of the potentials recorded between the neck and forehead (Fig. 3, CII-Forehead), when compared with potentials recorded between the inion and the neck (Fig. 3, Oz-CII), is consistent with the negative-positive complex being recorded by the cervical electrode from a generator in the upper cervical cord or medulla. The latency of the negative component recorded from the skin overlying the cervical cord is comparable to that reported by others using electrical stimulation of the nerve (Liberson and Kim, 1963; Matthews et al. 1974; Jones, 1977). These authors localized the generator of the component to the upper spinal cord, possibly to the dorsal column nuclei since the integrity of the dorsal columns themselves is essential for the detection of scalp-recorded, electrically evoked somatosensory potentials (Halliday and Wakefield, 1963; Giblin, 1964; Larson, Sances, and Christenson, 1966; Namerow, 1969). There is a report that mechanically evoked potentials are dependent, instead, on the ventrolateral tracts in the spinal cord (Nakanishi, Shimada, and Toyokura, 1974), and additional evidence is necessary to determine conclusively the generator of these mechanically evoked potentials.

The first major peak in the potentials evoked by the three types of stimuli at C4 referenced to the forehead corresponded in latency to the potentials recorded from the scalp overlying the somatosensory cortex, as previously reported by Dawson (1947), Goff et al. (1962), Allison, Goff, and Williamson (1974), and Cracco and Cracco (1976) with electrical stimulation, and by Kjellman et al. (1967), Franzén and Offenloch (1969), Larsson and Prevec (1970), and Nakanishi, Takita, and Toyokura (1973) with mechanical stimulation. The comparable amplitudes of the cortical potentials evoked by the three methods of stimulation, in contrast to the amplitude ratios in all other levels, may result from termination of electrically activated pathways at subcortical levels, giving rise to the relative amplitude loss of the electrically evoked potentials at the cortical level. Only careful scalp mapping correlated with recordings in patients with clearly demarcated lesions can resolve the generator sites for the various components of the evoked potentials.

The potentials evoked by each of the stimuli showed an increase in latency as the recording site moved rostrally, suggesting that the recordings represented a volley of action potentials propagating along the somatosensory pathway. The latencies of the potentials at various locations along the pathway may thus indicate the clinical state of the pathway and its particular capacity for conduction. The wide variability among subjects in the amplitudes of each of the potentials, renders absolute amplitudes unreliable as a clinical tool. The nerve conduction velocity obtained by measuring peak latency differences reflects the modal velocity of conduction in the nerve trunk. The peripheral nerve conduction velocities computed for the potentials evoked by the three types of stimuli were quite similar and comparable to previously reported values (Dawson and Scott, 1949; Bannister and Sears, 1962; Buchthal and Rosenfalck, 1966; McLeod, 1966; Liberson, Gratzer, Zales, and Wrabinski, 1966; Kemble and Peiris, 1967). The conduction velocities for the distal portion of the nerve were slower than the proximal portion of the nerve, which may be due to smaller diameter of the nerve fibers in the distal portion of the nerve (Mayer, 1963; Kemble, 1967).

The effect of age on peripheral nerve conduction velocities found in this study is consistent with both previously reported values in adults (Norris, Shock, and Wagman, 1953; Kemble, 1967) and with developmental studies of children from infancy through adolescence (Thomas and Lambert, 1960); Gamstorp and Shelburne, 1965). The lack of a significant effect of age on the conduction velocity of the distal peripheral nerve (digit-to-wrist) in response

to mechanical stimulation reinforces the impression that the mechanically evoked potentials recorded at the digit were primarily artifactual. This lack of effect contrasts sharply with the pronounced
slowing of nerve conduction velocity with age found for the potentials evoked by mechanical stimulation along the wrist-to-axilla
portion of the median nerve.

Differences between the mechanically and the electrically evoked potentials were in their amplitude, duration, complexity and
temporal dispersion after propagation (Fig. 3 and Table 1). The
higher amplitudes and shorter durations of the electrically evoked
potentials recorded along the median nerve, when compared with the
mechanically evoked potentials, suggest that the electrical stimulus activates more fibers more synchronously. However, the finding
that the potentials evoked by mechanical stimulation had little
temporal dispersion after conduction along the median nerve in the
arm compared to the electrically evoked potentials is consistent
with the mechanically evoked potentials being recorded from a relatively uniform fiber population. The relatively long duration of
these potentials recorded from the median nerve at the wrist was
probably due to mechanical factors underlying the coupling of the
stimulus to the skin and underlying tissue.

The measurement of the change in amplitude of the evoked potentials along the median nerve and spinal cord provides information about the fibers activited by the three stimuli. The ratio
of the amplitudes of the initial negativity recorded over the neck
compared to the amplitudes of the potentials recorded in the same
subject over the median nerve in the axilla (neck/axilla), was
0.15 ± 0.06 for electrical stimulation of the median nerve at the
wrist, 0.46 ± 0.23 for electrical stimulation of digital nerve,
and 0.73 ± 0.32 for mechanical stimulation of the finger. Because
the potentials recorded from both the axilla and the neck were of
comparable duration for the three types of stimulation, the amplitude ratio differences indicate a comparative loss of fibers contributing to the spinal cord potentials when evoked by electrical stimulation of the nerves (particularly the median nerve at the wrist)
were antrodromically conducting motor fibers which can not propagate
along the ascending pathways of the spinal cord past their synapses
in the anterior horn.

There were four prominent differences in the morphology of the
potentials evoked by electrical stimulation as compared to the mechanically evoked potentials. The first was the presence of a notch
in the positive potential recorded between the upper neck and forehead in response to electrical stimulation which was not found in
the potentials evoked mechanically. The second difference was the
occurrence of an initial negativity in the potentials recorded at
C4 referenced to the forehead with electrical stimulation that was

rarely recognizable in the mechanically evoked potentials (Fig. 3). The presence or absence of this negativity has been correlated with the functioning of the thalamus in humans (Domino, Matsuoka, Waltz, and Cooper, 1965; Noel and Desmedt, 1975). The third difference was a double-peaked major positivity in the cortical evoked potential observed in approximately half of the subjects with electrical but not with mechanical stimulation. The fourth difference was in the recordings obtained with the C4-Erb's point configuration in which the positive peak (latency 13 to 14 msec from electrical stimulation at the wrist) was split in some of the subjects and only in response to the electrical stimulus. This component (P2b Fig. 3) may derive from a generator slightly higher than the upper cerivcal region, possibly--as suggested by Cracco and Cracco (1976) and Jones (1977)--in the brainstem or midbrain. Thalamic contribution to this component cannot be ruled out, as depth recordings from the thalamus in humans have been reported with potentials at latencies corresponding to both this minor peak and the following trough (Goto, Kasaka, Kubota, Nakamura, and Narabayashi, 1968; Larson and Sances, 1968; Narabayashi, 1968; Matthews et al. 1970; Haider, Gangleberger, and Groll-Knapp, 1972; Fukushima, Mayanagi, and Bouchard, 1976). All of these changes may reflect differences in either the fiber pathways activated or their degree of synchrony resulting from the different types of stimuli used in this study.

Thus, we have shown that both mechanical stimulation of the fingernail and electrical stimulation of the digital or median nerves can evoke in humans a sequence of potentials from several levels of the sensory pathways. These recording methods may allow a detailed analysis of the function of the somatosensory pathway from receptor to cortex in clinical disorders leading to the definition of both the site and extent of the deficits.

SUMMARY

Somatosensory potentials evoked by mechanical as well as electrical stimulation were recorded by surface electrodes over (a) the digital nerves in the index finger, (b) the median nerve at the wrist, (c) the median nerve at the axilla, (d) the brachial plexus at Erb's point, (e) the cervical cord at CII, and (f) the scalp overlying the somatosensory cortex. Nerve conduction velocities were computed for two portions of the median nerve, and found to decrease with age. Three methods of stimulation were compared: (a) electrical stimulation of the nerve trunk at the wrist, (b) electrical stimulation of the index and digital nerves, and (c) mechanical stimulation of the fingernail.

Mechanically evoked potentials could be recorded from the same sites as the electrically evoked potentials. The mechanically evoked

potentials recorded from the digital electrodes were an artifact of
the finger movement. The combination of electrically and mechanically evoked potentials could prove useful in the assessment of
clinical disorders of somatosensory functions in man.

ACKNOWLEDGEMENTS

We are grateful to the volunteer subjects for their coopera-
tion, to Dr. Masa Ishijima for his help with monitoring the displacement, to Mrs. E´lane Wingerson for making the hand mold, and
to Mr. Douglas Politoske for his help with measurements and calculations.

REFERENCES

Allison, T., Goff, W.R., Williamson, P.D., & Van Gildern, J.C. On
    the neural origin of early components of the human somatosensory
    evoked potential. Proceedings of the international symposium on
    cerebral evoked potentials in man, Belgium, 1974 (in press).
Bannister, R.G., & Sears, T.A. The changes in nerve conduction in
    acute idiopathic polyneuritis. Journal of Neurology, Neuro-
    surgery and Psychiatry, 1962, 25, 312-328.
Buchthal, F., & Rosenfalck, A. Evoked action potentials and con-
    duction velocity in human sensory nerves. Brain Research,
    1966, 3, 1-122.
Cracco, R.Q. Spinal evoked response: peripheral nerve stimulation
    in man. Electroencephalography and Clinical Neurophysiology,
    1973, 35, 379-386.
Cracco, R.Q., & Cracco, J.B. Somatosensory evoked potential in
    man: far field potentials. Electroencephalography and Clinical
    Neurophysiology, 1976, 41, 460-466.
Dawson, G.D. Cerebral responses to electrical stimulation of peri-
    pheral nerve in man. Journal of Neurology, Neurosurgery and
    Psychiatry, 1947, 10, 134-140.
Dawson, G.D., & Scott, J.W. The recording of nerve action poten-
    tials through skin in man. Journal of Neurology, Neurosurgery
    and Psychiatry. 1949, 12, 259-269.
Domino, E.F., Matsuoka, S., Waltz, J., & Cooper, I.S. Effects of
    cryogenic thalamic lesions in the somesthetic evoked response
    in man. Electroencephalography and Clinical Neurophysiology,
    1965, 19, 127-138.
Franzén, O., & Offenloch, K. Evoked response correlates of psycho-
    physical magnitude estimates for tactile stimulation in man.
    Experimental Brain Research, 1969, 8, 1-18.
Fukushima, T., Mayanagi, Y., & Bouchard, G. Thalamic evoked poten-
    tials to somatosensory stimulation in man. Electroencephalo-
    graphy and Clinical Neurophysiology, 1976, 40, 481-490.
Gamstorp, I., & Shelburne, S.A. Peripheral sensory conduction in

ulnar and median nerves of normal infants, children and adolescents. Acta Paediatrica Scandinavica, 1965, 54, 309-313.

Giblin, D. R. Somatosensory evoked potentials in healthy subjects and in patients with lesions of the nervous system. Annals of the New York Academy of Science, 1964, 112, 93-142.

Gilliatt, R.W., & Sears, T.A. Sensory nerve action potentials in patients with peripheral nerve lesions. Journal of Neurology, Neurosurgery and Psychiatry, 1958, 21, 109-118.

Goff, W.R., Rosner, B.S., & Allison, T. Distribution of cerebral somatosensory evoked responses in normal man. Electroencephalography and Clinical Neurophysiology, 1962, 14, 697-713.

Goto, A., Kasaka, K., Kubota, R., Nakamura, R., & Narabayashi, H. Thalamic potentials from muscle afferents in the human. Archives of Neurology, 1968, 19, 302-309.

Haider, M., Gangleberger, J.A., & Groll-Knapp, E. Computer analysis of subcortical and cortical evoked potentials and of slow potential phenomena in humans. Confinia Neurology, 1972, 34, 224-229.

Halliday, A.M., & Wakefield, G.S. Cerebral evoked potentials in patients with dissociated memory loss. Journal of Neurology, Neurosurgery and Psychiatry, 1963, 26, 211-219.

Iragui-Madoz, V.J., & Wiederholt, W.C. Far field somatosensory evoked potentials in the cat: correlations with depth recording. Annals of Neurology, 1977, 1, 569-574.

Jones, S.J. Short latency potentials recorded from the neck and scalp following median nerve stimulation in man. Electroencephalography and Clinical Neurophysiology, 1977, 43, 853-863.

Kemble, F. Conduction in the normal adult median nerve: the effect of aging in men and women. Electromyography, 1967, 7, 275-288.

Kemble, F., & Peiris, O.A. General observations on sensory conduction in the normal adult median nerve. Electromyography, 1967, 7, 127-140.

Kjellman, A., Larsson, L.E., & Prevec, T. Potentials evoked by tapping recorded from the human scalp over the cortical somatosensory region. Electroencephalography and Clinical Neurophysiology, 1967, 23, 396.

Larson, S.J., Sances, A., Jr., & Christenson, P.C. Evoked somatosensory potentials in man. Archives of Neurology, 1966, 15, 88-93.

Larson, S.J., & Sances, A.,Jr. Averaged evoked potentials in stereotactic surgery. Journal of Neurosurgery, 1968, 28, 227-232.

Larsson, L.E., & Prevec, T.S. Somatosensory response to mechanical stimulation as recorded in human E.E.G. Electroencephalography and Clinical Neurophysiology, 1970, 28, 162-172.

Liberson, W.T., & Kim, K.C. Mapping evoked potentials elicited by stimulation of the median and peroneal nerves. Electroencephalography and Clinical Neurophysiology, 1963, 15, 721.

Liberson, W.T., Gratzer, M., Zales, A., & Wrabinski, B. Comparison of conduction velocities of motor and sensory fibres determined by different methods. Archives of Physical Medicine and Rehabilitation, 1966, 47, 17-23.

Lorente de Nó, R.   Analysis of the distribution of the action cur-
    rent of nerve in volume conductors. Studies of the Rockefeller
    Institute for Medical Research, 1947, 132, 384-482.
Matthews, G., Bertrand, G., & Broughton, R. Thalamic somatosensory
    evoked potential in Parksinsonian patients - correlation with
    unit response and thalamic stimulation. Electroencephalography
    and Clinical Neurophysiology, 1970, 28, 98-99.
Matthews, W.B., Beauchamp, M., & Small, D.G. Cervical somatosensory
    evoked responses in man. Nature, 1974, 252, 230-232.
Mayer, R.F. Nerve conduction studies in man. Neurology (Minneapolis)
    1963, 13, 1021-1030.
McLeod, J.G. Digital nerve conduction in the carpal tunnel syndrome
    after mechanical stimulation of the finger. Journal of Neurology,
    Neurosurgery and Psychiatry, 1966, 29, 12-22.
Nakanishi, T., Takita, K., & Toyokura, Y. Somatosensory evoked
    responses to tactile tap in man. Electroencephalography and
    Clinical Neurophysiology, 1973, 34, 1-6.
Nakanishi, T., Shimada, Y., & Toyokura, Y. Somatosensory evoked
    responses to mechanical stimulation in normal subjects and in
    patients with neurological disorders. Journal of the Neuro-
    logical Sciences, 1974, 21, 289-298.
Namerow, N. S. Somatosensory evoked responses following cervical
    cordotomy. Bulletin of the Los Angeles Neurological Society,
    1969, 34, 184-188.
Narabayashi, H. Functional differentiation in and around the ven-
    trolateral nucleus of the thalamus based on experience in human
    stereoencephalotomy. Johns Hopkins Medical Journal, 1968, 122,
    295-300.
Noel, P., & Desmedt, J. E. Somatosensory cerebral evoked potentials
    after vascular lesions of the brainstem and diencephalon. Brain,
    1975, 98, 113-128.
Norris, A. H., Shock, N. W., & Wagman, I. H. Age changes in the
    maximum conduction velocity of motor fibres of human ulnar nerves.
    Journal of Applied Physiology, 1953, 5, 489-593.
Sears, T. A. Action potentials evoked in digital nerves by stimu-
    lation of mechanoreceptors in the human finger. Journal of
    Physiology (London), 1959, 148, 30.
Thomas, J. E., & Lambert, E. H. Ulnar nerve conduction velocity and
    H-reflex in infants and children. Journal of Applied Physiology,
    1960, 15, 1-9.
Woodbury, J. W. Potentials in a volume conductor. In T. C. Ruch
    and J. F. Fulton (Eds.), Medical physiology and biophysics.
    Philadelphia: Saunders, 1960.

TACTILE AFFERENT UNITS WITH SMALL AND WELL DEMARCATED RECEPTIVE FIELDS IN THE GLABROUS SKIN AREA OF THE HUMAN HAND

Roland S. Johansson

Department of Physiology, University of Umea

S-901 Umea, Sweden

Microneurographic recordings have revealed that there are four distinct types of mechanoreceptive units in the glabrous skin area of the human hand (Knibestöl and Vallbo, 1970; Knibestöl, 1973, 1975; Johansson, 1978). They can most readily be distinguished on the basis of their adaption to sustained skin indentation and the properties of their cutaneous receptive fields. Figure 1 gives a schematic representation of the unit types with regard to these properties. The four types, which all have thick myelinated fibers (Aα) (Knibestöl, 1973, 1975; Hagbarth, Hongell, Hallin and Torebjörk, 1970) have striking similarities to four well described types in cats and subhuman primates (Iggo, 1963; Lindblom, 1965; Lindblom and Lund, 1966; Jänig, Schmidt and Zimmermann, 1968; Talbot, Darian-Smith, Kornhuber and Mountcastle, 1968; Iggo and Muir, 1969; Chambers, Andres, Duering and Iggo, 1972; Iggo and Ogawa, 1977). The human glabrous skin units have been accordingly denoted RA, PC, SA I, and SAII (Fig. 1). These abbreviations stand for rapidly adapting, Pacinian, slowly adapting type one and slowly adapting type two, respectively.

The two rapidly adapting unit types, the RA and the PC units, respond to skin indentation as long as the stimulus in in motion, i.e., these unit types exhibit only dynamic sensitivity. The two slowly adapting unit types are sensitive to the dynamic components of indentation but exhibit also a static response related to the amplitude of skin indentation (Fig. 1). In contrast to most of the rapidly adapting units, the dynamic response occurs only during increasing skin indentation. Measurements of amplitude thresholds with ramp indentations have shown that the rapidly adapting units (PC and RA) are the most sensitive of the four types (Johansson and

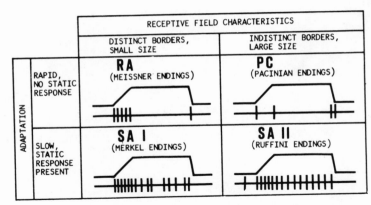

Fig. 1.   Types of mechanoreceptive units in the glabrous skin of
          the human hand classified on the basis of adaptation and
          receptive field properties. In this context, rapid
          adaptation is used to indicate that the neuronal re-
          sponse occurs only as long as the stimulus is in motion,
          whereas slow adaptation indicates that there is a steady
          impulse discharge even when the stimulus is held constant.
          The four unit types are denoted RA, PC, SA I and SA II
          units. These abbreviations stand for rapidly adapting,
          Pacinian, slowly adapting type I and slowly adapting type
          II, respectively. The morphological structures which
          are assumed to constitute their end-organs are given with-
          in brackets: (a) the Meissner corpuscles (RA-terminals)
          which are located in the dermal papillae, (b) the Merkel
          cell neurite complexes (SA I-terminals) at the tip of
          the intermediate epidermal ridges which project down to
          the dermis, (c) the spindle shaped Ruffini endings (SA II-
          terminals) located more deeply within the dermis, and
          finally (d) the Pacinian and smaller Paciniform corpuscles
          (PC-terminals) located more deeply within the dermis, and
          tissues. Diagrams below show schematically, the impulse
          discharge (lower trace) to ramp indentation of the skin
          (upper trace) for each type.

Vallbo, 1976; Vallbo and Johansson, 1976). Considering the extent
of the receptive fields as defined with manually held instruments,
e.g. small blunt glass probes and von Frey hairs, the RA and SA I
fields constitute relatively small and well defined skin areas of
approximately uniform sensitivity (Fig. 1). This area of high
sensitivity is typically circular, or slightly oval in shape, and
its size corresponds to a diameter of a few millimeters. A

detailed analysis of the sensitivity profile of receptive fields
demonstrates that there are a number of small zones of maximal
sensitivity within this area (Johansson, 1976a, 1978). The fields
of the PC and SA II units are significantly larger, and the field
boundaries are rather indistinct. They exhibit a single focus of
maximal sensitivity (Johansson, 1976a, 1978). The PC units respond readily to rapid taps and other mechanical transients of
remote parts of the hand, implying that their fields can be of
very large extent, e.g., covering a whole finger or the main part
of the hand (Knibestöl and Vallbo, 1970; Knibestöl, 1973). The SA
II units are sensitive to lateral skin stretching from remote skin
areas. The stretching response often shows a directional sensitivity (Knibestöl and Vallbo, 1970; Knibestöl, 1975; Johansson,
1976b, 1978).

The tentative correlation between unit type and structure of
the end organ, as indicated in Fig. 1 is based mainly on the functional similarity between units in the human skin and units identified with regard to type of end organ in other species (Lindblom
and Lund, 1966; Iggo and Muir, 1969; Lynn, 1969; Jänig, 1971; Munger,
Pubols and Pubols, 1971; Sakada, 1971; Chambers et al., 1972; Iggo
and Ogawa, 1977), and the fact that the four types of end organs
considered in Fig. 1 have been described in the glabrous skin of
the human hand (Cauna, 1954; Stilwell, 1957; Cauna and Mannan, 1958;
Miller, Ralston and Kasahara, 1958; Chouchov, 1973). Relations between properties of the receptive fields of the different unit types
and the structure of the end organs together with their location
in the skin and deeper structures, supporting this correlation,
have been discussed in previous reports (Johansson, 1976b, 1978).

Table 1

Innervation density (units/cm^2) of four kinds of mechanoreceptive
units in three different regions of the glabrous skin area of the
human hand. The skin of the terminal phalanx distal to the vortex
is referred to as the finger tip (Johansson and Vallbo, 1978).

	RA	SAI	PC	SA II
Finger tip	140.5	70.2	21.4	9.2[+]
Rest of finger	37.1	29.7	9.5	13.8
Palm	24.5	8.0	9.3	15.7

[+]SA II nail units excluded.

An important parameter concerning the tactile innervation is
the number and spatial distribution of mechanoreceptive units innervating various skin areas. These conditions have been analyzed
in the glabrous skin of the hand in terms of innervation densities
(Johansson and Vallbo, 1978). It was found that there is a slight
increase in the overall unit density from the palm to the main part
of the finger, and an abrupt increase from the main part of the
finger tip, i.e. the area distal to the vortex of the papillary
ridges. The relative densities in these three regions are 1.0,
1.6 and 4.2. It can be seen in Table 1 that these differences in
overall density are mainly accounted for by the RA and SA I units,
whereas the densities of the PC and SA II units are more uniform
over the entire glabrous skin area.

There are a number of findings indicating that the accurate
interpretation of the afferent information regarding tactile events
depends on the central integration of spatio-temporal impulse
patterns in the population of mechanoreceptive units (e.g. Armett,
Gray, Hunsperger and Lal, 1962; Fuller and Gray, 1966; Jänig, et al.,
1968; Talbot, et al., 1968; Johnson, 1974; Johansson and Vallbo,
1976). Therefore, in order to make inferences concerning the prin-
ciples involved when the afferent population transmits information
to the central nervous system, it seems that an approach which
emphasizes the function of the whole population of units, rather
than the characteristics of single units, is necessary. This is
particularly true if the afferent neuronal activity is to be combined with psychophysical findings, with the aim to illuminate the
manner in which the central nervous system processes the information in peripheral units before the perceptual experiences are
evoked. One of the most potent neuronal techniques which can be
used, in direct correlations between psychophysics and afferent
activity in man, is the percutaneous microneurographic technique
developed by Vallbo and Hagbarth (1968). However, when using this
technique, as well as other single unit techniques, one of the
major problems involved is related to the fact that only one different unit can be reliably recorded at a time. Thus, the recording
technique, per se, does not provide any direct information about
the number of units brought into play by the stimulation, nor about
the amount of activity in other individual units. So far, there
seems to be no way of obtaining this very important information, except by reconstructions of the whole population on the basis of the
properties of single units and the spatial organization of their
receptive fields. In the present communication, which deals with
such reconstructions, some estimates of the number of RA and SA I
units, which respond to localized skin indentations delivered to
the human hand, will be presented.

When a skin indentation is delivered, the number of units responding varies directly with the density of mechanoreceptive units
in the skin, and with the sizes of their receptive fields. This

number is the same as the number of receptive fields directly indented by the stimulus. Consequently, the spatial recruitment of units due to increasingly stronger stimuli can be described on the basis of an increase in the size of the receptive fields of the individual units with increasing stimulus intensity. The approach in the present study was to calculate the mean amount of overlap of receptive fields, as a function of the amplitude of skin indentation, and from these estimates deduce the mean number of units responding to localized skin indentations of various amplitudes.

METHODS

The calculations of the mean overlap of receptive fields within different skin regions were based on: (a) the density of units in the appropriate skin region, and (b) the distribution of receptive field sizes, within a representative unit sample, as a function of the indentation amplitude. The first of these two points has been considered earlier in this paper (Table 1). Regarding the relation between the indentation amplitude and the size of the receptive fields, once the threshold of the unit is reached, the fields of the RA and SA I units increase rapidly up to the size of the high sensitivity area of the field whereas any further increase occurs at a moderate rate (Johansson, 1976a). It has been shown that this relationship can be described by a simple power function, with power exponents well below unity (Johansson, 1978). Moreover, this relation can be approximated for the individual RA and SA I units on the basis of the indentation threshold (T_i) and the size of the field (a_i) as defined with a von Frey hair at 4 to 5 times threshold. The following equation describes the relation between field size, A_i, and indentation amplitude, I:

$$A_i(I) = a_i \left(\frac{I/T_i - 1}{I_{vF} - 1} \right)^b$$

(1)

The constant I_{vF} stands for the amplitude of indentation in multiples of threshold indentation, which on the average gives a receptive field equal in size to the field determined with von Frey hairs. b is the power exponent describing the function. The values of l_{vF} and b, which are empirically determined characteristics of the unit type, are 3.95 and 0.51 for the RA units and 4.24 and 0.65 for the SA I units. Strictly speaking, given these values of the constants, eqn. 1 refers to an indentation velocity of 4 mm/sec (Johansson, 1978). Thus, in order to determine the field size function ($A_i(I)$ in eqn. 1) for a sample of units, the size of the von Frey field and the indentation threshold were experimentally determined for 76 randomly isolated units with receptive fields in the glabrous skin area of the hand.

    Impulses were recorded from single mechanoreceptive afferents
in waking human subjects. A fine tungsten needle electrode was
inserted percutaneously in the median nerve on the upper arm
(Vallbc and Hagbarth, 1968). The recording electrode was adjusted
manually, in small steps, until single unit activity was discriminated from the background activity. The subjects were aged between
twenty and thirty years. The size of the receptive field was determined with a von Frey hair which provided a force of four or
five times the threshold force. A set of von Frey hairs, calibrated with a balance to provide the following forces when held
steadily, were used: 0.1 mN, 0.5 mN, 1 mN, 2 mN, 5 mN, 10 mN, 20
mN, 50 mN, and 100 mN. To determine the indentation thresholds,
stimuli of the same type were delivered as used when the sensitivity profiles of the receptive fields were investigated (cf.
Johansson, 1978). Triangular indentations were applied to the
skin with a moving coil stimulator which has previously been described (Westling, Johansson and Vallbo, 1976). The probe, which
was made of gold, had a diameter of 0.4 mm and a hemispherical
tip. An indentation velocity of 4 mm/sec was routinely used. When
a stable unit was encountered a zone of maximal sensitivity within
its receptive field was defined, under microscopic observation at
a magnification of 25 X, and the stimuli were delivered into this
zone during the threshold measurement. The threshold was defined
as the indentation amplitude at which the probability for one nerve
impulse was about 0.5.

    The unit samples (55 RA and 21 SA I units) were representative,
in that there were no statistically significant differences between them, and much larger samples from the corresponding skin
areas, with regard to von Frey receptive field sizes and force
thresholds (Vallbo and Johansson, 1978). In concordance with
earlier studies, it was appropriate to divide the RA sample into
three subsamples collected from the finger tip, the rest of the
finger and the palm, as the fields were smaller the more distal
the region (Vallbo and Johansson, 1978). On the other hand, there
were no regional differences in the case of the SA I units implying that the whole sample could be regarded as representative
for any of the three skin regions.

RESULTS

    Figure 2 shows the field size functions, obtained according to
eqn. 1 of RA units in the finger tip (A) and of SA I units (B). A
common finding was that the majority of the receptive fields within
each of the four unit samples (RA finger tip, RA rest of finger,
RA palm, SA I), constitute a rather homogenous group with regard
to extent of the field size functions. It appears, from Fig. 2,
that there were, however, a few units which had particularly large

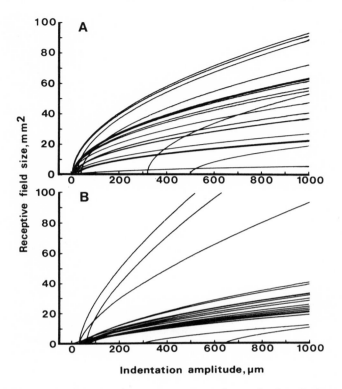

Fig. 2.   Receptive field size as a function of the indentation
          amplitude. Each curve represents an individual unit and
          is a power function according to eqn. 1 in text. A, 23
          RA units in the finger tip. B, 21 SA I units, distributed
          over the whole glabrous skin area.

receptive fields, or particularly high thresholds. The threshold
amplitude for the individual unit corresponds to a field size of
zero, in the diagrams.

     From the above section, it is quite clear that the number of
receptive fields overlapping any point on the skin is not fixed
but is dependent on the stimulus intensity. By using the derived
field size functions, examples of which are shown in Fig. 2, together with the appropriate density values described earlier (Table
1), the mean amount of receptive field overlap was estimated, as a
function of the indentation amplitude, for the following three skin
regions: (a) the finger tip, (b) the remaining part of the finger
and (c) the palm. This division has been considered in detail in

an earlier report (Johansson and Vallbo, 1978) (Table 1). The mean
size of the receptive fields was calculated for a certain amplitude
value. This value was then multiplied by the density of units in
order to obtain the mean overlap corresponding to the particular
amplitude. This procedure was repeated for very small amplitude
increments throughout the whole amplitude range, giving the overlap as a function of stimulus amplitude (Fig. 3). A formal description of the calculation is given by the following equation:

$$R = \frac{D}{n} \sum_{i=1}^{n} A_i(I) \tag{2}$$

where R stands for the mean overlap, I for the indentation amplitude and A_i (I) for the field size of the individual unit as a
function of the indentation amplitude (cf. eqn. 1).   D is the
density of units and n is the size of the sample (Table 1). In the
case of the RA units, the density values used were corrected for
the proportion of units with velocity thresholds above 4 mm/sec,
implying that the values, upon which the calculations were based,
were 94.8 percent of those shown in Table 1 (5.2 percent of the
RA units have velocity thresholds above 4 mm/sec, Johansson and
Vallbo, 1976).

     The diagrams in Fig. 3 show the results of separate calcu-
lations for the RA and SA 1 units. The three diagrams refer to
the finger tip, the main part of the finger and the palm. The
abscissae give the indentation amplitude and the ordinate the mean
receptive field overlap. A comparison between the different curves
reveals that the overlap is higher the more distal the region, and
that the RA population had the higher overlap of receptive fields,
throughout the whole amplitude range, in any skin region. The
overlap of RA fields in the main part of the finger and the palm
were very similar because the effect of the smaller fields in the
finger region (cf. Vallbo and Johansson, 1978) was approximately
cancelled by the higher innervation density (Table 1).

     The amount of overlap of receptive fields, as shown in the
diagrams of Fig. 3, is equivalent to the mean number of units excited by localized point stimuli. Therefore, these diagrams illustrate, not only the overlap, but also the number of units recruited
by point indentations, as a function of indentation amplitude. For
instance, indentations of an amplitude as low as 50 µm would on the
average excite 12 RA units at the finger tips and about 5 RA units
in the remaining part of the finger, and in the palm. The mean
number of SA I units excited would be less than one in the palm and
the main part of the finger, and only 2 at the finger tip at this
identation amplitude. Considering stronger stimuli, a localized
indentation of 0.5 mm would excite, on the average, 50 RA and 25

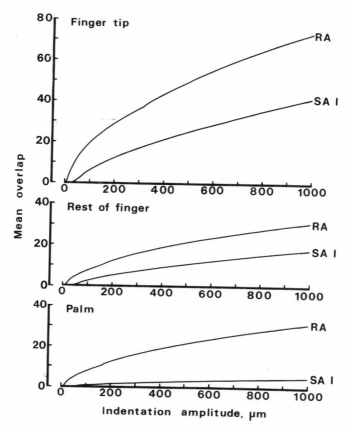

Fig. 3.   Estimated mean overlap of receptive fields of RA and SA I
          units in three different regions of the glabrous skin
          area of the human hand.

SA I units in the finger tip, but only three SA units in the palm.
Finally, an indentation of 1 mm would excite 74 RA units in the
finger tip, about 30 in the remaining part of the finger and the
palm. The corresponding values for the SA I population are 42, 18,
and 5.

DISCUSSION

     The problem of the present study was to estimate the overlap
of receptive fields in the various parts of the glabrous skin
area of the human hand, and from these estimates predict the

number of units participating in the transmission of information
concerning weak tactile stimuli, of minimal spatial extent, delivered to the skin. The estimates were based on data gathered
by single unit analysis and concerned the RA and SA I units. It
seems likely that these units account for the pronounced acuity
of the tactile sense in the human hand (see below).

Two basic parameters in the calculations are the innervation
density (Table 1) and the equation describing the relation between
the indentation amplitude and the size of the receptive field of
the individual units (eqn. 1). The experimental findings underlying the density data have been discussed in other contexts
(Johansson and Vallbo, 1978). As to the equation, it is largely
based upon experimental data obtained with indentations of relatively low amplitudes (below 25 multiples of the threshold of the
unit) (Johansson, 1978), implying that some of the present calculations are partly based on extrapolations in this respect. Therefore, the reliability of the inference concerning the number of
units recruited, as a function of indentation amplitude, is higher
the lower the amplitude. Strictly speaking, the estimates are
valid only for indentations with a velocity of 4 mm/sec since the
underlying sample parameters were collected with such stimuli.
Likewise, the field size functions underlying the calculations were
gathered with a small probe with a hemispherical tip, implying that
the point stimuli, considered in the results, actually refer to
that type of stimulation.

The interpretation of the mean values describing the receptive
field overlap (Fig. 3) is dependent on the actual distribution of
the receptive fields within the skin region considered. On the
assumption that the distribution of units is uniform within the
skin region, with regard to density and size of the fields, the
mean value of the overlap would be representative for any locus of
the region. This assumption seems reasonable, since there is
nothing to suggest a pronounced spatial segregation in these respects (cf. Johansson and Vallbo, 1978).

The present results reveal that there is a pronounced overlap
of SA I, and particularly RA receptive fields, even for tactile
stimuli of weak intensities. This indicates that, under most
stimulus conditions, a large number of RA and SA I units are engaged in transmitting the tactile message, besides the single units
recorded from when using the microneurographic technique. An organization with overlapping receptive fields seems to be well
suited, not only for spatial analysis, but also for analysis of the
intensity of stimuli by recruitment of units. In several earlier
reports, concerning the intensity aspects of skin indentations, the
response intensity of individual efferent units has been emphasized
(eg. Werner and Mountcastle, 1965; Mountcastle, et al., 1966;

Harrington and Merzenich, 1970; Knibestöl and Vallbo, 1976), whereas
the information encoded by the recruitment of units due to increasingly stronger stimuli has been given less consideration. The present inference of the total number of RA and SA I units excited,
as a function of indentation amplitude, indicates that the recruitment of units per se provides a considerable amount of information
about the amplitude of indentation: the functions are strictly
monotonic and negatively accelerated. However, since information
is very likely transmitted to the central nervous system in terms
of patterns of impulses in populations of mechanoreceptive units
with different functional properties, there are several quantities
related to the indentation amplitude. It seems to be an open
question which quantities the central nervous system relies upon
for the analysis of the indentation amplitude.

The fact that there are four types of mechanoreceptive units,
which have very distinctive functional characteristics, in the
glabrous skin suggests differential functional roles, for the four
types, in tactile sensibility. It is well known, from every day
experiences, that the tactile acuity increases in the proximodistal direction of the hand and is particularly well developed at
the finger tips. A pronounced gradient in the same direction has
also been shown in psychophysical tests to determine the capacity
of detailed spatial analysis (e.g. Weber, 1835; Weinstein, 1968;
Vallbo and Johansson, 1978). The fact that the pronounced proximodistal gradient in the overall unit density is accounted for mainly
by the RA and SA I units, and that the receptive fields of these
units are well suited for encoding mechanical events with a high
degree of spatial selectivity, indicate that these two types of
units account for the essential information concerning the detailed
spatial features of tactile stimuli (Vallbo and Johansson, 1978).
The multiple end-organs of these unit types (Meissner and Merkel
endings) are located close enough to provide a sharply defined
cutaneous receptive field with practically uniform sensitivity.
At the same time, the endings are scattered well enough to allow
a large number of such units to interdigitate (Johansson, 1978).
It seems that such an arrangement which renders possible overlapping
of sharply defined receptive fields of one rapidly and one slowly
adapting unit type, both with high dynamic sensitivity, is well
suited for the detailed analysis of mechanical events of the skin
surface, with maximal efficiency with regard to the number of peripheral units. An example illustrating the close concordance between tactile acuity and the density of RA and SA I units is to be
found in tactile reading with the fingers. It has been noted that
only a limited area of the fingers can be used to recognize letters
presented via the Optacon (a reading aid for the blind) (Hill,
1974). This area is the distal 12-15 mm of the finger pad, i.e.
the area of extremely high densities of RA and SA I units (Table
1).

There are several findings that emphasize the role of the RA
units as the most important afferent units in tactile acuity, in
addition to the fact that they have the highest density. For instance, single impulses in one, or very few, RA units in the fingers are detected by the subject, and the transmission of these
single impulses in the central nervous system may be practically
free from noise, as there is a 1:1 relation between individual impulses and correct psychophysical detection (Vallbo and Johansson,
1976). A temporally tight coupling between impulse activity in
RA units and in cortical neurones (SI) has been demonstrated in
the hand of the monkey (Mountcastle, Talbot, Sakata and Hyvärinen,
1969), suggesting that the RA units account for detailed temporal
analysis of mechanical events on the glabrous skin area of the
primate hand (cf. LaMotte and Mountcastle, 1978). Moreover, it
has been shown that the encoding of stimulus intensity in the discharge of individual RA units, in the foot pad of the cat, yields
much greater information transmission (30 bits/sec) than has been
found for all other types of skin mechanoreceptive units (Dickhaus,
Sassen and Zimmermann, 1976).

The tentative conclusion that the main role of the PC and SA
II units in tactile sensibility does not lie in detailed spatial
analysis, is based mainly on the following findings: the PC and SA
II units have obscure cutaneous receptive fields, as defined with
skin indentations; they are approximately evenly distributed on the
glabrous skin, and their density is considerably lower than the RA
and SA I densities in the skin regions of the fingers. The fact
that the end-organs of these units (Pacinian and Ruffini endings)
are more deeply and widely distributed within the structures of
the hand than the RA and SA I endings (Meissner and Merkel endings),
which are superficially located in the skin (e.g. Stilwell, 1957;
Miller et al., 1958), agrees with the view that they have functions
other than detailed analysis of events restricted to the skin surface. The role of the PC units has been considered in may other
investigations, and it seems clear that they can provide information about high frequency transients and vibrations of objects in
contrast with the hand (e.g. Talbot, et al., 1968; Verrillo, 1968;
Merzenich and Harrington, 1969; Mountcastle, LaMotte and Carli,
1972). Taking into account the high sensitivity and the very wide
receptive fields of these units, it seems likely that they also
can respond to joint movements and muscle contraction. No direct
experimental evidence has been presented regarding the functional
role of the SA II units. It has been suggested that their primary
function is to provide detailed information on the direction, the
magnitude and the rate of change of the tensions within the skin,
as well as between the skin and deeper and less flexible structures
of the hand (Johansson, 1978). Such information should be of significance for the evaluation of shearing forces between the skin
and a handheld object. They may also participate in subserving the

sensation of cutaneous pressure (Harrington and Merzenich, 1970) and in proprioception due to their response to joint movement (Knibestöl and Vallbo, 1970; Knibestöl, 1975).

SUMMARY

Two types of low threshold mechanoreceptive units in the glabrous skin are of the human hand - one rapidly adapting (RA) and one slowly adapting (SA I) - have small and well demarcated receptive fields. In contrast, the other two types found in this area (PC and SA II) have large fields with indistinct borders. There are several findings that indicate that the RA and SA I units account for the pronounced tactile acuity of the hand. For instance, these units have receptive fields which can provide distinct information concerning localization of a stimulus, and the densities of these units are particularly high in skin regions where the tactile acuity is high, i.e. the tips of the fingers.

The mean value of the receptive field overlap was estimated as a function of indentation amplitude for the RA and SA I unit populations in different glabrous skin regions of the hand. The estimates were based on data gathered by single unit analysis. The reconstructions take into account (1), that sizes of the receptive fields increase with increasing stimulus amplitude, (2), that the sensitivity as well as the rate of growth of receptive field size, varies from one unit to another, and (3), that the density of units varies between skin regions. The values arrived at can be directly used to deduce the mean number of RA and SA I units excited by point indentations of various amplitudes. The inference indicates that, even for rather small amplitudes, a large number of RA and SA I units are engaged in transmitting the tactile message, and this number increases monotonically with amplitude; reaching a number greater than 100 units for a point indentations of 1 mm amplitude delivered to the finger tip. In addition to the RA and SA I units, a number of SA II, and particularly PC units, may be brought into play by most tactile stimuli.

ACKNOWLEDGEMENTS

This study was supported by grants from the Swedish Medical Research Council (project no. 04X-3548), and the University of Umea (Reservationsanslaget för främjande av ograduerades forskares vetenskapliga verksamhet).

REFERENCES

Armett, C. J., Gray, J. A. B., Hunsperger, R. W., & Lal, S. The transmission of information in primary receptor neurons and second-order neurones of a phasic system. Journal of Physiology (London), 1962, 164, 395-421.

Cauna, N.   Nature and functions of the papillary ridges of the
    digital skin. Anatomical Record, 1954, 119, 449-468.
Cauna, N. & Mannan, G. The struture of human digital Pacinian
    corpuscles (Corpuscula Lamellosa) and its functional signifi-
    cance. Journal of Anatomy, 1958, 92, 1-20.
Chambers, M. R., Andres, K. H., v. Duering, M., & Iggo, A.   The
    structure and function of the slowly adapting type II mechano-
    receptor in hairy skin. Quarterly Journal of Experimental
    Physiology, 1972, 57, 417-445.
Chouchov, Ch. N. The fine structure of small encapsulated re-
    ceptors in human digital glabrous skin. Journal of Anatomy,
    1973, 114, 25-33.
Dickhaus, H., Sassen, M., & Zimmermann, M. Rapidly adapting cutan-
    eous mechanoreceptors (RA): coding, variability and informa-
    tion transmission. In Y. Zotterman (Ed.), Sensory functions
    of the skin in primates (Vol. 27). Oxford: Pergamon Press,
    1976.
Fuller, D. R. G. & Gray, J. A. B. The relation between mechanical
    displacements applied to a cat's pad and the resultant impulse
    patterns. Journal of Physiology (London), 1966, 182, 465-483.
Hagbarth, K.-E., Hongell, A., Hallin, R. A., & Törebjork, H. E.
    Afferent impulses in median nerve fascicles evoked by tactile
    stimuli of the human hand. Brain Research, 1970, 24, 423-442.
Harrington, R. & Merzenich, M. M. Neural coding in the sense of
    touch: Human sensation of skin indentation compared with the
    responses of slowly adapting mechanoreceptive afferents in-
    nervating the hairy skin of monkeys. Experimental Brain Re-
    search, 1970, 10, 251-264.
Hill, J. W. Limited field of view in reading lettershapes with
    the fingers. In F. A. Geldard (Ed.), Conference of vibro-
    tactile communication. Austin, TX.: The Psychonomic Society,
    1974.
Iggo, A. An electrophysiological analysis of afferent fibers in
    primate skin. Acta Neurovegetativa, 1963, 24, 225-240.
Iggo, A. & Muir, A. R. The structure and function of a slowly
    adapting touch corpuscle in hairy skin. Journal of Phy-
    siology (London), 1969, 200, 703-796.
Iggo, A. & Ogawa, H. Correlative physiological and morphological
    studies of rapidly-adapting units in the cat's glabrous skin.
    Journal of Physiology (London), 1977, 266, 275-296.
Jänig, W. Morphology of rapidly and slowly adapting mechanorecep-
    tors in the hairless skin of the cat's hind foot. Brain Re-
    search, 1971, 28, 217-231.
Jänig, W., Schmidt, R. F., & Zimmermann, M. Single unit responses
    and the total afferent outflow from the cat's foot pad upon
    mechanical stimulation. Experimental Brain Research, 1968,
    6, 100-115.

Johansson, R. S. Receptive field sensitivity profile of mechano-sensitive units innervating the glabrous skin of the human hand. Brain Research, 1976a, 104, 330-334.

Johansson, R. S. Skin mechanoreceptors in the human hand: Recep-tive field characteristics. In Y. Zotterman (Ed.), Sensory functions of the skin in primates. Oxford: Pergamon Press, 1976b.

Johansson, R. S. Tactile sensibility in the human hand: Receptive field characteristics of mechanoreceptive units in the glab-rous skin area. Journal of Physiology (London), 1978, 281, 101-123.

Johansson, R. S. & Vallbo, Å. B. Skin mechanoreceptors in the human hand. An inference of some population properties. In Y. Zotterman (Ed.), Sensory functions of the skin in primates. Oxford: Pergamon Press, 1976.

Johansson, R. S. & Vallbo, Å. B. Tactile sensibility in the human hand: relative and absolute densities of four types of mechano-receptive units in the glabrous skin area. Journal of Phy-siology (London), 1978, In press.

Johnson, K. O. Reconstruction of population to a vibratory stimulus in quickly adapting mechanoreceptive afferent fiber population innervating glabrous skin of the monkey. Journal of Neuro-physiology, 1974, 37, 48-72.

Knibestöl, M. Stimulus-response functions of rapidly adapting mechanoreceptors in the human glabrous skin area. Journal of Physiology (London), 1973, 232, 427-452.

Knibestöl, M. Stimulus-response functions of slowly adapting mechanoreceptors in the human glabrous skin area. Journal of Physiology (London), 1975, 245, 63-80.

Knibestöl, M. & Vallbo, Å. B. Single unit analysis of mechano-receptor activity from the human glabrous skin. Acta Phy-siologica Scandinavica, 1970, 80, 178-195.

Knibestöl, M. & Vallbo, Å. B. Stimulus response functions of pri-mary afferents and psychophysical intensity estimation on mechanical skin stimulation in the human hand. In Y. Zotter-man (Ed.), Sensory functions of the skin in primates. Oxford: Pergamon Press, 1976.

LaMotte, R. H. & Mountcastle, V. B. Neural processing of tempor-ally-ordered somesthetic input: remaining capacity in monkeys following lesions of the parietal lobe. In G. Gordon (Ed.), Active touch: the mechanism of recogntion of objects by mani-pulation: A multi-disciplinary approach. Oxford: Pergamon Press, 1978.

Lindblom, U. Properties of touch receptors in distal glabrous skin of the monkey. Journal of Neurophysiology, 1965, 28, 966-985.

Lindblom, U. & Lund, L. The discharge from vibration-sensitive re-ceptors in the monkey foot. Experimental Neurology, 1966, 15, 401-417.

Lynn, B. The nature and location of certain phasic mechanorecep-
    tors in the cat's foot pad. Journal of Physiology (London),
    1969, 201, 768-773.
Merzenich, M. M., & Harrington, T. The sense of flutter-vibration
    evoked by stimulation of the hairy skin of primates: Com-
    parisons of human sensory capacity with the responses of
    mechanoreceptive afferents innervating the hairy skin of
    monkeys. Experimental Brain Research, 1969, 9, 236-260.
Miller, M. R., Ralston III, H. J., & Kasahara, M. The pattern of
    cutaneous innervation of the human hand. American Journal of
    Anatomy, 1958, 102, 183-217.
Mountcastle, V. B., LaMotte, R. H., & Carli, G. Detection thresh-
    olds for stimuli in humans and monkeys: Comparison with
    threshold events in mechanoreceptive afferent nerve fiber in-
    nervating the monkey hand. Journal of Neurophysiology, 1972,
    35, 122-136.
Mountcastle, V. B., Talbot, W. H., & Kornhuber, H. H. The
    neural transformation of mechanical stimuli delivered to the
    monkey's hand. In A.V.S. deReuck & J. Knight (Eds.), Touch,
    heat and pain. London: Ciba Foundation, Churchill, 1966.
Mountcastle, V. B., Talbot, W. H., Sakata, H., & Hyvärinen, J.
    Cortical neuronal mechanism in flutter-vibration studied in
    unanesthetized monkeys: Neuronal periodicity and frequency
    discharge. Journal of Neurophysiology, 1969, 32, 452-484.
Munger, B. L., Pubols, L. M., & Pubols, B. H. The Merkel rete
    papilla - a slowly adapting sensory receptor in mammalian
    glabrous skin. Brain Research, 1971, 29, 47-61.
Sakada, S. Response of Golgi-Mazzoni corpuscles in the cat peri-
    ostea to mechanical stimuli. In R. Dubner & Y. Kawamura
    (Eds.), Oral-facial sensory motor mechanisms. New York:
    Appleton, 1976.
Stilwell, Jr., D. L. The innervation of deep structures of the
    hand. American Journal of Anatomy, 1957, 101, 75-92.
Talbot, W. H., Darian-Smith, I., Kornhuber, H. H., & Mountcastle,
    V. B. The sense of flutter-vibration: Comparison of the
    human capacity with response patterns of mechanoreceptive
    afferents from the monkey hand. Journal of Neurophysiology,
    1968, 31, 301-334.
Vallbo, Å. B., & Hagbarth, K.-E. Activity from skin mechanorecep-
    tors recorded percutaneously in awake human subjects. Experi-
    mental Neurology, 1968, 21, 270-289.
Vallbo, Å. B., & Johansson, R. S. Skin mechanoreceptors in the
    human hand: Neural and psychophysical thresholds. In Y.
    Zotterman (Ed.), Sensory functions of the skin in primates.
    Oxford: Pergamon Press, 1976.
Vallbo, Å. B., & Johansson, R. S. Tactile sensory innervation of
    the glabrous skin of the human hand. In G. Gordon (Ed.),
    Active Touch: The mechanism of recognition of objects by
    manipulation. Oxford: Pergamon Press, 1978.

Verrillo, R. T.   A duplex mechanism of mechanoreception.   In D. R. Kenshalo (Ed.),   The skin senses.   Springfield, Ill.: Thomas, 1968.

Weber, E. H.   Über den Tastsinn.   Archiv der Anatomie und Physiologie, 1835, 152-159.

Weinstein, S.   Intensive and extensive aspects of tactile sensitivity as a function of body part, sex and laterality.   In D. R. Kenshalo (Ed.), The skin senses. Springfield, Ill.: Thomas, 1968.

Werner, G., & Mountcastle, V. B.   Neural activity in mechanoreceptive cutaneous afferents: stimulus-response relations. Weber functions, and information transmission.   Journal of Neurophysiology, 1965, 28, 359-397.

Westling, G., Johansson, R. S., & Vallbo, Å. B.   A method for mechanical stimulation of skin receptors.   In Y. Zotterman (Ed.), Sensory functions of the skin in primates.   Oxford: Pergamon Press, 1976.

DISCUSSION

DR. IGGO: As I indicated when I introduced Dr. Johansson, he had some fine details to give us and now I think we have an opportunity to question him about his results.

DR. HENSEL: Have you done any morphological studies concerning the structures underlying your receptive fields.

DR. JOHANSSON: No, we have not.

DR. ZOTTERMAN: I would like to ask you what your opinion is about the depth in the skin of these different receptors, if we go to the Pacinian corpuscles, which we can see with the naked eye. They are apt to be entirely exposed in the cat's mesentery and there, already in Adrian's lab in 1926, I recorded from the fiber from single Pacinian corpuscles and we, Gernandt and I (1946), described that later in the early 1940's. Those were quite exposed and you can see them in the mesentery. It's enough to "poof", like that, to stimulate them. Their threshold is frightfully low but in the skin you do not stimulate them by that, I suppose.

DR. JOHANSSON: No, we do not, but it would be possible to more or less directly stimulate some of the Meissner corpuscles if the superficial layer of the epidermis is sliced off immediately after the receptive field of the unit recorded from had been determined.

DR. ZOTTERMAN: Yes, but not the Pacinian that are deeply located as they are in the cat. They are rather deep, at the tendons or right behind the tendons. They must have a much higher threshold, and in that case the receptive fields must be much, much broader because of their deep situation. There must be some relation between the depth of the situation and the area of the receptive field, is that so?

DR. JOHANSSON: Yes, there are studies by Jänig (1971), who showed that if you slice off the corneal layer, the receptive fields will be smaller and the threshold slightly lower. That is, the distance between the skin surface and the end-organ is smaller than the receptive field will be smaller, so it fits very well with what you say. These were Meissner corpuscles but it may be the same with the Pacinian corpuscle.

DR. JÄRVILEHTO: I wonder about the types of receptors, whether the situation for the glabrous skin is really so simple. For the hairy skin we often have difficulty in classifying receptors, at least, many receptors in the hairy skin. There seem to be transitional forms. How many receptors have you found that do not fit the classification that you show now?

DR. JOHANSSON: In a sample of approximately 400 units we have
found 5 per cent which were difficult to fit into the appropriate
subgroup of rapidly or slowly adapting units. However, we are not
sure that they all are intermediate types, simply due to scanty
information.

DR. JÄRVILEHTO: Let us say that many slowly adapting fibers have
different thresholds for the dynamic response and the static
response, what is the criterion that you use for slowly adapting
fibers, for example?

DR. JOHANSSON: It is simply that the fiber can keep on discharging
during sustained indentation. We used glass probes and von
Frey hairs and if you make an indentation with the glass probe or
a heavy von Frey hair, for instance 10 g, then you will readily
see the differences between rapidly and slowly adapting units.

DR. JÄRVILEHTO: Have you found such slowly adapting fibers that
if you use a larger stimulus area you hardly get a response, but
if you use small stimulus area then you get a response?

DR. JOHANSSON: Yes, one type shows that behavior.

DR. JÄRVILEHTO: Which type is this, is this an SA I or SA II?

DR. JOHANSSON: SA I.

DR. IGGO: That fits in with the evidence of the hairy skin of the
cat, but for the SA I, if the probe is glued onto the skin,
directly on top of the receptor and then pressed into the skin,
that stimulus is much less effective than if, with the skin free,
the probe is pushed onto the receptor surface. So deformation
does seem to be a factor of importance in exciting the SA I.

DR. JOHANSSON: That phenomenon can be viewed as some sort of
lateral inhibition mechanism in the periphery. If you have a
block indentation, those SA I units with their receptive field
located at the edge of the block will respond at a very high rate
whereas those with the field completely covered will hardly be
excited. This can be viewed as a contour or edge sharpening
around the block coded in the afferent message to the CNS.

DR. FRANZÉN: First, I would like to congratulate Dr. Johansson
for a very nice study. It is very useful for understanding the
coding mechanism. We did a study using tactile stimuli, the same

as Dr. Lindblom talked about this morning. It could be just a
coincidence, but the average psychophysical function had a slope
of about 0.6 plus some dispersion. Maybe it agrees too well with
your data. Your recruitment functions, however, look very much
like our psychophysical data. The stimulus we used was a very
short pulse, as you did, but had a higher velocity than yours.
As far as we understand the single RA unit, the fiber gives only
1 spike out although the intensity of the stimulus is increased.
It is maybe too simple of a story, but maybe this psychophysical
function mirrors the recruitment function and will fit your data
very nicely.

DR. LINDBLOM: Let me briefly emphasize that your curves were
from one set of receptors but our curves were from all types of
receptors. With the deformation, the PCs will also be recruited
so the question is whether you could add them to your intensity
function and still get the same result.

DR. JOHANSSON: If you consider the PC population separately, the
function will not be the negatively accelerated function that has
a power exponent of less than 1. It will be a positively
accelerated curve because of the shapes of the PC receptive
fields.

DR. VERRILLO: Do you have any intention of attempting to do
similar studies with sinusoidal stimuli? The stimulus you use is
very complicated, physically, and sinusoids are much simpler
things to deal with.

DR. JOHANSSON: It would be nice to use sinusoids, but it is a
question of priority. For the moment, however, there are other
things which are of higher priority in my mind.

DR. IGGO: There is one topic I would like to raise in general
discussion. It arose out of a presentation earlier today and is
in response to comments made to me after the session. It has to
do with the ethics of certain kinds of animal experiments. This
is a very difficult and sensitive area. I raise it here because
I think we may have the opportunity, at a meeting like this, of
having people contribute who are more familiar, than the
experimentalist, with the situation in the clinic and the
operating theater, and with reports of some patients who have
experienced certain kinds of surgical treatment. The topic is the
use of an unanesthetized, immobilized, animal preparation for the
purposes of recording from the central nervous system. The
situation is one in which there is no access to the animal's
experience apart from that recorded by the microelectrodes or by

looking at other parameters, such as the EEG or arterial pressure.
I wonder whether there is anybody who has any knowledge of what
human subjects experience in such conditions.

DR. TOREBJÖRK: It happens, by mistake, that patients who undergo
certain types of surgery are immobilized by neuromuscular
blocking agents before they get their anesthesia. It also may
occur that the patient may awaken from the general anesthesia
before the neuromuscular blocking agent, such as suxametonium,
has disappeared. This is a very unpleasant procedure with pain
experienced in the muscles. I do not know if EEGs have been
made on patients during these states, but if EEG recordings should
have been made they probably would have been desynchronized.

DR. WHITSEL: As an experimentalist with training in pharmacology,
I would like to point out that there are depolarizing and non-
depolarizing neuromuscular blocking agents; Syncurine (succinylcholine) and decamethonium are depolarizing drugs whereas
gallamine blocks neuromuscular transmission by combining with
acetylcholine receptive sites but does not produce membrane
depolarization. Most depolarizing drugs produce intense and
prolonged activation of muscle spindle afferents (Albuquerque, et
al., 1968) and afferents innervating a variety of chemoreceptors
and mechanoreceptors. The intense peripheral afferent activation
produced by depolarizing drugs would appear to account for some
(the afferent barrage can outlast the neuromuscular block), if
not all, of the uncomfortable sensory experiences you describe
under the condition of emergence from general anesthesia. Of
course emergence of anesthesia is also not totally devoid of
unpleasant but characteristic sensory experiences. I wonder if
anyone could comment on the reactions a person might have to being
placed into an instrument in which head movements are prevented
by chambers or attaching bolts fixed to the skull as is necessary
to obtain stabilty during recordings from single neurons in the
waking or alert animal. Since that must be rather unpleasant and
could therfore potentially influence sensory neuron responsiveness,
I would welcome the comments of experimentalists or clinicians
in the room with experience with this approach.

DR. IGGO: One needs to be careful not to say that two blacks
make a white, but this is a rather delicate topic and I think
that, now that we are here, we should take the opportunity for
comment. It seems quite likely that the future will yield more
movement in the direction of using unanaesthetized animals for the
very reasons that Dr. Whitsel showed in his work, where the
behavior of these units may be, not entirely different, but
actually different under anaesthesia.

DR. STARR: There are two issues, one of paralysis and one of
immobility without paralysis, and I think that the main reason
the gallamine paralysis was introduced was because we wished to
work with preparations that did not require anaesthesia. It seems
to me that the precautions that you have taken are really quite
normal and routine. There is an experience that many of you may
have had in terms of paralysis. That occurs when you awakened
early in the morning and know that you are perfectly awake yet
have been unable to move. You have just awakened from the stage
of REM sleep. You still have your central inhibitory processes
going and you are unable to move, but the main thing is the fear,
the experience is anxiety. Once you explain to people what they are
going through they can deal with this information and they are no
longer afraid. This, then is a reply to what a human experiences
when he is immobilized. There are two examples that I know of in
the literature of paralysis in normal people who have subjected
themselves for studies to disprove Bickford's hypothesis that
everything that is coming from the head is muscle. They were
assured of what was going on and handled it very well. Of course
they were paid and therefore were not very involved in the
experiment. One could argue that the animals are not involved and
therefore are perhaps improperly treated. But I really think that
paralysis, by itself, is not a difficult situation. In neurosurgery
we have a procedure where we immobilize heads of individuals who
have had broken necks. Initially, this is very uncomfortable
but then everyone adapts to it. It really depends upon intent of
the experiment.

DR. ZOTTERMAN: I can only tell you about a prominent physiologist
who tells me about having been paralyzed during a knee operation.
Of course, he had spinal anaesthesia and on top of that, for
some reason, he had curare as well. That was Alex von Muralt from
Switzerland. He told me that it was a very peculiar feeling. If
you awaken sometime with the circulation in your arm blocked, it
just hangs there and you cannot move it. It is a funny feeling,
you know that the arm no longer belongs to you. It is just
something outside yourself when you have no sensation from it.
The same occurs when both of your legs are paralyzed after spinal
anaesthesia. That part of the body no longer belongs to you, it
has disappeared from your consciousness.

DR. HENSEL: I would like to make two comments on your question.
The first comment is I remember that a colleague of mine in
Heidelberg, many years ago, volunteered to undergo complete
immobilization without anaesthesia. He reported that this was a
very fearful and dreadful experience. It had been necessary to
apply artificial respiration in that state and I wonder if this,
per se, might not also influence the activity of the central nervous

system, perhaps as much as some kinds of anaesthesia. The second comment on this topic is a recent experience of Dr. Lorenz who is working in experimental surgery in Marburg. They immobilized rats by putting them in plaster of paris casts so they could not move. Even after a few hours they found multiple ulcers in their stomachs induced by the immobilization. So it seems that immobilization, per se, might be of considerable stress for the animal. It would be worthwhile to consider whether this stress would interfere with the functions of the central nervous system. It is an unproven belief that keeping an animal immobilized without anaesthesia will give an undisturbed picture of the function of the central nervous system.

DR. IGGO: This discussion was not really opened other than in a very general sense. It is not directed at any particular person or set of experiments. It is just that the comment was made to me and I think it has been useful to air the problems that are associated with the matter.

DR. WHITSEL: One brief comment, please. I totally agree that this type of forum is appropriate for discussion of the ethics and acceptability of the data obtained using a given preparation. However, I would also plead that the data we submit to bear on the issue raised today be evaluated critically and with scientific criteria just as severe as those we use when examining data bearing on questions dealing less with ethical and more with biological issues. A quite useful series of papers on the effects of neuromuscular blocking agents (depolarizing and non-depolarizing agents) on unanesthetized man was published by K. R. Unna and his colleagues in the early 1950's.

REFERENCES

Albuquerque, E., Whitsel, B. L., & Smith, C. M. Patterns of muscle spindle afferent stimulation by alkylammonium compounds. Journal of Pharmacology and Experimental Therapeutics, 1968, 164, 191-201.

Gernandt, B. & Zotterman, Y. Intestinal pain: An electrophysiological investigation on mesenteric nerves. Acta Physiologica Scandinavica, 1946, 12, 56-72.

Jänig, W. Morphology of rapidly adapting mechanoreceptors in the hairless skin of the cat's hindfoot. Brain Research, 1971, 28, 217-231.

Pelikan, E. W., Unna, K. R., MacFarlane, D. E., Cazort, R. J., Sadove, M. S., & Nelson, J. T. Evaluations of curarizing drugs in man. II. Journal of Pharmacology and Experimental Therapeutics, 1950, 99, 215-225.

Unna, K. R. & Pelikan, E. W. Evaluation of curarizing drugs in man.
    VI. Critique of experiments on unanesthetized subjects.
    Annals of New York Academy of Science, 1951, 54, 480-492.

Unna, K. R., Pelikan, E. W., MacFarlane, D. W., Cazort, R. J.,
    Sadove, M. S., & Nelson, J. T. Evaluation of curarizing
    drugs in man. Journal of American Medical Association, 1950,
    144, 448-451.

Unna, K. R., Pelikan, E. W., MacFarlane, D. W., Cazort, R. J.,
    Sadove, M. S., Nelson, J. R., & Drucker, A. P. Evaluation
    of curarizing drugs in man. I. Journal of Pharmacology and
    Experimental Therapeutics, 1950, 98, 318-329.

Unna, K. R., Pelikan, E. W., MacFarlane, D. W., & Sadove, M. S.
    Evaluation of curarizing drugs in man. IV. Journal of
    Pharmacology and Experimental Therapeutics, 1950, 100, 201-
    329.

PSYCHOPHYSICAL MEASUREMENTS OF ENHANCEMENT, SUPPRESSION, AND SURFACE GRADIENT EFFECTS IN VIBROTACTION

Ronald T. Verrillo, Institute for Sensory Research
Syracuse University, Syracuse, New York 13210

George A. Gescheider, Department of Psychology
Hamilton College, Clinton, New York 13323

Twelve years ago at the First International Symposium on the Skin Senses held in Tallahassee (Kenshalo, 1968), it was proposed that the pattern theory of mechanoreception was not sufficient to explain the results of an extensive series of psychophysical experiments (Verrillo, 1968). At that time it was demonstrated that our perception of repetitive mechanical stimuli is mediated by at least two types of end organs in cutaneous tissue and their accompanying neural systems (Verrillo, 1963, 1966a,b, 1968). The duplex model was consistent, in part, with the limited knowledge we had at that time of the physiological response of specific end organs (Sato, 1961). Subsequent experimentation performed in other laboratories later verified or supported this model (Harrington and Merzenich, 1970; Lindblom, 1965; Merzenich and Harrington, 1969; Talbot et al., 1968). The development of techniques for microneurography in humans (Vallbo and Hagbarth, 1968) gave strong support for the position that at least two neural systems subserve our appreciation of vibration on the skin (Järvilehto, Hämäläinen, and Laurinen, 1976; Knibestöl and Vallbo, 1970; Knibestöl, 1973; Konietzny and Hensel, 1977; and others).

The early research concerning a duplex model focused primarily on the psychophysical threshold response of human subjects. More recently our attention has shifted to the investigation of suprathreshold responses within each system and possible interactions between systems. We should like to start with several figures which briefly summarize the threshold data of the original model, then go to examine several suprathreshold phenomena, and finally to end with our most recent experiments in which we explored aspects of gradient or edge effects as they are reflected in the psychophysically measured responses of humans.

THRESHOLD EXPERIMENTS

Let us begin with some of our early results that will constitute the basis for what follows. Figure 1 shows the threshold of detection on the thenar eminence for a number of sinusoidal frequencies and for different sizes of contactor. In these experiments a rigid surround prevented the spread of vibrations across the surface of the skin. The gap between contactor and surround was kept constant at 1.0 mm for all contactor sizes. Note that in all but the smallest contactor sizes the shape of the frequency function is U-shaped in the upper frequencies and relatively flat at lower frequencies. As the contactor gets smaller the break-point frequency between the flat and U-shaped portion increases. For the smallest contactor sizes the threshold becomes independent of frequency. Note also the inverse relationship between threshold and contactor size: as contactor size increases, the overall position of the U-shaped portion of the curve decreases. The two-limbed curves imply that the mechanism responsible for a threshold response across frequencies is not unitary. It is apparent that at least two mechanisms are involved: one that is dependent upon frequency and contactor area, and another that is independent of both frequency and area.

The next figure (Fig. 2) illustrates these phenomena in a different way by showing the same data plotted as a function of contactor area. The slopes of the curves for higher frequencies is approximately -3.0 dB per doubling of contactor area. At these frequencies spatial summation is strongly evident. The low frequencies (25 and 40 Hz) show no such dependence upon contactor size. Other experiments (Gescheider, 1976; Verrillo, 1966a) showed that only at high frequencies are temporal effects observed that are consistent with Zwislocki's theory of temporal summation (Zwislocki, 1960). Thus, we may hypothesize at this point that cutaneous tissue contains at least two receptor systems: one that is capable of spatial and temporal summation, and one that is capable of neither phenomenon.

At the time that these results were reported, several physiological studies (Hunt, 1961; Sato, 1961; Scott, 1951; Loewenstein, 1958) had shown that the Pacinian corpuscle could be activated by high-frequency mechanical stimulation. It was reasonable to suggest, therefore, that this receptor was a likely candidate to account for the temporal and spatial summation. It was logical also to expect that an area of the body devoid of Pacinian corpuscles should not show these characteristics. According to the anatomical literature the dorsal surface of the tongue was such a site. Threshold measurements made on the dorsal tongue are shown in Fig. 3 plotted as a function of frequency and compared to similar data obtained from the thenar eminences of the same subjects. It is apparent

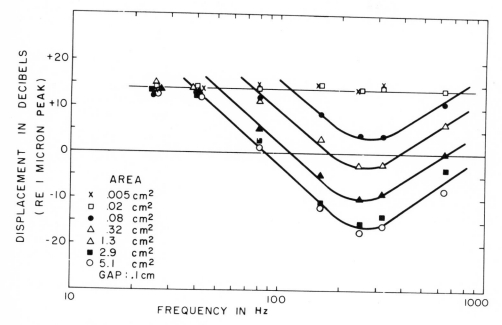

Fig. 1.   Thresholds of detection for different contactor areas
plotted as a function of frequency. At low frequencies
the threshold is independent of contactor size and for
small contactor sizes the threshold is independent of
frequency. (Verrillo, 1963)

that the threshold for vibration on the tongue is independent of
frequency. The data shown in Fig. 4 from the same subjects illustrate that the threshold for vibration on the tongue is also independent of contactor size. In addition, no temporal summation
effects could be demonstrated on the dorsal surface of the tongue
(Verrillo, 1966b).

   The preceding four graphs strongly suggest that cutaneous
tissue contains at least two mechanoreceptor systems, one that in-
tegrates energy over time and space and another that does not.
They further show that temporal and spatial summation is not found
in a part of the body (dorsal tongue) that is devoid of Pacinian
corpuscles. Thus, the Pacinian corpuscle becomes the most likely
end organ responsible for spatial and temporal summation in cutaneous tissue. Many other experiments in our laboratory and in
others, both psychophysical and physiological, have supported this
view. A comparison of some results from these experiments is
shown in Fig. 5. The basic psychophysical function is shown in the

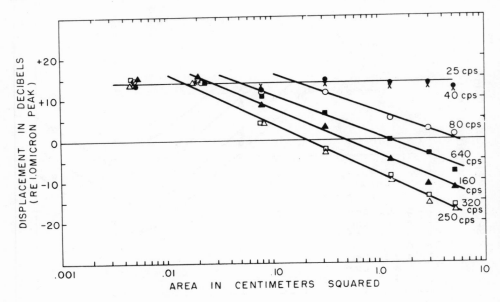

Fig. 2.   The data of Fig. 1 replotted as a function of contactor
area.   The slopes of -3 dB/doubling of area show spatial
summation at the higher frequencies.   At low frequencies
spatial summation was not observed.   (Verrillo, 1963)

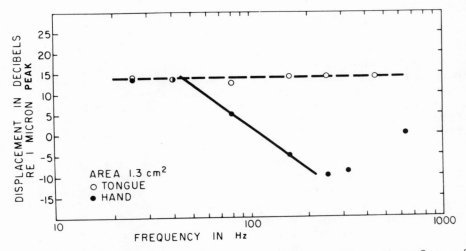

Fig. 3.   Thresholds of detection measured on the dorsal surface of
the tongue and on the thenar eminence as a function of frequency.   On the surface of the tongue the threshold is independent of frequency.   (Verrillo, 1966b)

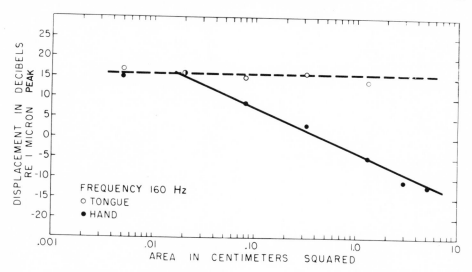

Fig. 4.   Comparison of vibrotactile thresholds measured on the dorsal surface of the tongue and the thenar eminence plotted
as a function of contactor area. Spatial summation is
not evident on the surface of the tongue. (Verrillo,
1966b)

lower curve. It is flat in the lower frequencies, decreases with
a slope of approximately -12 dB to a maximum sensitivity at about
250 Hz, and then rises again in the upper frequencies to complete
the U-shaped portion of the function. These basic psychophysical
curves were published by Verrillo (1963, 1968) and later replicated by Gescheider (1976). The physiological recordings from
Pacinian corpuscles follow closely the shape of the function at
higher frequencies. Only Sato (1961) stimulated the corpuscle
directly and recorded directly from its nerve fiber. Talbot et al.
(1968), Merzenich and Harrington (1969), and Mountcastle et al.
(1972) all stimulated the intact monkey skin and recorded from a
proximal portion of the peripheral neuron. There is a remarkable
correspondence of shape in the U-shaped portion of these curves.
Differences in the vertical position of the curves is probably due
to differences in the criterion for threshold used in different
laboratories.

SUPRATHRESHOLD EXPERIMENTS

    The basic experiments relating to the duplex model of mechano-
reception were concerned primarily with threshold events. But, in
the course of a normal day's activities we do not often encounter

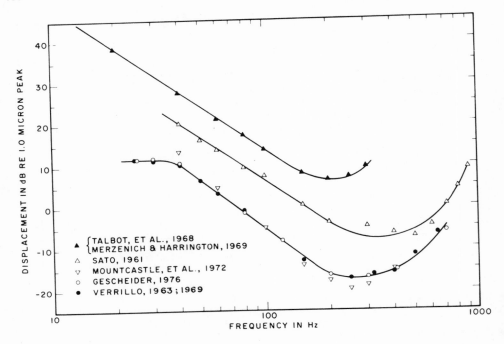

Fig. 5.   Vibrotactile thresholds from two psychophysical experi-
          ments compared with electrophysiological measurements from
          Pacinian corpuscles. Note the close correspondence of
          shape and slope (-12 dB/doubling of frequency) in the data
          from the two types of experiments.

threshold stimuli. It becomes important, therefore, to explore our
model at suprathreshold levels of stimulation. The reasons for
doing so are twofold. First, we are interested in the theoretical
aspects of neural functioning, particularly those mechanisms which
underlie the neural coding of intensity. The approach to this problem must include not only the response of individual nerve fibers
but also a precise description of how stimulus parameters affect
the responses of intact organisms, especially humans. The second
reason for doing these experiments involves more practical or at
least immediate considerations. A not uncommon experience in
clinical practice is the patient who may or may not show a sensory
deficit at threshold, but gives responses at suprathreshold levels
of stimulation that indicate neural pathology. We must know more
about the normal suprathreshold functions if we are to diagnose
with precision the underlying pathology. Another practical aspect
of the research lies with the ever increasing attempts to utilize

the cutaneous surface as a surrogate channel of communication for
persons with severe sensory deficits, as in deafness and blindness.
Adequate communication demands that the signals be delivered at
suprathreshold levels of stimulation, so it becomes imperative that
we understand how the systems function at these levels. Now let us
proceed with the experiments.

In a recent series of auditory experiments Zwislocki and his
associates showed that two fundamentally different sensory processes, enhancement and summation, could be differentiated by psychophysical means (Zwislocki and Ketkar, 1972; Zwislocki, Ketkar,
Cannon, and Nodar, 1974; Zwislocki and Sokolich, 1974). These processes were later shown to be operative for vibrotactile stimuli
(Verrillo and Gescheider, 1975). We will be concerned here only
with the phenomenon known as enhancement.

The stimulus paradigm for these experiments is shown in Fig. 6.
A pair of short sinusoidal bursts of vibration are presented with
a variable time interval between the bursts. This is followed at
750 msec by a third (comparison) burst. The burst pair is carefully matched by the subject for subjective intensity at a sensation level of 24 dB. The subject is then asked to match the
subjective intensity of the third burst to that of the second,
first without the first burst to establish a base line for the
effect and then in the presence of the first burst as the test
match. Any difference between the control and the test matches
may be attributed to the effect of the first burst upon the subjective intensity of the second. Many auditory and vibrotactile

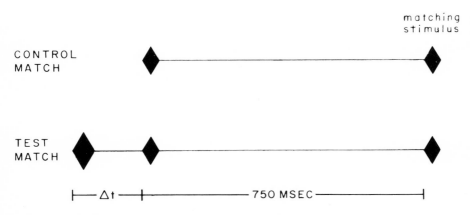

Fig. 6. Paradigm for measuring enhancement. The burst pair com-
         prises the first and second bursts in the test match.
         (Gescheider et al., 1977)

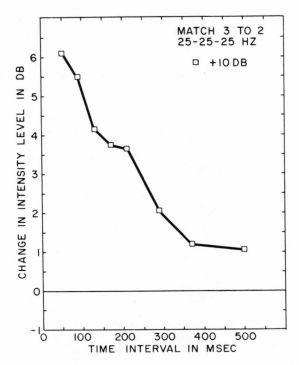

Fig. 7.   Enhancement effect within the non-Pacinian system.   Change
           in the intensity level of the third burst (enhancement)
           when matched to the second burst of a preceding pair as a
           function of the time interval between the first two bursts.
           The first burst was set at 10 dB above the intensity of
           the second burst.   (Modified from Verrillo and Gescheider,
           1975).

experiments have confirmed this statement.

        A series of experiments was conducted to investigate enhance-
ment effects within both the Pacinian and non-Pacinian systems and
to determine if interactions between the systems could be detected.
Figure 7 shows the results when all three bursts had a frequency
of 25 Hz, that is, all bursts were within the non-Pacinian system.
Note that the first burst is raised 10 dB above the second burst
after the subjective-intensity match was performed by the subject.
The increase in the intensity of the first burst was found to be
necessary in both auditory (Zwislocki and Sokolich, 1974) and
vibrotactile (Verrillo and Gescheider, 1975) experiments.   Enhancement effects are negligible when the initial pair of stimuli
are at the same intensity.   It is apparent from Fig. 7 that in the

low-frequency system there is a strong enhancement effect that
diminishes with the time interval between the first and second
burst until it is nil at about 500 msec. This means that the presence of the first burst increases the subjective intensity of the
second burst, the phenomenon that is called enhancement.

The experiment was repeated using 300 Hz stimuli for all three
bursts which means that the Pacinian system would be activated. The
results shown in Fig. 8 closely approximate those of the non-
Pacinian system shown in Fig. 7. We may conclude then that enhancement effects may be demonstrated within both the Pacinian and
non-Pacinian systems.

We must now ask the question, do the two systems interact at
the suprathreshold levels at which we are working? An experiment

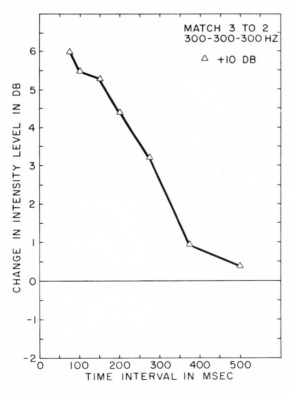

Fig. 8. Enhancement effect within the Pacinian system. Same as
          Fig. 7. (Modified from Verrillo and Gescheider, 1975)

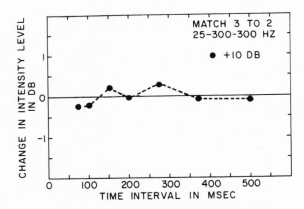

Fig. 9.   Enhancement effect reduces to nil when the first burst
          activates the non-Pacinian system (25 Hz) and the second
          the Pacinian system (300 Hz). The two systems do not
          appear to interact to produce an enhancement effect.
          (Modified from Verrillo and Gescheider, 1975)

was conducted using widely separated frequencies for the burst pair
so that the first stimulus was in the non-Pacinian system (25 Hz)
and the second was within the frequency range of the Pacinian system (300 Hz). The comparison burst was set at 300 Hz. The results (Fig. 9) show that the enhancement effect disappears when
the first and second stimuli activate the non-Pacinian and Pacinian
systems respectively. The two systems do not appear to interact
in a way that produces an enhancement effect. This result is consistent with auditory experiments in which a maximum enhancement
effect was found when the burst-pair frequencies were in the same
critical band; and, when the frequencies were in widely separated
critical bands, the enhancement effect disappeared (Zwislocki et
al., 1974; Zwislocki and Sokolich, 1974). The cutaneous mechanoreceptor systems appear to function in an analogous manner to auditory critical bands.

     Our final experiment in this series explored the frequency
effect in a more systematic fashion. Two experiments were performed. In the first the frequency of the first stimulus was
varied and the frequency of the second and third bursts activated
the Pacinian system (100 Hz). In the second, the first stimulus
again was varied and the frequency of the second and third bursts
activated the non-Pacinian system (25 Hz). The time interval between the first and second bursts was set at 150 msec. According
to the duplex model and armed with the results in Fig. 9, we predicted a maximum enhancement effect when the frequencies in the
first two bursts are confined to either the Pacinian or non-Pacinian

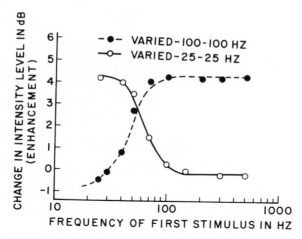

Fig. 10.   Change in the intensity level of the third burst when
matched to the second burst of the preceding pair as a
function of the frequency of the first burst. The frequency of the second and matching (third) bursts was
either 25 or 100 Hz. The curves are theoretical predictions. (Modified from Gescheider et al., 1977)

system and no effect when the frequencies are separated between
systems. The results shown in Fig. 10 confirm this prediction.
For a second stimulus of 100 Hz (Pacinian system), enhancement was
at a maximum when the frequency of the first stimulus was also within
the range of the Pacinian system. When the frequency of the first
stimulus was decreased below 70 Hz, the amount of enhancement
dropped off rapidly to nil at 25 Hz. The opposite effect was observed when the second stimulus was 25 Hz (non-Pacinian system).
In this case the amount of enhancement was maximal at low frequencies, and as the frequency of the first stimulus was increased
the amount of enhancement decreased sharply and was negligible
above 100 Hz.

The symbols in this figure represent data points from the two
experiments. The solid and dashed lines are theoretical predictions
based upon the duplex model of mechanoreception. The theoretical
predictions are derived from two items of information about each
system: (1) the effective intensity difference between the first
and second stimuli of the pair at each frequency, and (2) the relationship between enhancement and the intensity difference between
the pair when Δt was 150 msec. Effective intensity difference is
the effective intensity of the first burst minus the effective
intensity of the second. Effective intensity is defined as the

difference in decibels between the stimulus intensity and the threshold of the appropriate system. Figure 11 illustrates the calculation of these values at 40, 80, and 150 Hz for both systems.

In the non-Pacinian system (Fig. 11a) the intensity of the first stimulus above that of the system threshold (heavy line) is determined at each frequency. Examples are shown at 40 Hz = 21 dB;

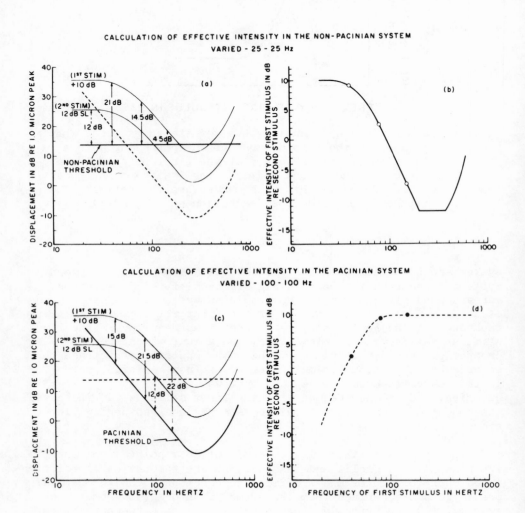

Fig. 11.   Calculation of effective intensity differences within the Pacinian and non-Pacinian systems from threshold curves of the duplex model. Illustrations are given at 40, 80, and 150 Hz for both systems. See text for explanation.

80 Hz = 14.5 dB; and 150 Hz = 4.5 dB. These values represent the effective intensity of the first stimulus within the non-Pacinian system. From these the effective intensity of the second stimulus (12 dB) at 25 Hz is subtracted. The differences are plotted as a function of frequency (Fig. 11b). When all frequencies are calculated, the resultant curve is the effective intensity difference between the first and second stimuli of the burst pair.

A similar procedure is followed for the Pacinian system (Fig. 11c) except that the effective intensities now represent the difference at each frequency between the intensity of the first stimuli and the Pacinian-system threshold (heavy curve). Examples are given at three frequencies: 40 Hz = 15 dB; 80 Hz = 21.5 dB; and 150 Hz = 22 dB. Substracting the effective intensity of the second stimulus (12 dB) yields the curve of effective intensity difference for the Pacinian system (Fig. 11d).

Having derived these curves, we may now proceed to predict the enhancement curves shown in Fig. 10. The procedure for making this prediction is illustrated in Fig. 12. The theoretical effective-intensity-difference curves from Fig. 11 are both presented in Fig. 12a and an illustrative example at 80 Hz (thin line with arrows) is given. A simple linear transposition is made (Fig. 12b) of the intensity axis in Fig. 12a to the abscissa of Fig. 12c. Figure 12c is an experimentally determined function relating enhancement and intensity difference between the burst pair obtained for a Δt of 150 msec. Thus, the effective intensity difference of 3.5 dB at 80 Hz in Fig. 12a is transposed through Fig. 12b to a value of 1.5 dB on the ordinate of Fig. 12c which is projected as a predicted value at 80 Hz in Fig. 12d. The predicted functions for enhancement in the Pacinian and non-Pacinian systems shown in Fig. 12d were generated by repeating this procedure for many frequencies. It is clear from the close approximation of data points and theoretical curves in Figs. 10 and 12d that the duplex model is sufficient to predict responses to suprathreshold stimulation.

One of the difficulties encountered in the measurement of enhancement effects is that at very short time intervals between the first two bursts the subject may be unable to resolve the separate stimuli. Because of the difficulty in separating the pair, the subject may match not to the subjective intensity of the second burst alone but rather to the sum of both the first and second bursts combined. In order to overcome this problem we did a series of experiments in which the first two stimuli were separated in space on the body surface (Verrillo and Gescheider, 1976). In one set of experiments the first stimulus of the burst pair was presented to the distal pad of the middle finger. The second member of the pair and the comparison burst were presented to the thenar eminence of the same hand. The experiment was repeated twice;

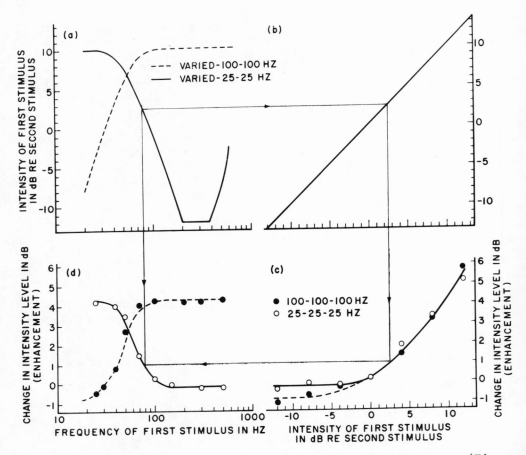

Fig. 12.   Transform from the effective intensity differences (Fig.
            11), based on the duplex model, to the predicted enhance-
            ment functions (Fig. 10).   An example at 80 Hz is shown.
            (Gescheider et al., 1977)

once using 300 Hz for all three bursts, and again using 25 Hz
throughout.   The results of both experiments are shown in Fig.
13 plotted as a function of the time interval between the members
of the burst pair.   As the time interval approaches zero there is
a marked suppression of the second stimulus by the first; that is,
the stimulus on the thenar became more difficult to perceive when
it was preceded by a stimulus delivered to the finger.   Note that
the second burst was impossible to perceive when the burst pair
was presented simultaneously.   However, at approximately 50 msec
the enhancement effect starts to dominate the response and reaches

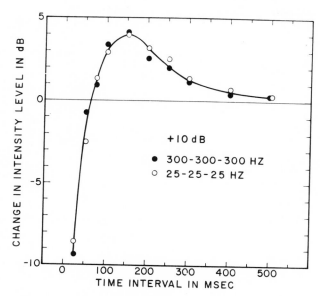

Fig. 13. Change in the intensity level of the third burst when matched to the subjective intensity of the second burst of a preceding pair (enhancement) as a function of the time interval between the bursts of a pair. The first burst was delivered to the distal pad of the middle finger; the second and third bursts to the thenar eminence, all on the right hand. The intensity level of the first burst was set at 10 dB above that of the second. Pacinian (300 Hz) and non-Pacinian (25 Hz) systems are compared. (Verrillo and Gescheider, 1976)

a maximum at about 150 msec where it begins a gradual decline. The results in both the Pacinian (300 Hz) and non-Pacinian (25 Hz) systems were so alike that a single curve could be drawn to represent both sets of data.

We next decided to repeat the experiment at two sites more widely separated on the body surface. We chose the ventral aspect of the right thigh for the first stimulus. The second and comparison stimuli were presented to the thenar eminence on the same side. The results may be seen in Fig. 14. Although there is a reduction in the suppression effect when compared to the finger-thenar condition (Fig. 13), a substantial degree of suppression is still evident at these two widely separated sites on the body. A striking difference is seen between the finger-thenar and thigh-thenar conditions when the time interval was increased. Beyond 60 msec the

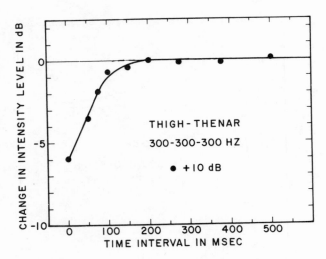

Fig. 14. Same as Fig. 13 except that the first burst was delivered
          to the ventral right thigh and the second and third
          bursts to the right thenar eminence. (Modified from
          Verrillo and Gescheider, 1976)

stimulus delivered to the thigh had no effect, neither suppression
nor enhancement, on the subjective intensity of the stimulus at the
thenar eminence.

As a resumé of the foregoing experiments, Fig. 15 shows a comparison of the results for identical site (thenar-thenar), closely
separated sites (finger-thenar), and widely separated sites (thigh-
thenar) of stimulation. The results support the hypothesis that
when the burst pair is delivered to the same site at short time intervals, fusion of stimuli may occur and the subject may be responding to the sum of the pair rather than to the second stimulus
alone. This can be seen in the continual increase of the enhancement effect at very short time intervals. However, when the possibility of fusion and confusion is reduced by the spatial separation
of the first two bursts, the enhancement effect is reduced or eliminated at short time intervals and another phenomenon, suppression,
dominates the response.

The preceding three figures (Figs. 13, 14, and 15) demonstrate
that suppression is a characteristic of both cutaneous mechanoreceptive systems. We decided next to examine possible interactions
between the systems using widely separated frequencies for the burst
pair (25 and 300 Hz). This procedure resulted in a substantial
reduction of suppression in both the finger-thenar and the thigh-

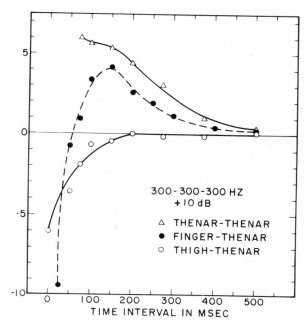

Fig. 15.   Results obtained when the burst pair was delivered to
different parts of the body compared to same site stimulation. (Verrillo and Gescheider, 1976).

thenar experiments and the complete elimination of the enhancement
effect (Fig. 16).

It may be concluded that both the Pacinian and non-Pacinian
systems exhibit the phenomenon of suppression when both components
of the stimulus configuration are presented within a single system.
The effect is severely reduced or eliminated, however, when both
systems are excited within a time span of approximately 100 msec.

GRADIENT EFFECTS

Because of its relatively large size and accessibility, the
Pacinian corpuscle has been the most thoroughly investigated of the
cutaneous receptor end organs. By comparison, our knowledge of the
non-Pacinian receptors is sparse. Lindblom (1965) first suggested
that in glabrous skin low-frequency sensation was probably mediated
by Meissner corpuscles. However, we suspect that the flat psychophysical curve is a composite of several functions that represent

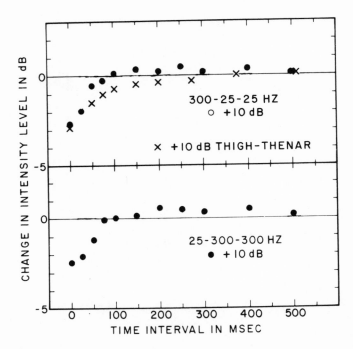

Fig. 16. Change in the intensity level of the third burst when
          matched to the subjective intensity of the second burst
          of the preceding pair, as a function of the time interval
          between the bursts of the pair. Frequencies were selected
          so that the members of the burst pair activated different
          mechanoreceptor systems. Thenar-thenar and thigh-thenar
          (upper graph) data are shown. (Modified from Verrillo
          and Gescheider, 1976)

more than a single end organ. We know that this system does not
summate energy over time or space, it does not respond differentially at threshold to differences in frequency, and the size of its
receptive field is relatively small (Johansson, 1976). What then
is its function? The following experiments may shed some light on
this question.

First, let us return to a study reported in 1962 (Verrillo,
1962). We have seen that when we increase contactor size and use a
rigid surround to prevent the spread of vibrations across the skin,
the low-frequency threshold response remains constant for all contactor areas. However, if we keep the size of the contactor constant (.113cm^2) and increase the size of the rigid surround, the

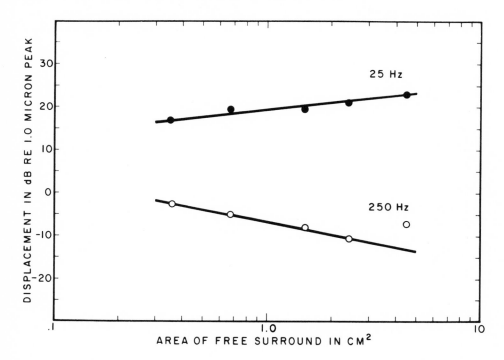

Fig. 17. Vibrotactile threshold for two frequencies as a function
of the area of the free surround measured with a contractor of constant size (.113 cm^2). (Modified from
Verrillo, 1962)

threshold at 25 Hz is no longer constant; it rises as the size of
the free surface of skin gets larger (Verrillo, 1962). This can be
seen in Fig. 17. Note that the 250-Hz thresholds decrease with
the area of the free surround. This is due to spatial summation
in the Pacinian system. The decreasing sensitivity in the low-
frequency system, however, had no explanation at the time.

Another curious effect was observed in 1963 (Verrillo, 1963)
when we used an annular contactor with a non-vibrating center which
produced a double gradient on the skin, one on either side of the
vibrating annulus. When compared to a contactor having the same
circumference but without a rigid center (single gradient), the
high frequencies produced higher thresholds, proportional to the
decrease in the overall area stimulated; but at low frequencies
(25 and 40 Hz) the threshold response improved by about 3.0 dB
(Fig. 18). Again, we had no ready explanation for this result.

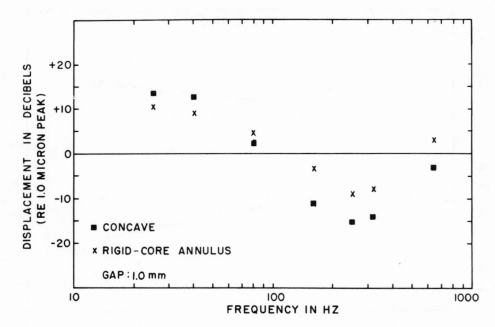

Fig. 18.   Comparison of threshold measurements made with a solid
           contactor and with a vibrating annulus having a rigid
           core and surround.   (Modified from Verrillo, 1963)

In a recent series of experiments we systematically tested the
effect of the rigid surround on thresholds and the effect appeared
again; larger gaps between the vibrating contactor and the rigid
surround resulted in greater sensitivity at higher frequencies
and a loss of sensitivity at low frequencies (Gescheider, Capraro,
Frisina, Hamer, and Verrillo, 1978). It was suggested by Gescheider
and his co-workers that the low-frequency system may be involved
in the detection of gradients or edges.

    Now, if we take a closer look at the old data (Verrillo, 1962,
Fig. 10; Verrillo, 1963, Fig. 5), several things become apparent.
When the 1962 data for 25 Hz are replotted as a function of the gap
between contactor and surround, instead of area, the resulting
slope is +3 dB/doubling of gap distance. That is, as the distance
of the surround, which produces a gradient, from the contactor
doubled, the sensitivity decreased by 3 dB. Since the 3 dB slope
appeared to be a function only of the distance of the edge of the
rigid surround from the contactor and because the non-Pacinian system does not summate over space, we reasoned that a single point

may be as effective an edge as an entire surround.

Several experiments were designed in which the configuration of the edge was varied and in which a single, small non-vibrating probe (.005 cm^2) was substituted in place of the entire surround. In the first experiment two disks (surrounds) were used, one in which the edge was a very abrupt right angle in cross section and another in which the edge was rounded into a soft curve thus producing a more gentle gradient. As a counterpart, small probes were substituted for the surround, one having a right-angled profile and another having a rounded tip. No surround was used when measurements were made with the probe. The distance between the edge of the contactor and the edge of the disk or probe was always 7.4 mm. The contactor size was .32 cm^2 for these and the following experiments.

The results are shown in Fig. 19 in which the height of the bars represents absolute threshold in decibels. The clear bars above the zero line are results using a 25 Hz stimulus and the hatched bars below the zero line are thresholds measured for a 250 Hz stimulus. Note that in the first set of bars those discontinuities having a sharp edge, whether it was a disk completely surrounding the contactor or a single probe, both yielded approximately the same threshold (within 1.0 dB). The diminished gradients produced by rounded edges, represented in the second set of bars, resulted in thresholds approximately 3.0 dB higher, but again there was little difference between the disk and the probe. The 250 Hz results show no difference between the sharp and rounded edges. The third column is the threshold without surround or probe. This condition produced the highest thresholds at 25 Hz (no gradient) and the lowest thresholds at 250 Hz (spatial summation).

The next experiment utilized a probe at half the distance between the edge of the contactor and the edge of the surround. The results are shown in the last (far right) set of bars in Fig. 19. The "NO PROBE" condition is identical to the "DISK" experiment shown at the far left and the thresholds were within 0.5 dB of each other. However, the inclusion of the probe resulted in a 3.0 dB improvement of threshold. The probe had little effect on the results at 250 Hz. The response at low frequencies then is dominated by the surface discontinuity that is nearest to the source of the vibration and the response at high frequencies by the area of the stimulated surface.

The final experiment included a replication of the study (Verrillo, 1962) in which thresholds were determined for a frequency of 25 Hz using disks of increasing diameter or gap distance. The experiment was then repeated substituting the single probe positioned at the same distances from the edge of the .32 cm^2

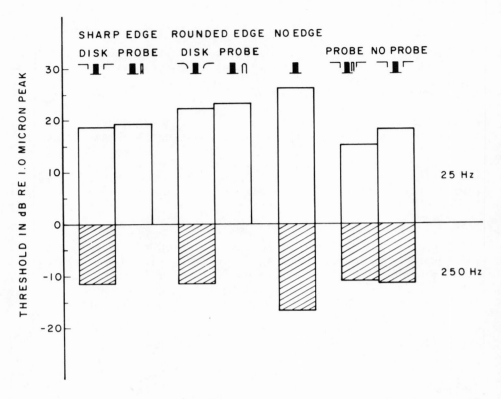

Fig. 19.   Vibrotactile thresholds measured at 25 and 250 Hz using
           a variety of "edge" conditions. Diagrams above each bar
           show the stimulus configuration for the threshold shown
           in the bars. See text for explanation of stimulus con-
           figurations.

contactor. No surround was used when the thresholds were measured
with the probe. The results of both experiments are shown in Fig.
20 along with the thresholds obtained by Verrillo in 1962 replotted
as a function of gap distance. At 25 Hz the threshold for detection
increases with a slope of 3 dB per doubling of the linear distance
of free skin between the edge of the contactor and a gradient on
the skin produced by a circular disk concentric to the contactor or
by a single point. Not shown in the figure are the results using a
frequency of 250 Hz which shows an increase of sensitivity as the
gap distance between contactor and surround increases. This effect
may be attributed to spatial summation since the increasing gap
distance also results in an increased area of stimulation.

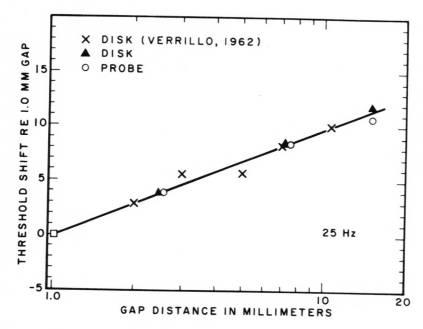

Fig. 20.   Threshold shift in decibels referred to the threshold
using a 1.0 mm gap plotted as a function of the distance
from the edge of the contactor to the edge of the rigid
surround or to a single, small probe on the skin.
Measurements were made at 25 Hz. The data for 25 Hz from
Fig. 17 are replotted for comparison.

        We interpret the results shown in Figs. 19 and 20 as strong
evidence that the non-Pacinian receptors function primarily as
detectors of gradients or edges. Reducing the gradient by presenting a less-distinct edge (sharp vs. rounded edge, Fig. 19) results in decreased sensitivity. Placing the edge at increasing
distances from the vibrating contactor also produces a decrease in
sensitivity (Fig. 20). When two edges are present on the skin, the
non-Pacinian response is determined by the closer edge (Fig. 19,
far right bars). In addition, it is apparent that any discontinuity,
regardless of its geometric configuration, may create an edge
sufficient to affect the response of the system. This is illustrated by the data which compares disks and single probes (Fig. 20).
On the other hand, the response of the Pacinian system is determined primarily by the total area of stimulation (Fig. 19, far
right bars).

The response of the non-Pacinian receptors appears to be influenced primarily by discontinuities of stimulation on the skin's
surface. The more distinct the discontinuity, the greater the
effect on the response of the system and consequently the lower the
psychophysical threshold. Because of these properties, it is
reasonable to expect that the non-Pacinian receptors are most likely
involved in the perception of spatial patterns on the surface of
the skin. We are in agreement with Lindblom (1965) who suggested
that non-Pacinian receptors are primarily responsible for spatial
discriminative sensibility. Our experiments may be regarded as
preliminary investigations of these effects.

ACKNOWLEDGMENTS

    This work was supported by Grant NS-09940 from the National
Institutes of Health, U.S. Department of Health, Education, and
Welfare.

REFERENCES

Gescheider, G. A. Evidence in support of the duplex theory of
    mechanoreception. Sensory Processes, 1976, 1, 68-76.
Gescheider, G. A., Caparo, A. J., Frisina, R. D., Hamer, R. D., &
    Verrillo, R. T. The effects of a surround on vibrotactile
    thresholds. Sensory Processes, 1978, 2, 99-115.
Gescheider, G. A., Verrillo, R. T., Capraro, A. J., & Hamer, R. D.
    Enhancement of vibrotactile sensation magnitude and predic-
    tions from the duplex model of mechanoreception. Sensory
    Processes, 1977, 1, 187-203.
Harrington, T. & Merzenich, M. M. Neural coding in the sense of
    touch. Experimental Brain Research, 1970, 10, 251-264.
Hunt, C. C. On the nature of vibration receptors in the hind limb
    of the cat. Journal of Physiology, (London), 1961, 155, 175-186.
Järvilehto, T., Hämäläinen, H., & Laurinen, P. Characteristics of
    single mechanoreceptive fibres innervating hairy skin of the
    human hand. Experimental Brain Research, 1976, 25, 45-61.
Johansson, R. Skin mechanoreceptors in the human hand: Receptive
    field characteristics. In Y. Zotterman (Ed.) Sensory functions
    of the skin in primates. (Vol. 27),New York: Pergamon, 1976.
Kenshalo, D. R. (Ed.) The skin senses. Springfield, Ill: Thomas,
    1968.
Knibestöl, M. Stimulus-response functions of rapidly adapting
    mechanoreceptors in the human glabrous skin area. Journal of
    Physiology, (London), 1973, 232, 427-452.
Knibestöl, M. & Vallbo, Å. B. Single unit analysis of mechano-
    receptor activity from the human glabrous skin. Acta Phy-
    siologica Scandinavica, 1970, 80, 178-195.

Konietzny, R. & Hensel, H. Response of rapidly and slowly adapting mechanoreceptors and vibratory sensitivity in human hairy skin. Pflügers Archiv, 1977, 368, 39-44.

Lindblom, U. Properties of touch receptors in distal glabrous skin of the monkey. Journal of Neurophysiology, 1965, 28, 966-985.

Loewenstein, W. R. Generator processes of repetitive activity in a Pacinian corpuscle. Journal of General Physiology, 1958, 41, 825-845.

Merzenich, M. M. & Harrington, T. The sense of flutter-vibration evoked by stimulation of the hairy skin of primates: Comparison of human sensory capacity with the responses of mechanoreceptive afferents innervating the hairy skin of monkeys. Experimental Brain Research, 1969, 9, 236-260.

Mountcastle, V. B., LaMotte, R. H., & Carli, G. Detection thresholds for stimuli in humans and monkeys: Comparison with threshold events in mechanoreceptive afferent nerve fibers innervating the monkey hand. Journal of Neurophysiology, 1972, 35, 122-136.

Sato, M. Response of Pacinian corpuscles to sinusoidal vibration. Journal of Physiology, (London), 1961, 159, 391-409.

Scott, D. Response of Pacinian corpuscles to oscillatory stimulation. Federation Proceedings, 1951, 10, 123.

Talbot, W. H., Darian-Smith, I., Kornhuber, H. H., & Mountcastle, V. B. The sense of flutter-vibration: Comparison of the human capacity with response patterns of mechanoreceptive afferents in the monkey hand. Journal of Neurophysiology, 1968, 31, 301-334.

Vallbo, Å. B. & Hagbarth, K.-E. Activity from skin mechanoreceptors recorded percutaneously in awake human subjects. Experimental Neurology, 1968, 21, 270-289.

Verrillo, R. T. Investigation of some parameters of the cutaneous threshold for vibration. Journal of the Acoustical Society of America, 1962, 34, 1768-1773.

Verrillo, R. T. The effects of a surround on vibrotactile threshold. Journal of the Acoustical Society of America, 1963, 35, 1962-1966.

Verrillo, R. T. Vibrotactile sensitivity and the frequency response of Pacinian corpuscles. Psychonomic Science, 1966, 4. 135-136 (a).

Verrillo, R. T. Specificity of a cutaneous receptor. Perception and Psychophysics, 1966, 1, 149-153 (b).

Verrillo, R. T. A duplex mechanism of mechanoreception. In D. R. Kenshalo (Ed.), The skin senses. Springfield, Ill.: Thomas, 1968.

Verrillo, R. T. & Gescheider, G. A. Enhancement and summation in the perception of two successive vibrotactile stimuli. Perception and Psychophysics, 1975, 18, 128-136.

Verrillo, R. T. & Gescheider, G. A. Effect of double ipsilateral
    stimulation on vibrotactile sensation magnitude. Sensory Pro-
    cesses, 1976, 1, 127-137.
Zwislocki, J. J. Theory of temporal summation. Journal of the
    Acoustical Society of America, 1960, 32, 1046-1060.
Zwislocki, J. J. & Ketkar, I. Loudness enhancement and summation
    in pairs of short sound bursts. Journal of the Acoustical
    Society of America, 1972, 51, 140(A).
Zwislocki, J. J., Ketkar, I., Cannon, M. W., & Nodar, R. H. Loud-
    ness enhancement and summation in pairs of short sound bursts.
    Perception and Psychophysics, 1974, 16, 91-100.
Zwislocki, J. J. & Sokolich, W. G. On loudness enhancement of a
    tone burst by a preceding tone burst. Perception and Psycho-
    physics, 1974, 16, 87-90.

DISCUSSION

DR. JOHANSSON: Your suppression experiments are very interesting. You delivered the first stimulus ("Masker") to the finger tip and tested the effect on the thenar. Have you done the reverse?

DR. VERRILLO: No, we have not.

DR. JOHANSSON: If you will remember the communication I had yesterday on the innervation densities, it may be interesting to see if the distal part of the fingers, so to speak, dominate the palm.

DR. VERRILLO: We did just finger-thenar and then thigh-thenar comparisons.

DR. GESCHEIDER: The stimuli were matched on the subjective amplitude, so maybe, in a sense, that takes care of it.

DR. VERRILLO: There would not be a difference in the subjective amplitude of the two places, because they are matched before we started. We present the two stimuli and the subject has to match them up so they are within one dB of each other before we start the experiment. However, that does not invalidate your question; it is a good one and we should do it.

DR. STARR: This reminds me of the clinical test that Maurice Bender devised for testing cortical function. This is the face-hand test in clinical neurology in which two places on the body are touched simultaneously. Most normal people will extinguish the more distal spot. People with lesions, most likely in the parietal cortex, will consistently, after many, many trials, still extinguish. I'm struck by this finger-thenar and thigh-thenar as being that kind of model.

DR. VERRILLO: In the clinical situation, the distal stimulus is extinguished, and here it is the proximal one that is extinguished, so they must have lesions in a different place.

DR. STARR: But, you see, you are able to control the timing of the situation very carefully. We can not do that clinically.

DR. LINDBLOM: You also have in clinical situations sometimes, as with parietal lobe lesions, a sensory extinction over one side. Have you made any bilateral experiments?

DR. VERRILLO: No, we have not done contralateral experiments. That is on the agenda.

DR. KIRMAN: I wonder if it follows from this that if you stimulated the skin with a high frequency stimulator of some kind with sharp contours, you would get poor spatial resolution. Is that a prediction?

DR. VERRILLO: I would get poor spatial resolution at high frequencies, because the Pacinian corpuscles are all over the place and they are very, very sensitive; you get spatial summation, but the spatial resolution is, I think, in the non-Pacinian system.

DR. KIRMAN: What about the Optacon research that uses 230 Hz?

DR. VERRILLO: They did that for greater sensitivity, incidentally, they do not have to make the bimorphs move very far.

DR. KIRMAN: But would you predict that they would get better spatial resolution if they lowered the frequency to, say, 20 Hz.

DR. VERRILLO: It is a possibility, I think it should be tried.

DR. LINDBLOM: I think it is an important point that you use sine wave stimulation. If you used short pulses that would be different in this context.

DR. HENSEL: Have you any idea about the physical events that occur in your setup? If you have a probe and a surrounding gap, and so on, I think there might be rather complicated physical events with wave reflection and standing waves and interferences. Have you ever tried to figure this out?

DR. VERRILLO: Yes, that will be our next series of experiments. The wave length of a 25 Hz stimulus is approximately 7.2 cm on the skin, which is long. We are using 1.5 cm as our largest gap. It appears then, that there is probably a standing wave.

DR. FRANZÉN: With regard to what you said about the Optacon system, I think they tried it out in Bliss's laboratory and found that 250 Hz was, indeed, the best frequency although this contradicts what we know. It could equally well be that the system that has a good spatial resolution is, sort of, kicked on.

DR. LINDBLOM: I never understood why the high frequency of the Optacon system gave such good spatial resolution. Perhaps it has to do with the curves Dr. Verrillo has shown when he started his paper. The small contactor activated the non-Pacinian system. It is a question of lowering the mechanical impedance of the system so that the stimulus gets down to the Pacinians. If you have a small contactor and indent the skin you may at first stimulate the intercutaneous receptors and the mechanical impedance will remain relatively high and prevent the stimulus from getting down to the Pacinian corpuscles. That would answer the question of why you get such a flat curve and why you get such good spatial resolution with the Optacon system.

DR. VERRILLO: That would apply to the Optacon system because it has a very low mechanical impedance source. The mechanical impedance of our vibrator is very high, so the impedance of the skin does not affect our response, in any way.

DR. LINDBLOM: Do you use a preindentation also?

DR. VERRILLO: I am not sure how to answer that, except to note that it is static. The impedance of our vibrator is high and we can get a maximum displacement of about 1.2 cm with it. I am convinced that the impedance of the skin is not a factor in the results that we got. With respect to the Optacon system, they are using very light piezoelectric crystal type vibrators and if you start shaking them much more than what they are designed for they will break.

VIBROTACTILE FREQUENCY CHARACTERISTICS AS DETERMINED BY ADAPTATION AND MASKING PROCEDURES

George A. Gescheider, Department of Psychology,
Hamilton College, Clinton, New York 13323

Ronald T. Verrillo, Institute of Sensory Research
Syracuse University, Syracuse, New York 13210

It is a well established fact that when all the smallest contactors are used to stimulate glabrous or hairy skin the vibrotactile threshold is a U-shaped function of frequency with the lowest values at approximately 250-300 Hz (Békésy, 1939; Gescheider, 1976; Gilmer, 1935; Hugony, 1935; Sherrick, 1953; Verrillo, 1962, 1963, 1966a). In some of these studies there was a tendency for the psychophysical threshold curve to become flat at low frequencies. The sharpest discontinuities in the threshold function were first reported by Verrillo (1963). When vibration was applied to the thenar eminence of the hand for 1.0 sec through contactors that were 2.9 cm^2 or larger, the function was flat out to 40 Hz whereupon threshold began to decrease at a rate of 12 dB/octave until maximum sensitivity was reached at approximately 250 Hz.

Examples of threshold functions for two subjects are seen in Fig. 1. The stimulus was applied to the thenar eminence in 1.0-sec bursts through a .75 cm^2 contactor. The vibratory stimulus was confined to the area of the contactor through the use of a rigid surround consisting of a heavy plate with a hole through which the contactor of the vibrator was positioned to make contact with the surface of the skin. The gap between the contactor and the surround was 1.0 mm. Vibration amplitude expressed in decibels re: 1.0 µm peak displacement of the contactor was measured with a calibrated accelerometer mounted on the moving element of the vibrator. The two subjects produced similar results with thresholds below about 50 Hz being independent of frequency and thresholds above 50 Hz being a U-shaped function of frequency.

183

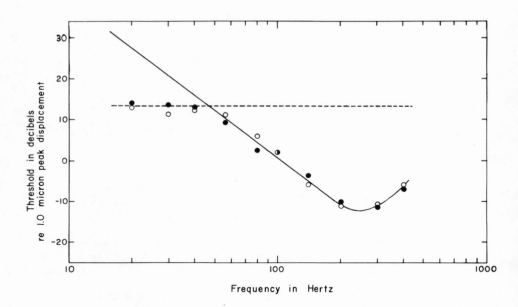

Fig. 1. Vibrotactile thresholds as a function of frequency. For
         each of the two subjects the data points represent the
         average of three measurements. The horizontal line and
         the U-shaped curve represent hypothesized neural thres-
         holds of the non-Pacinian and Pacinian systems respectively.

The horizontal dashed line and the solid U-shaped curve were
fitted to the data of Fig. 1 to suggest the operation of two independent sensory systems which mediate the detection of vibration.
Each function represents the hypothetical neural threshold for the
system, and according to this notion the psychophysical threshold
at a particular frequency should be determined by the system with
the lower threshold. It can be seen in Fig. 1, however, that although psychophysical thresholds may be determined by one neural
system, stimuli above the psychophysical threshold, if made sufficiently intense, can excite both systems. This model of vibrotactile sensitivity was originally presented with supporting data
in 1963 by Verrillo although originally Békésy (1939), based on
his observation of bisegmented threshold function, had suggested
that two processes may be involved in detecting vibrotactile
stimuli.

The duplex theory of vibrotactile sensitivity has been supported by electrophysiological data obtained by recording from
cutaneous nerve fibers. Verrillo (1966b), in comparing his

psychophysical threshold data with the electrophysiological tuning curves of Sato (1961) for single Pacinian corpuscles in cat, proposed that this receptor was the neural element mediating the U-shaped portion of the psychophysical threshold function. The cutaneous receptors mediating the detection of low-frequency vibration have not been positively identified, although it has been suggested that, in glabrous skin, Meissner corpuscles are involved (Lindblom, 1965). Lindblom (1966) and Lindblom and Lund (1966) recorded discharges from two types of sensory fibers in monkey foot and Mountcastle and his associates (e.g., Mountcastle, LaMotte and Carli, 1972; Talbot, Darian-Smith, Kornhuber and Mountcastle, 1968) have shown strong correlations between electrophysiological tuning curves of two populations of mechanoreceptors in monkey and the two segments of the psychophysical threshold function.

The relatively flat frequency characteristic of the non-Pacinian system and the U-shaped characteristic of the Pacinian system frequently have been inferred from results obtained by a variety of psychophysical procedures, but in most cases the evidence is indirect. For example, it has been found that the flat segment of the threshold curve is extended to higher frequencies by reducing contactor size (Gescheider, 1976; Gescheider, Capraro, Frisina, Hamer and Verrillo, 1978; Verrillo, 1963) or stimulus duration (Gescheider, Verrillo, Capraro and Hamer, 1977). It has been assumed that these results are due to the elevation of thresholds for small or short duration stimuli of the spatially and temporally summating Pacinian system coupled with an insensitivity of the non-Pacinian system to changes in contractor size or stimulus duration. The results are consistent with a duplex model in which one system, the non-Pacinian, is not capable of spatial or temporal summation and the Pacinian system is. However, they do not constitute independent psychophysical evidence for the tuning characteristics of the two systems. The tuning characteristics of the two systems along with their energy summation properties were hypothesized to account for the data.

Support for the proposed tuning characteristics of the two systems has come from studies in which correlations have been observed between psychophysical thresholds and differences in the anatomy of the receptors thought to mediate stimulus detection. Verrillo (1966c) found psychophysical thresholds for vibration of the dorsal surface of the tongue to be independent of frequency. Since there are no Pacinian corpuscles on the dorsal surface of the tongue, it was proposed that the frequency response of the non-Pacinian receptors in this tissue was flat. The U-shaped threshold function, characteristic of Pacinian corpuscles, however, was found when psychophysical thresholds were measured for the ventral surface of the tongue where Pacinian-like receptors (Golgi-Mazzoni corpuscles) are found. In addition, thresholds on glabrous skin

in which both Pacinian and non-Pacinian receptors are found are
correlated with anatomical changes that occur in these receptors
with age. Thresholds along the U-shaped segment of the psychophysical function tend to increase with the age of subjects, whereas at lower frequencies the flat segment of the function is not influenced by age (Frisina and Gescheider, 1977; Verrillo, 1977a;
Verrillo, 1977b). Cauna (1965), by examining skin samples from
over 200 individuals ranging in age from birth to 93 years, demonstrated that throughout life lamellae are added to Pacinian corpuscles, and consequently they become larger and distorted in
shape. The lamellae surrounding the nerve fiber are built up like
the layers of an onion and are separated by viscous fluid. The
lamellated corpuscle surrounding the nerve fiber has been found to
modify the mechanical stimulus but not to contribute to the neural
excitatory process directly (Lowenstein and Rathkamp, 1958).
According to Mendelson and Lowenstein (1964), the corpuscle acts
as a high-pass mechanical filter attenuating steady or slowly
changing displacements but permitting stimulation of the nerve by
rapid changes. The psychophysical finding that it is only the U-
shaped segment of the threshold function which becomes elevated
with age is consistent with the hypothesis that this U-shaped segment is mediated by Pacinian corpuscles which, with age, increase
in their capacity to attentuate the mechanical stimulus.

     An illustration of the duplex model of vibrotactile sensitivity
as it applies to the experimental findings discussed thus far is
seen in Fig. 2. The horizontal dashed line represents the threshold function of the non-Pacinian system, a system that does not
change in sensitivity as the stimulus size, stimulus duration, or
age of the subjects changes. On the other hand, the U-shaped
functions, representing the thresholds of the Pacinian system, are
raised or lowered as the size or duration of the stimulus or the
age of the subjects is changed.

     The argument presented thus far for a flat tuning character-
istic of the non-Pacinian system and a U-shaped characteristic for
the Pacinian system is based on three experimental findings. (a)
The effects of contactor size and stimulus duration, because they
were specific to the U-shaped segment of the threshold curve, imply
that only the Pacinian system is capable of spatial and temporal
summation and that the tuning characteristic of this system is U-
shaped whereas it is flat for the non-Pacinian system. (b) The
tuning curves of quickly adapting fibers innervating the monkey's
hand are either U-shaped and correspond closely in shape to the
high-frequency segment of the psychophysical threshold function or
are relatively flat and correspond to the low-frequency segment of
the threshold functions. (c) Flat psychophysical functions are
obtained when the stimulus is applied to tissue containing no
Pacinian corpuscles, and changes in the anatomy of Pacinian

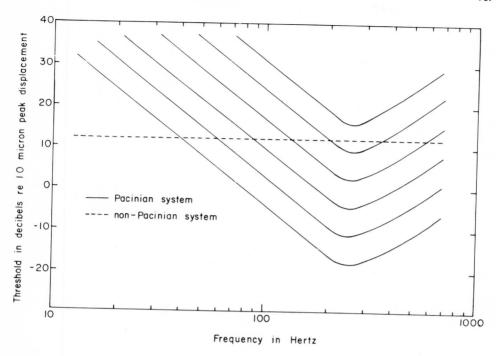

Fig. 2.   Illustration of the duplex model of mechanoreception. The
non-Pacinian system, being frequency independent and in-
capable of spatial or temporal summation, has a fixed
threshold as the frequency, area, and duration of the
stimulus are varied. The sensitivity of this system does
not change with age. The threshold of the Pacinian system is a U-shaped function of frequency which, because of
spatial and temporal summation, can be lowered or raised
depending on stimulus area and duration. The sensitivity
of this system decreases with age. (Gescheider, Capraro,
Frisina, Hamer, and Verrillo, 1978).

corpuscles with age are correlated with changes in psychophysical
thresholds along the U-shaped segment of the threshold curve.

    Although these findings constitute a strong case in support
of the hypothesized tuning characteristics of the two vibrotactile
systems, additional direct psychophysical measurement of these
characteristics would be desirable. To this end we have employed
two procedures, each of which was designed to isolate one system
so that its tuning curve could be measured over a wide range of

frequencies. In one procedure selective adaptation was used to
elevate the threshold of the other could be measured over a wider
range of frequencies. In the other procedure psychophysical tuning
curves analagous to those measured in audition were determined by
measuring the intensities of masking stimuli of variable frequency
needed to mask a weak test stimulus.

SELECTIVE ADAPTATION

Experiments were conducted to measure the tuning characteristics of one system over a wide frequency range by elevating the
threshold of the other system through selective adaptation. Thresholds on the thenar eminence were measured before and after 10 min
of exposure of either a 10 Hz or 250 Hz adapting stimulus. Stimuli
were delivered through a 2.9 cm^2 (10 Hz adapting stimulus) or a
3.0 cm^2 (250 Hz adapting stimulus contactor). A concentric rigid
surround with a 1.0 mm gap prevented surface waves from radiating
beyond the immediate vicinity of the contactor. The duration of
the test stimulus was 1.0 sec, and its rise-decay time was adjusted
to 100 msec to prevent transients. Thresholds were determined by
the Békésy tracking method, and measurements of vibration amplitude
were made by using a calibrated accelerometer mounted on the moving
element of the vibrator. All measurements were expressed in decibels re: 1.0 μm peak displacement of the contactor. The subject
and vibratory apparatus were located in a sound-proofed booth and
the subject wore earphones that delivered band-limited random
noise to mask the sound of the vibrator.

Figure 3 shows the psychophysical threshold as a function of
frequency before and after the presentation of 10 Hz adapting
stimuli of various intensities. The solid symbols are measurements made before adaptation and the open symbols represent thes-
holds measured during 30 sec following the adaptation period. All
data points are the median values of four subjects. In agreement
with earlier studies (e.g. Gescheider, 1976; Verrillo, 1963) the
unadapted threshold function obtained with a 2.9 cm^2 contactor has
two distinct segments. Thresholds do not change with changes in
frequency below 40 Hz, but above 40 Hz thresholds decrease at a
rate of 12 dB/octave. Thresholds measured after adaptation form a
family of curves that also imply the existence of two distinct
system for the detection of vibrotactile stimuli. Each curve has
a flat branch, the level of which increases as the intensity of
the adapting stimulus was increased from 6 to 20 dB SL. Thresholds
along these segments of the curves were presumably mediated by the
neural activity of non-Pacinian receptors, which was affected in
varying amounts depending on the intensity of the adapting stimulus.
Each curve also has a branch which decreases at a rate of 12 dB/
octave. Pancinian corpuscles are thought to determine detection
thresholds along this branch of the curve. When the adapting
stimulus was 30 dB SL, only the Pacinian portion of the curve was

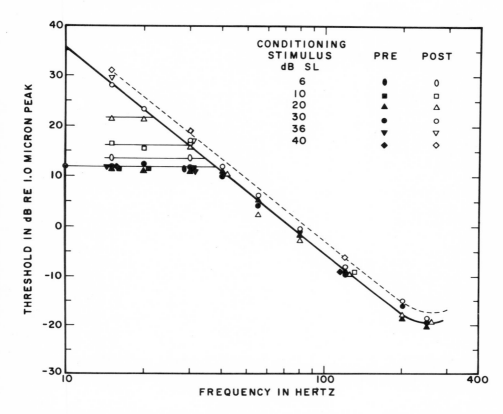

Fig. 3.   Vibrotactile thresholds as a function of frequency. Closed
          symbols represent thresholds obtained prior to adaptation.
          Open symbols represent thresholds measured for a 30 sec
          period following stimulation for 10 min by a 10 Hz adapting
          stimulus. The adapting stimulus was delivered at intensity
          levels ranging from 6 to 40 dB above threshold (Verrillo
          and Gescheider, 1977).

present. It can be seen that the 10 Hz adapting stimulus had no
systematic effect on the sloping portion of the curve for adapting
levels of up to 30 dB SL.

     It appears that by selective adaptation of the non-Pacinian
system it is possible to elevate its threshold sufficiently so that
the threshold of the Pacinian system can be measured over a range
of 15 to 250 Hz. Thus, we were able to determine by psychophysical
measurement that the Pacinian threshold function has a constant
slope on the order of -12 dB/octave down to 15 Hz. This finding

agrees with physiological measurements of neural thresholds in
the Pacinian system (e.g., Talbot et al., 1968).

When the 10 Hz adapting stimulus was raised to a sensation
level of 40 dB, the threshold of the Pacinian as well as the non-
Pacinian system was substantially exceeded and there was evidence
of adaptation in both systems. This effect is shown in Fig. 3 by
the dashed line connecting the open diamonds at 15, 30, and 120
Hz. It can be seen that the effect is a parallel shift of thresholds with respect to the unadapted Pacinian threshold curve.
The fact that thresholds along this U-shaped curve were uniformly elevated is evidence that a single system mediated all
thresholds along the curve. On the other hand, if the U-shaped
portion of the curve was mediated by more than one system, we
would expect a greater threshold shift at frequencies close to
that of the 10 Hz adapting stimulus than at higher frequencies.

A second adaptation experiment was conducted to see whether
or not the Pacinian segment of the threshold function could be
elevated by the application of a 250 Hz adapting stimulus. Thresholds were measured before and after the 10 min application of a
250 Hz adapting stimulus at an intensity approximately 35 dB above
the threshold of the Pacinian system and approximately at the
threshold of the non-Pacinian system (15 dB re: 1.0 μm peak).
Under these conditions the Pacinian thresholds should be substantially elevated so that a greater portion of the non-Pacinian
segment of the threshold curve would be exposed.

The threshold measurements obtained before and after adaptation are seen in Fig. 4. The data for individual subjects were in
close agreement, and therefore median data for four subjects are
presented. Before adaptation, the threshold function was nearly
flat between 15 and 40 Hz and decreased at a rate of 12 dB/octave
between 40 and 200 Hz. Adaptation had the effect of uniformly
raising the sloping portion of the curve by about 10 dB and, as a
consequence, the flat portion was extended to about 70 Hz. It
appears that adaptation raised the threshold of the Pacinian system
but did not affect the sensitivity of the non-Pacinian system.

The selective-adaptation procedure, although highly successful
in isolating the tuning characteristics of the Pacinian system, was
only partially successful when applied to the problem of examining
the tuning characteristics of the non-Pacinian system. Under no
conditions were we able to observe the flat, low-frequency branch
of the threshold curve beyond about 70 or 80 Hz. Subsequent
studies have shown that 250 Hz adapting stimulus, when increased
in intensity above the 35 dB SL level used in this study, produced
adaptation along both branches of the threshold curve and consequently the flat segment still extends only to about 70 Hz.

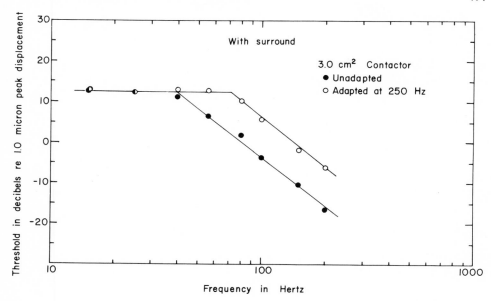

Fig. 4.   Vibrotactile thresholds before and after adaptation by a
250 Hz stimulus applied for 10 min at an intensity level
of approximately 35 dB above threshold (Gescheider,
Capraro, Frisina, Hamer, and Verrillo, 1978).

In order to obtain a clearer picture of the tuning characteristic of the non-Pacinian system and to confirm the results obtained
with selective adaptation, a series of experiments was conducted
using a masking procedure analogous to that used in audition to
obtain psychoacoustic tuning curves.

In audition an electrophysiological tuning curve consists of
a graph in which sound pressure necessary to bring the response of
a neuron to a constant level is plotted against stimulus frequency
(e.g., Kiang, 1965).   In the psychoacoustic analog a tuning curve
is a plot of the intensity of masking tones of varied frequency
needed to mask a weak test tone of constant frequency (e.g.,
Zwicker, 1974).   Because psychophysical tuning curves often correspond closely in form to tuning curves for single neurons, they have
become very useful in the analysis of tuning characteristics of the
human auditory system.   The successful use of this procedure in
audition prompted an attempt to measure vibrotactile tuning curves
by the same method (Labs, 1978).   It was reasoned that when the
frequency and intensity of a vibrotactile test stimulus is adjusted
to excite only one of the two sensory systems, then the intensity

of masking stimuli of varied frequency needed to mask this test
stimulus could constitute the tuning characteristic of the system.

SIMULTANEOUS MASKING

   In the first experiment a simultaneous masking procedure was
employed in which the masking stimulus was on continuously and a
200 msec test stimulus was presented every 2700 msec. The subject's task was to regulate the intensity of the masking stimulus
so that it barely masked a test stimulus that was fixed in frequency and fixed in intensity at 10 dB above his unmasked absolute
threshold. The subject used a modified Békésy tracking procedure
to continuously track the level of the masking stimulus necessary
to mask the test stimulus. Within each session a tuning curve was
obtained by employing this procedure for a wide range of masker
frequencies with a single test stimulus. This procedure was repeated three times for each test stimulus frequency with each of
five subjects.

   Sinusoidal electrical signals for the masking and test stimuli
were generated by two separate function generators and after amplification and timing were mixed before the input to the vibrator.
The size of the contactor was 0.75 cm^2 and a rigid surround was
used to restrict vibration of the skin to the immediate area of the
contactor. The subject was located in a sound-proofed booth that
isolated him from extraneous sound and vibration. Narrow-band
noise centered around the frequency of the vibrotactile stimuli was
presented through earphones to mask the sound of the vibrator.

   A modified Békésy tracking procedure, XN-N tracking, developed
by Gescheider, Herman, and Phillips (1970) was used because of its

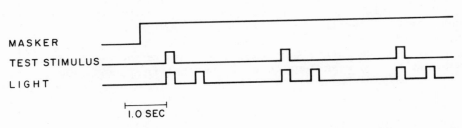

Fig. 5. Timing relationships in the simultaneous masking procedure
         of masking stimulus and observation interval light (Labs,
         Gescheider, Fay, and Lyons, submitted for publication).

freedom from possible contaminating influences of the subject's decision criterion. During the tracking period the subject was presented with pairs of 200 msec observation intervals indicated by a light emitting diode. The first observation contained the test stimulus plus the masker and the second contained only the masker. The observation intervals were separated by 500 msec and the pair was presented every 2700 msec (Fig. 5). The subject was instructed to allow the intensity of the masker to increase until the vibratory sensations in the two observation intervals felt the same, at which time he should push a hand switch which allowed the intensity of the masker to decrease until he could first feel different sensations in the two observation intervals. Using this decision rule the subject tracked continuously for a 1 to 2 min period at the end of which the intensity of the masker corresponding to the average value on the recording attenuator was measured.

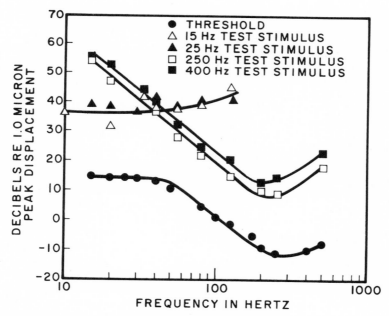

Fig. 6. Absolute thresholds and masking functions measured with the simultaneous masking procedure for test stimulus frequencies of 15, 25, 250, and 400 Hz. Data points are the median results from five subjects (Labs, Gescheider, Fay, and Lyons, submitted for publication).

The results for individual subjects were in close agreement and therefore an absolute threshold curve and psychophysical tuning curves were constructed from the medians of the five subjects (Fig. 6). The characteristic bisegmented absolute threshold curve was obtained in this experiment and the break point appears to be at about 50 Hz.

The masking procedure was highly successful in psychophysically isolating the frequency response characteristics of the Pacinian system. The tuning curves for test stimulus frequencies of 250 Hz and 400 Hz both exhibited the characteristic U shape of the Pacinian system, and the slope of the function was approximately -12 dB/octave between 15 and 250 Hz. These data are in close agreement with the psychophysical functions of the Pacinian system obtained by selective adaptation (Fig. 3) and with electrophysiological data obtained from single afferent fibers innervating Pacinian corpuscles (e.g., Mountcastle et al., 1972; Sato, 1961; Talbot et al., 1968).

The masking procedure was only partially successful in isolating the frequency response characteristics of the non-Pacinian system. Although the curves for the 15 Hz and 25 Hz test stimuli were relatively flat between 10 and 80 Hz, beyond 80 Hz the function began to increase at a rate so rapid that measurements of the masking stimulus were often impossible at frequencies above 125 Hz.

Subsequent experiments have shown that the relative difficulty of masking a low frequency test stimulus with a simultaneously presented high frequency masker is due to a facilitation of the detectability of the test stimulus by the masker. The absolute thresholds for a 15 Hz test stimulus were lower by 10 to 15 dB when this stimulus was presented simultaneously was an intense (30 to 45 dB SL) 250 Hz stimulus than when it was presented alone. One possible explanation for this result is that a weak 15 Hz test stimulus, when simultaneously presented with an intense 250 Hz stimulus, produces a detectable disruption of the synchronous neural firing set up by high intensity 250 Hz vibration. If this is the case, the simultaneous masking procedure is inadequate for measuring the high frequency end of the non-Pacinian tuning curve. Since the disruptive effects of the test stimulus on the neural response to the masker can occur only when the two stimuli are simultaneously presented, it was thought that this problem could be eliminated by using a forward masking procedure in which the masker and test stimulus are separated in time.

FORWARD MASKING

A forward masking procedure was employed to determine masking functions for test stimulus frequencies of 15, 65, and 250 Hz.

The temporal sequence of stimuli is illustrated in Fig. 7. The
masking stimulus was 500 msec in duration, and 25 msec after its
termination a 10 dB SL test stimulus was presented during a 200
msec observation interval. The observation interval was presented
to the subject by the light emitting diode. After 650 msec a
second masking stimulus was presented, followed 25 msec later by a
second observation interval containing no test stimulus. This sequence was repeated every 2700 msec as the subject tracked the intensity of the masking stimulus necessary to mask the test stimulus.
Subjects were instructed to use the XN-N tracking procedure as in
the simultaneous masking experiment.

Absolute thresholds and psychophysical tuning curves for 15 Hz
and 250 Hz test stimuli are seen in Fig. 8. Three sets of measurements were made on each subject for each condition, and the data
points in Fig. 8 represent medians for three subjects. The masking
function for the 250 Hz test stimulus was U-shaped with a slope of
approximately -11 dB/octave between 20 and 250 Hz indicating
Pacinian mediation for the detection of the test stimulus. Furthermore, this slope is nearly identical to that of the threshold
function between 60 and 250 Hz. Thus, the frequency response
characteristics of the Pacinian system are in close agreement when
determined by absolute threshold after selective adaptation, simultaneous masking, forward masking and physiological recordings.

The masking function for the 15 Hz test stimulus was flat between 20 and 400 Hz and slightly elevated at 10 Hz. This nearly
flat function is in remarkable agreement with the flat frequency
characteristic postulated for the non-Pacinian system in the duplex
model (Fig. 2) and closely resembles the flat threshold functions
obtained with small contactors on glabrous (Gescheider, 1976;
Verrillo, 1963) or hairy skin (Verrillo, 1966a), or when the dorsal

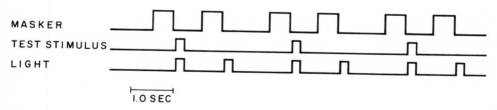

Fig. 7. Timing relationships in the forward masking procedure of
        masking stimulul, test stimulus, and observation interval
        light (Labs, Gescheider, Fay, and Lyons, submitted for
        publication).

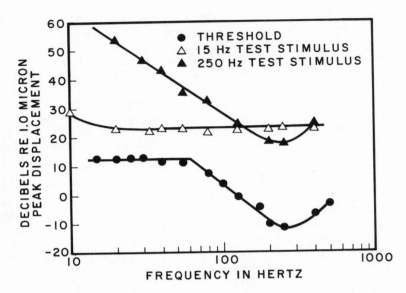

Fig. 8.   Absolute thresholds and masking functions measured with
the forward masking procedure for test stimulus frequencies of 15 and 250 Hz.   Data points are the median results
of three subjects (Labs, Gescheider, Fay, and Lyons,
submitted for publication).

surface of the tongue is vibrated (Verrillo, 1966c).

It appears that the masking function obtained when the test
stimulus excites only one system reflects the tuning characteristics
of that system. The effect on the masking function of exciting
both systems with the test stimulus was studied by using a 65 Hz
test stimulus at 10 dB above absolute threshold. It can be seen
from the threshold function of Fig. 8 that this stimulus should
activate both systems equally. According to the duplex model, the
masking function for this test stimulus should be a composite of
the masking functions for the 15 Hz and 250 Hz test stimuli. The
masking function for the 65 Hz test stimulus should not be a tuning
curve for any sensory system because the test stimulus does not
serve to isolate a single system by activating it exclusively.
Nevertheless, this function is predictable from the two masking
functions in which the systems were isolated. The results in Fig.
9 show that the data obtained for the 65 Hz test stimulus could be
accounted for with reasonable accuracy by the tuning curves measured
for 15 Hz and 250 Hz test stimuli. The 15 Hz and 250 Hz tuning
curves of Fig. 8 are redrawn in Fig. 9. The solid line portion of

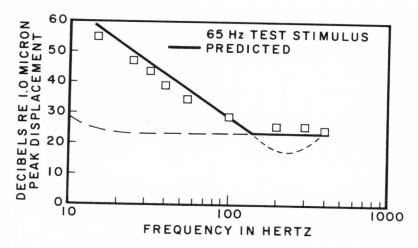

Fig. 9.   Masking function measured with the forward masking pro-
          cedure for a 65 Hz test stimulus. Data points are the
          median results of three subjects. The curves fitted to
          the data in Fig. 8 for 15 Hz and 250 Hz test stimuli are
          reproduced in this figure. The solid function, a com-
          bination of segments of the 15 Hz and 250 Hz masking
          functions, is the predicted composite of masking function
          for the 65 Hz test stimulus (Labs, Gescheider, Fay, and
          Lyons, submitted for publication).

the two tuning curves is the predicted masking function for the 65
Hz test stimulus. This predicted function defines the intensity of
the masking stimulus at a particular frequency needed to mask the
neural activity of both receptor systems and consequently mask
detection of the test stimulus. Notice that at low frequencies
the masking stimulus will first mask the non-Pacinian system and
with further increases of intensity eventually the Pacinian system
will also be masked. The reverse is true for a high frequency
masking stimulus. In this case the Pacinian system is masked
first, followed by masking of the non-Pacinian system as masker
intensity is increased. The confirmation of the predicted masking
function for the 65 Hz test stimulus where two systems are excited
argues strongly for the validity of the tuning curves obtained
when the test stimuli excited only one system.

     It is notable that the psychophysical tuning curve for the
non-Pacinian system is not in exact agreement with physiologically
measured tuning curves for non-Pacinian, rapidly adapting fibers
that innervate the monkey hand (Talbot et al., 1968). These fibers

were found to be tuned at about 30 Hz and for lower or higher frequencies the threshold increased at a rate of 4 or 5 dB/octave.
The nearly flat psychophysical tuning curve of our study resembles
more the flat threshold functions obtained psychophysically with
small contactors or the threshold function obtained on the dorsal
surface of the tongue where there are no Pacinian receptors. The
difference between the psychophysical and physiological results
may depend on the use of the rigid surround to confine the stimulus
to the area of the contactor. In the physiological studies, rigid
surrounds were not used. Consistent with this hypothesis is the
fact that the low frequency branch of the absolute threshold
function is not flat but instead has a slope of approximately 4 or
5 dB/octave when a surround is not used (Gescheider, Capraro,
Frisina, Hamer and Verrillo, 1978; Mountcastle et al., 1972;
Talbot, et al., 1968).

To test the hypothesis that the non-Pacinian system becomes
tuned when a surround is not used, an experiment was conducted in

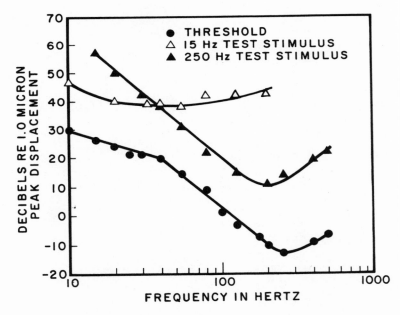

Fig. 10.   Absolute thresholds and masking functions measured with
           with the forward masking procedure for test stimulus fre-
           quencies of 15 and 250 Hz. No rigid surround was used.
           Data points are the median results of three subjects (Labs,
           Gescheider, Fay, and Lyons, submitted for publication).

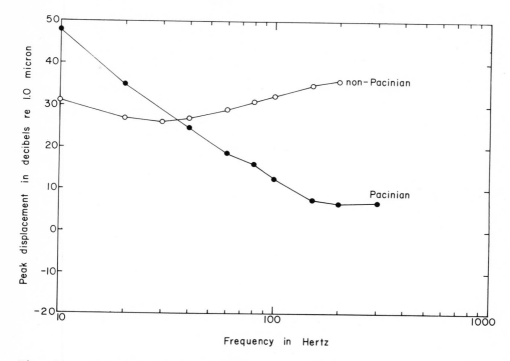

Fig. 11.   Average entrainment thresholds for Pacinian and rapidly
           adapting afferents innervating glabrous skin of the mon-
           key hand (Talbot et al., 1968). These curves are essen-
           tially identical to the results of Mountcastle et al.
           (1972) except for sensitivity level. Data averaging was
           done by Russell Hamer.

which psychophysical tuning curves were measured without the use of
a rigid surround. Masking functions were obtained for 15 Hz and
250 Hz test stimuli. Three subjects participated in this experiment and the medians of their data are seen in Fig. 10. As in
earlier studies the absolute threshold function without rigid
surround had two branches each with a non-zero slope. The slopes
of the low and high frequency branches were approximately 5 dB/
octave and 13 dB/octave, respectively. The masking function for
the 250 Hz test stimulus had the characteristic form of the
Pacinian system. Thus, removal of the surround does not appear to
have any obvious effects on the form of the tuning curve for the
non-Pacinian system. The tuning curve for the 15 Hz stimulus
appears to be slightly more tuned when the surround is not used
than when it is used as in the previous experiment. Unfortunately,
because of distortion problems with the vibrator at high inten-

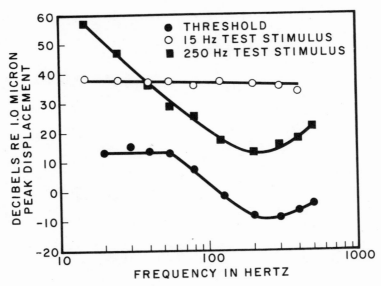

Fig. 12. Absolute thresholds and masking functions measured when the masking stimulus was on the index fingertip and the test stimulus was on the thenar eminence of the same hand. Test stimuli were either 15 or 250 Hz. Data points represent the average results of two subjects (based on data from Labs, Gescheider, Fay, and Lyons, submitted for publication).

sities and high frequencies, data for the psychophysical tuning curve could not be obtained above 200 Hz. In spite of this limitation it seems safe to conclude that there is reasonably close agreement between the forms of physiological and psychophysical tuning curves for the non-Pacinian system when they are obtained under somewhat comparable stimulus conditions. Physiological tuning curves plotted as the medians of several single fiber recordings taken from Talbot et al. (1968) are presented in Fig. 11 for comparison with the psychophysical of Fig. 10.

The final experiment was concerned with the problem of masking functions obtained when the test stimulus and the masking stimulus were applied at different sites. It was thought that the results might have implications for the neural locus of the masking process upon which psychophysical tuning curves are based. In this experiment the test stimulus was applied to the thenar eminance and the masking stimulus was applied to the index fingertip. The contactors on both locations were 0.75 cm^2 and rigid surrounds were used. A 500 msec masking stimulus was presented to the index fingertip, and 150 msec after its onset a 200 msec test stimulus was presented to the thenar eminence. A second masking stimulus was presented alone 650 msec after the termination of the first masking stimulus (SN-N tracking).

The average results for two subjects are seen in Fig. 12. It appears that the shapes of the 15 Hz and 250 Hz tuning curves were very much the same under the conditions of this experiment as when the two stimuli were presented to the same skin area successively in the forward masking procedure. The results of this experiment suggest that the masking process that underlies the measurement of psychophysical tuning curves is not exclusively at the receptor level. The close correspondence of receptor and psychophysical tuning curves, however, indicates that the frequency response characteristics of both the non-Pacinian and Pacinian systems are probably determined primarily at the receptor level.

ACKNOWLEDGEMENTS

    This work was supported in part by Grant NS 09940 from the National Institutes of Health, U. S. Department of Health, Education, and Welfare (Syracuse University); and by faculty research funds from Hamilton College.

REFERENCES

Békésy, G. von. Über die Vibrationsempfindung. Akustische Zeitschrift, 1939, 4, 316-334.
Cauna, N. The effects of aging on the receptor organs of the human dermis. In W. Montagna (Ed.), Advances in biology of skin (Vol.6), Aging. New York: Pergamon, 1965.
Frisina, R. D., & Gescheider, G. A. Comparison of child and adult vibrotactile thresholds as a function of frequency and duration. Perception and Psychophysics, 1977, 22, 100-103.
Gescheider, G. A. Evidence in support of the duplex theory of mechanoreception. Sensory Processes, 1976, 1, 68-76.
Gescheider, G. A., Capraro, A. J., Frisina, R. D., Hamer, R. D., & Verrillo, R. T. A comparison of vibrotactile thresholds measured with and without rigit surround. Sensory Processes, 1978, 2, 99-115.
Gescheider, G. A., Herman, D. D., & Phillips, J. N. Criterion shifts in the measurement of tactile masking. Perception and Psychophysics, 1970, 8, 433-436.
Gescheider, G. A., Verrillo, R. T., Capraro, A. J., & Hamer, R. D. Enhancement of vibrotactile sensation magnitude and predictions from the duplex model of mechanoreception. Sensory Processes, 1977, 1, 187-203.

Gilmer, B. von H. The measurement of the sensitivity of the skin
    to mechanical vibration. Journal of General Psychology, 1935,
    13, 36-61.
Hugony, A. Uber die Empfindung von Schwingungen mittels des Tast-
    sinner. Zeitschrift für Biologie, 1935, 96, 548-553.
Kiang, N. Y. S. Discharge patterns of single fibers in the cat's
    auditory nerve. Cambridge, Mass.: M.I.T. Press, 1965.
Labs, S. M. Psychophysical tuning curves in vibrotaction. Un-
    published Masters Thesis, Loyola University of Chicago, 1978.
Labs, S. M., Gescheider, G. A., Fay, R. R., & Lyons, C. Psycho-
    physical tuning curves in vibrotaction. (submitted for publica-
    tion).
Lindblom, U. Properties of touch receptors in distal glabrous skin
    of the monkey. Journal of Neurophysiology, 1965, 28, 966-985.
Lindblom, U. The relationship of skin displacement of receptor
    activation. In A.V.S. deReuck & J. Knight (Eds.), Touch,
    heat, and pain. Boston: Little, Brown, 1966.
Lindblom, U., & Lund, L. The discharge from vibration-sensitive
    receptors in the monkey foot. Experimental Neurology, 1966,
    15, 401-417.
Lowenstein, W. R., & Rathkamp, R. The sites for mechanoelectric
    conversion in a Pacinian corpuscle. Journal of General Physio-
    logy, 1958, 41, 1245-1265.
Mendelson, M., & Lowenstein, W. R. Mechanisms of receptor adapta-
    tion. Science, 1964, 144, 554-555.
Mountcastle, V. B., LaMotte, R. H., & Carli, G. Detection thresh-
    olds for stimuli in humans and in monkeys: Comparison with
    threshold events in mechanoreceptive afferent fibers innerva-
    ting the monkey hand. Journal of Neurophysiology, 1972, 35,
    122-136.
Sato, M. Response of Pacinian corpuscles to sinusoidal vibration.
    Journal of Physiology (London), 1961, 159, 391-409.
Sherrick, C. E. Variables affecting sensitivity of the human skin
    to mechanical vibration. Journal of Experimental Psychology,
    1953, 45, 273-282.
Talbot, W. H., Darian-Smith, I., Kornhuber, H. H., & Mountcastle,
    V. B. The sense of flutter-vibration: Comparison of the
    human capacity with response patterns of mechanoreceptive af-
    ferents from the monkey hand. Journal of Neurophysiology,
    1968, 31, 301-334.
Verrillo, R. T. Investigation of some parameters of the cutaneous
    threshold for vibration. Journal of the Acoustical Society
    of America, 1962, 34, 1768-1773.
Verrillo, R. T. Effect of contactor area on the vibrotactile
    threshold. Journal of the Acoustical Society of America, 1963,
    35, 1962-1966.
Verrillo, R. T. Effect of spatial parameters in the vibrotactile
    threshold. Journal of Experimental Psychology, 1966a, 71,
    570-575.

Verrillo, R. T.   Vibrotactile sensitivity and the frequency re-
    sponse of Pacinian corpuscles. Psychonomic Science, 1966b,
    4, 135-136.
Verrillo, R. T.   Specificity in a cutaneous receptor. Perception
    and Psychophysics, 1966c, 1, 149-153.
Verrillo, R. T.   Comparison of child and adult vibrotactile thres-
    holds. Psychonomic Bulletin, 1977a, 9, 197-200.
Verrillo, R. T.   Effects of age on vibrotactile thresholds and on
    receptor morphology. Paper presented at the 18th annual
    meeting of the Psychonomic Society, Washington, D. C., 1977b.
Verrillo, R. T., & Gescheider, G. A.   Effect of prior stimulation
    on vibrotactile thresholds. Sensory Processes, 1977, 1,
    191-300.
Zwicker, E.   On a psychoacoustical equivalent of tuning curves.
    In E. Zwicker & E. Terhardt (Eds.), Facts and models in hearing.
    New York: Springer, 1974.

DISCUSSION

DR. CRAIG: A student, Mark Yama, in my laboratory is doing some work with adaptation, and has a result somewhat consistent with this model. He is using a high frequency adaptor and measuring spatial summation with a high frequency stimulus by varying the size of the test contactor, and at preadaptation for high frequencies, as you and Ron (Verrillo) have shown, you get nice spatial summation. Postadaptation, you raise the threshold and knock out spatial summation; that is- the curves look very flat at high frequencies as you change contactor area after adaptation. The results are consistent with your notion of the two receptor systems.

DR. DREYER: Have you put your masking stimulus any farther away from the test site than almost adjacent?

DR. GESCHEIDER: The farthest distance is fingertip to thenar. We have not varied that distance yet; however, one interesting thing we observed in comparing the level of the tuning curves for the two systems is that there appears to be virtually no significant difference between the level of the tuning curve if we used the high frequencies when we test the Pacinian system. That might be expected due to the summating properties of that system. In the case of the low frequency system, however, when we used the 15 Hz test stimulus, it takes a much greater masking stimulus and the tuning curve is elevated perhaps 10, 15, or even 20 dB, if you move the masking stimulus out to the finger tip. But experiments that systematically vary that distance between the two stimuli are for the future.

DR. HENSEL: Your model fits quite nicely into some results Konietzny and I have found with direct comparison of the tuning curves of rapidly adapting mechanoreceptors in hairy skin of the human hand, and the vibration threshold. It looks almost the same. I will not go into details now, because I will be showing some of the results this afternoon.

DR. JOHANSSON: I would like to comment on the interpretation of the aging effect on your curves. You thought it was some sort of aging of the Pacinian corpuscles, and you referred to Cauna. In fact, both the Pacinian and Meissner corpuscles change quite dramatically and quite similarly; they grow bigger and more lobulated with age (Cauna, 1965). If you assume that the non-Pacinian system are the Meissner, you cannot say that the Pacinian system is more dramatically changed with age than the non-Pacinian system. I have an alternative interpretation. Another thing that happens with age is that the number of myelinated fibers decrease about 0.5 to 1 percent per year after the age of 20 (eg. Gardner, 1940). That implies that the density decreases with age, and, as the Pacinian system seems to be a spatial summation system, when you have a lower density than the threshold curve, it will be elevated. But the Meissner system is not a spatial summation system and would remain.

DR. GESCHEIDER: That is an interesting interpretation, and we have actually thought of that also. It may be a combination of structural changes as well as the reduced number of fibers. I am not sure about the filtering characteristics of the Meissner system, and it seems that there is more known about the filtering characteristics of the Pacinian system and how important the lamellae are for the filtering. That is what made us feel that increasing the number of lamellae of Pacinian corpuscles would have a very significant effect on the sensitivity of that receptor. I am just not sure about the Meissner, but that may also be true for them.

DR. VERRILLO: It is a good question, and I think you answered part of your own question by saying that the Meissners do decrease in number and there is not as dramatic a structural change according to Cauna (1965). More recent work (Andres & During, 1973) shows a different structure for the Meissner than that depicted by Cauna. But in the Pacinian corpuscle change in the number of lamellae, and possibly in the thickness and the mass of these lamellae, with age. That fits the notion of changing the filter characteristics of the Pacinian corpuscle with age. It may fit these data; I do not know yet whether that particular formulation is going to work out. However, it is the first hunch that we had, by which you might be able to predict the psychophysical results as a function of age. If we can use the Lowenstein and Skalak (1966) model, slightly modified, of a bandpass filter and adding elements to that filter could possibly produce the kind of age effects that we found psychophysically.

REFERENCES

Andres, K. H. & Düring, M. von. Morphology of cutaneous receptors. In A. Iggo (Ed.), Handbook of sensory physiology, (Vol. 2): Somatosensory system. Berlin: Springer-Verlag, 1973.

Cauna, N. The effects of aging on the receptor organs of the human dermis. In W. Montagna (Ed.), Advances in biology of skin, (Vol. 6): Aging. New York: Pergamon, 1965.

Gardner, E. Decrease in neurons with age. Anatomical Record, 1940, 77, 529-536.

Loewenstein, W. R. & Skalak, R. Mechanical transmission in a Pacinian corpuscle. Journal of Physiology (London), 1966, 182, 346-378.

THERMO-TACTILE INTERACTIONS: SOME INFLUENCES OF TEMPERATURE ON TOUCH

Joseph C. Stevens

John B. Pierce Foundation Laboratory and Yale University

New Haven, Connecticut 06519

Although psychophysical interactions and confusions among the dermal sense-modalities and their adequate stimuli have cropped up from time to time over the last century, they have tended, in my opinion, to receive less attention and follow-up research than they deserve. Sometimes the various modalities appear to behave with remarkable independence from one another, as for example when the skin is mapped for punctiform sensibility by needles, horse-hairs, and tiny thermal contactors. These hardly mimic the stimuli of everyday life, however, nor has the physiological meaning of the dermal "spot" maps ever come under agreement by students of the senses. In any case, since the time of von Frey the study of a given dermal sense has tended to proceed as if the others never existed, and stimulation has often tended to be unrealistically microscopic and monodimensional.

Various sensory interactions have come under renewed study recently in the Pierce Foundation Laboratory. These studies have antecedents that trace back as far as the mid-nineteenth century, but the old data prove generally too scarce to be more than suggestive. This paper deals with the influence of temperature on three aspects of touch: (a) punctate sensitivity; (b) vibrotactile sensitivity, and (c) magnitude of sensation.

Punctate Touch Sensitivity

Tactile sensitivity to punctate (hair) stimulation of the finger-tip came under study in five subjects at eight skin temperatures between $10°$ and $43°C$. During a given threshold measurement, skin temperature was held constant by means of a combination of convective cooling and warming with a heat lamp, whose output was

controlled by a thermostat on the skin, near the site of stimulation.

Figure 1 is a plot of the threshold pressures, showing that
punctate sensitivity is remarkably independent of skin temperature
between 25° and 43°C. A slight loss of sensitivity may occur at
temperatures of 40° and higher. A loss in sensitivity also occurs
when the skin is lower than about 20°C. This sensory loss in the
cold also shows up in tactile acuity, as measured by a person's
capacity to resolve a gap between two edges (Mackworth, 1953; Mills,
1956; Morton and Provins, 1960; Provins and Morton, 1960). Such
loss may be the result of receptor or nerve cold block. Cold block
alone fails, however, to explain the temperature related losses
that characterize vibrotactile sensitivity, the subject to which
we now turn.

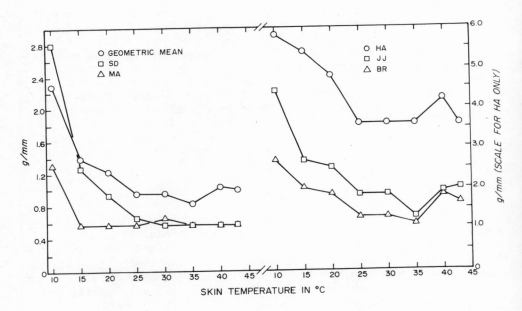

Fig. 1.   Pressure thresholds to punctate sensitivity as a function
           of skin temperature for five subjects and their average
           (geometric means). The threshold is expressed as force/
           radius in grams per millimeter. N.B.: The right-hand
           ordinate applies to the data of subject HA only.
           (Stevens, Green, and Krimsley, 1977)

Vibrotactile Sensitivity

This study, which grew out of pioneer work of Weitz (1941), was undertaken by Green (1977) to explore how sensitivity might depend on skin temperature and on several frequencies of vibration. Two subjects were tested extensively with a tiny vibrator at the hairless region between the base of the thumb and the index finger, the hand and arm being immersed in a temperature-controlled bath.

Figure 2 shows how threshold amplitude varied with skin temperature (20° to 42°C) at two representative frequencies--30 Hz (relatively low) and 250 Hz (relatively high). As Weitz had earlier found, sensitivity at high frequencies depends strongly on temperature. Interestingly, sensitivity peaks at about 36°C, considerably warmer than the normal temperature of the region stimulated, and on either side of 36°C sensitivity falls off steadily. In contrast, observe that the threshold amplitude for low frequency stimulation turned out to be remarkably independent of skin temperature between 20° and 40°C.

A parsimonious explanation of the difference between low and high frequency behavior lies in the duplex mechanoreceptor hypothesis of Verrillo (1968), which posits, on the basis of a large variety of psychophysical data, a high-frequency receptor system (probably the Pacinian corpuscles), which we might presume to be temperature-sensitive, and a low frequency receptor system, which we might presume to be relatively temperature-insensitive. Electrophysiological studies (Inman and Peruzzi, 1961; Ishiko and Lowenstein, 1961) do show that the behavior of Pacinian corpuscles is temperature-sensitive, but the threshold curve in Fig. 2 may turn out to take its exact shape from an interplay of neural, mechanical, and/or vasomotor factors.

Magnitude of Touch Sensation

It is in the realm of touch magnitude that the influence of temperature reveals itself most curiously (Stevens and Green, 1978). The first observation appears to be that of the great German physiologist Weber in 1846. Weber noted that a cold Thaler (a coin slightly smaller than a U.S. dollar) resting on the forehead feels heavier than two warm Thaler stacked one on the other. Weber conjectured that cold might intensify touch magnitude and warm inhibit it. This view was correctly refuted by Szabadföldi (1865), who claimed that both warm and cold intensify touch sensation. After that, only sporadic interest seemed to attach to the subject until 1962, when Jones, Singer, and Twelker (1962) attacked the problem with fresh methodology and came out with data that seemed to refute both Weber and Szabadföldi, i.e., no statistically significant effect of either warming or cooling on touch magnitude.

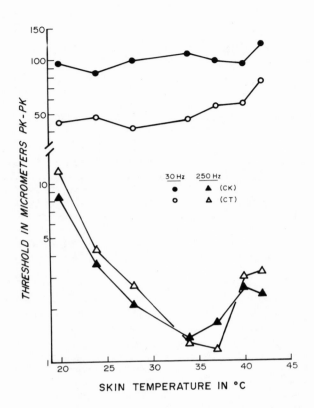

Fig. 2.   Vibratory thresholds of two subjects to low (30 Hz) and
          high (250 Hz) frequencies as functions of skin temperature.
          The threshold amplitude is measured in micrometers, peak
          to peak.   (Green, 1977)

This negative outcome probably reflects the use of a tiny stimulus
contactor: 0.4 cm^2. With stimuli that small we, too, failed to
produce reliable effects. But with large contactors the intensification effect of cooling on touch is profound and unmistakable. Warming appears to have little or no effect on the forehead but on the
forearm has a clearly demonstrable effect (though less dramatic than
cooling).

     Our experiments have typically called upon subjects (15 to 20
per experiment) to make magnitude estimations of the heaviness of
aluminum weights or the apparent force with which an aluminum contactor was pressed onto the skin, as measured by a tension gauge.
The various contactors were heated or cooled in regulated water

baths. The weights or blocks were quickly dried and applied to the skin for about 3 sec at a time. The subjects were told to estimate only the perceived heaviness or force, to ignore temperature, and to avoid any conjectures about what effect temperature might have on perceived heaviness. Cold, neutral (i.e., close to the skin temperature), and warm stimuli were systematically alternated so as to avoid serious drift in the skin temperature from normal. Experience has taught us this need and has prompted us to plan future research to assess more exactly how temperature adaptation of the skin might disrupt or facilitate interaction.

Figure 3 shows the geometric means of apparent heaviness of various weights placed on the forehead. The warm weights (45°C) received almost exactly the same average estimates as the neutral ones (33°C), but the cold objects received much higher estimates, at extremely high levels of statistical confidence. In the light of Fig. 3, Weber's contention that a single cold <u>Thaler</u> felt heavier than two warm ones is hardly an exaggeration; for in Fig. 3, 5 gm cold approximately matches 20 gm warm or neutral.

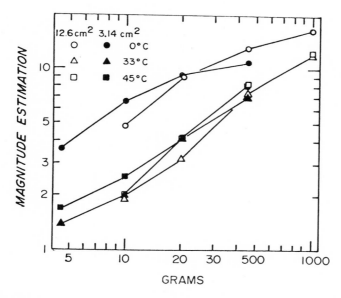

Fig. 3. Magnitude estimation of apparent heaviness of cold, warm, and neutral weights placed on the forehead. Each point stands for a geometric mean of 40 estimates from 20 subjects.

It should be pointed out that 0°C and 45°C were selected for this study because they produce warmth and cold sensations of roughly equal magnitude (Stevens and Stevens, 1960). Hence the interaction cannot readily be explained by supposing that a subject consciously or unconsciously sums a thermal sensation with a touch sensation! It should also be pointed out that area of contact made little difference in this experiment (3.14 vs 12.6 cm^2); area does matter, however, when it gets small enough. Finally, it may be noted that the influence of cooling tends to diminish, percentage-wise, with increasing weight, as shown by the slight convergence of the functions in Fig. 3.

Figure 4 shows the results of a very similar experiment on the volar forearm. Again area (3.14, 12.6, 29 cm^2) turned out to have relatively minor importance, cold stimuli received impressively higher estimates of heaviness than neutral ones, and warm ones also received higher estimates than neutral ones, generally at highly

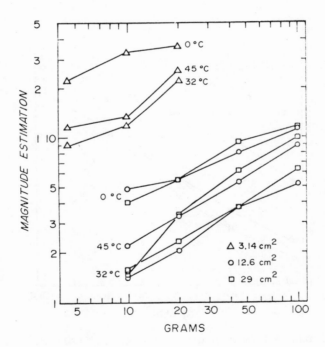

Fig. 4. Magnitude estimation of apparent heaviness of cold, warm, and neutral weights placed on the forearm. Each point stands for the geometric mean of 40 estimates from 20 subjects.

reliable levels of statistical confidence. The influence of warm, though less striking than cold, can be large: e.g., the 50 gm warm stimuli approximately matched the 100 gm neutral stimuli for apparent heaviness. The striking difference between forehead and forearm with regards to warmth and touch interaction poses an interesting physiological puzzle, and suggests a possible neurological difference between those two skin regions. These are the only two body regions that we have so far had time to investigate.

Figure 5 shows an experiment conducted under my direction by Daniel Schwartzman. Here the estimates of perceived force are plotted as a function of temperature, with force in gm, as measured on the tension gauge, as the parameter. Note that the interactions tend to increase systematically as temperature departs more and more from neutral and also that the apparent interactions tend to fade as the force of application increases more and more.

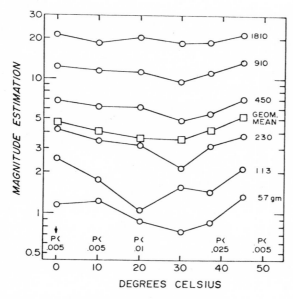

Fig. 5. Magnitude estimation of perceived force of 36 different combinations of temperature and force of application on the forearm. Each circle stands for the geometric mean of 30 estimates from 15 subjects. The squares show the grand geometric mean across force levels.

Finally, Fig. 6 shows the outcome of an experiment, conducted under my direction by Sandra Onofrio and Ellen Sorman, to compare the effects of two stimuli of radically different size: 29 cm^2 vs 0.4 cm^2. The large stimuli produced statistically significant cool and warm intensification, but the small stimuli failed to reveal any interaction, perhaps because the small stimuli arouse too small a population of receptors or too few types of receptors to produce a stable enough response.

What can be said concerning the neurological locus of the thermal intensification of touch magnitude? The simplest conjecture places the interaction in the periphery, where mechanoreceptive afferents may fire "non-adequately" to cooling and warming. Numerous studies have revealed many mechanoreceptors that show enhanced spontaneous firing rates on cooling (Darian-Smith, Johnson, and Dykes, 1973; Douglas, Richie, and Straub, 1960; Hensel, 1966; Hensel and Zotterman, 1951; Hunt and McIntyre, 1960; Iggo, 1960; Knibestöl and Vallbo, 1970; Poulos and Lende, 1970; Tapper, 1965). Thus concomitant cooling during mechanical stimulation could be perceived as intensified touch sensation. Warm intensification may elude such simple explanation, however, because moderate

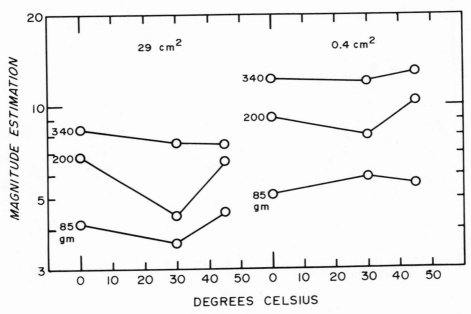

Fig. 6. A comparison of magnitude estimations of perceived force of small and large stimuli at various temperature and force levels. Each point stands for the geometric mean of 30 estimates from 15 subjects. Data are for forearm.

warming usually leaves mechanoreceptors unaffected (Bessou and
Perl, 1969; Burton, Terashima, and Clark, 1972; Hensel and Zotterman, 1951) or may even inhibit them (Chambers, Andres, Duering,
and Iggo, 1972; Iggo, 1969; Rowe and Sessle, 1972). Kenton, Crue,
and Carregal (1975) did, however, observe some mechanoreceptive
fibers whose response to mechanical stimulation rose with concomitant warming between 34° and 43°C. Another possible explanation
of warm intensification might be the recruitment of polymodal nociceptors, which respond rather unselectively to multiple forms of
energy. The relative concentration of these C-fibers could con-
ceivably explain the difference between the forehead and forearm.
C-fibers in humans have been reported more often in hairy than in
glabrous skin (Torebjörk, 1974); it is therefore possible that the
relatively hairy forearm may have more C-fibers than the forehead.

It can be instructive and challenging to seek parallels between psychophysical and neurophysiological data. Certainly the
psychophysicist should have been much earlier prompted by neurological studies, dating back over a quarter of a century, to search
for and find the prominent interactions that appear at the conscious
level. The search for parallels can also be stymied by the failure
to stimulate multidimensionally. By this I mean, for example, that
an experimenter may be content simply to demonstrate that a given
neuron will fire to more than one form of energy, when what might
really help would be to measure its dynamic response as joint
functions of, say, temperature and skin indentation. Among other
things, such parametric assessment permits the investigator to
stipulate how temperature and degree of mechanical stimulation can
be traded one for the other to preserve any given amount of neural
activity from weak to strong.

After nearly a century of differentiating the dermal sense-
modalities, the time may have come to take more seriously their
interrelations and interactions. The ones I have described here
are fairly simple and probably reflect relatively straightforward
peripheral effects such as nerve block, vasomotor activity, and
imperfect receptor selectivity. We stand, though a longer way from
resolving a far more profound and mysterious interaction: how do
the spatiotemporal patterns of dermal neural activity together with
subdermal and proprioceptive signals combine and transform themselves into perception of unitary objects "projected" outside of
the skin?

SUMMARY

Warming and cooling the skin can affect (a) the sensitivity to
punctate (hair) touch stimulation, (b) the sensitivity to vibrotactile stimulation, and (c) the magnitude of touch sensation. As
assessed by threshold measurements, sensitivity to punctate and

low-frequency stimulation is remarkably constant over a wide range of skin temperature, falling precipitously only below about 20°C. In contrast, sensitivity to high frequencies peaks at 36°C and falls markedly with cooler or warmer skin temperature. The magnitude of touch sensations, as assessed by the method of magnitude estimation, can be strongly intensified by concomitant cooling of the skin. Concomitant warming can also intensify a touch sensation aroused in the forearm but not, apparently, in the forehead. In any case, cooling always has a stronger effect than warming. The degree of intensification depends on several variables: (a) the greater the temperature difference from neutral, the greater is the intensification; (b) the stronger the mechanical stimulation, the smaller is the proportional degree of thermal intensification; (c) the areal size of stimulation is relatively unimportant except that very small areas (0.4 cm^2) prove to be disadvantageous to revealing intensification. These various thermo-tactile interactions are reviewed in the light of current knowledge and speculation concerning the peripheral mechanoreceptors and their neural attachments.

ACKNOWLEDGEMENT

Preparation of this paper was aided by Grant No. BNS76-24341 from the National Science Foundation.

REFERENCES

Bessou, P., & Perl, E. R. Response of cutaneous sensory units with unmyelinated fibers to noxious stimuli. Journal of Neurophysiology, 1969, 32, 1025-1043.

Burton, H., Terashima, S., & Clark, J. Response properties of slowly adapting mechanoreceptors to temperature stimulation in cats. Brain Research, 1972, 45, 401-416.

Chambers, M. R., Andres, K. H., Duering, M. von & Iggo, A. The structure and function of the slowly adapting type II mechanoreceptor in hairy skin. Quarterly Journal of Experimental Physiology, 1972, 57, 417-445.

Darian-Smith, I., Johnson, K. O., & Dykes, R. "Cold" fiber population innervating palmar and digital skin of the monkey; Responses to cooling pulses. Journal of Neurophysiology, 1973, 36, 325-346.

Douglas, W. W., Ritchie, J. M., & Straub, R. W. The role of non-myelinated fibres in signalling cooling of the skin. Journal of Physiology (London), 1960, 150, 266-283.

Green, B. G. The effect of skin temperature on vibrotactile sensitivity. Perception and Psychophysics, 1977, 21, 243-248.

Hensel, H. Classes of receptor units predominantly related to thermal stimuli. In A. V. S. DeReuck & J. Knight (Eds.), Touch, heat and pain. Boston: Little, Brown, 1966.

Hensel, H., & Zotterman, Y. Response of mechanoreceptors to ther-
    mal stimulation. Journal of Physiology (London), 1951, 115,
    16-24.
Hunt, C. C., & McIntyre, A. K. Properties of cutaneous touch re-
    ceptors in cat. Journal of Physiology (London), 1960, 153,
    88-98.
Iggo, A. Cutaneous mechanoreceptors with afferent C fibres.
    Journal of Physiology (London), 1960, 152, 337-353.
Iggo, A. Cutaneous thermoreceptors in primates and sub-primates.
    Journal of Physiology (London), 1969, 200, 403-430.
Inman, D. R., & Peruzzi, P. The effects of temperature on the
    responses of Pacinian corpuscles. Journal of Physiology
    (London), 1961, 155, 280-301.
Ishiko, N., & Loewenstein, W. R. Effects of temperature on the
    generator and action potentials of a sense organ. Journal of
    General Physiology, 1961, 45, 105-124.
Jones, F. N., Singer, D., & Twelker P. A. Interactions among
    the somesthetic senses in judgments of subjective magnitude.
    Journal of Experimental Psychology, 1962, 64, 103-109.
Kenton, B., Crue, B. L., & Carregal, E. J. A. Quantitative measures
    of the thermal reactivity of cutaneous mechanoreceptors.
    Neuroscience Letters, 1975, 1, 321-326.
Knibestöl, M., & Vallbo, A. B. Single unit analysis of mechano-
    receptor activity from the human glabrous skin. Acta Physio-
    logica Scandinavica, 1970, 80, 178-195.
Mackworth, N. H. Finger numbness in very cold winds. Journal of
    Applied Physiology, 1953, 5, 533-543.
Mills, A. W. Finger numbness and skin temperature. Journal of
    Applied Physiology, 1956, 9, 447-450.
Morton, R., & Provins, K. A. Finger numbness after acute local
    exposure to cold. Journal of Applied Physiology, 1960, 15,
    149-154.
Poulos, D. A., & Lende, R. A. Response of trigeminal ganglion
    neurons to thermal stimulation of oral-facial regions. I.
    Steady-state response. Journal of Neurophysiology, 1970, 33,
    508-517.
Provins, K. A., & Morton, R. Tactile discrimination and skin tem-
    perature. Journal of Applied Physiology, 1960, 15, 155-160.
Rowe, M. J., & Sessle, B. J. Responses of trigeminal ganglion and
    brain stem neurones in the cat to mechanical and thermal stimu-
    lation of the face. Brain Research, 1972, 42, 367-384.
Stevens, J. C., & Green, B. G. Temperature-touch interaction:
    Weber's phenomenon revisited. Sensory Processes, 1978, 2,
    206-219.
Stevens, J. C., Green, B. G., & Krimsley, A. S. Punctate pres-
    sure sensitivity: Effects of skin temperature. Sensory
    Processes, 1977, 1, 238-243.
Stevens, J. C., & Stevens, S. S. Warmth and cold: Dynamics of
    sensory intensity. Journal of Experimental Psychology, 1960,
    60, 183-192.

Szabadföldi, M.   Beiträge zur Physiologie des Tastsinnes.   Unter-
    suchungen zur Naturlehre des Menschen und der Thiere, 1865,
    9, 624-631.
Tapper, D. N.   Stimulus-response relationships in the cutaneous
    slowly-adapting mechanoreceptor in hairy skin of the cat.
    Experimental Neurology, 1965, 13, 364-385.
Torebjörk, H. E.   Afferent C units responding to mechanical thermal
    and chemical stimuli in human non-glabrous skin.   Acta Physio-
    logica Scandinavica, 1974, 92, 374-390.
Verrillo, R. T.   A duplex mechanism of mechanoreception.   In
    D. R. Kenshalo (Ed.), The skin senses. Springfield, Ill:
    Thomas, 1968.
Weber, E. H.   Der Tastsinn und das Gemeingefühl.   In R. Wagner
    (Ed.), Handwörterbuch der Physiologie, 1846, 3, 481-588.
Weitz, J.   Vibratory sensitivity as a function of skin tempera-
    ture.   Journal of Experimental Psychology, 1941, 28, 21-36.

DISCUSSION

DR. ZOTTERMAN: Dr. Hensel and I may have some words to say. Hensel came to me in 1950 when we were studying cold fibers in the cat. We found afferent fibers that were dual modality fibers, responding as well to mechanical stimuli as to cooling. We both were quite aware that this could offer some kind of explanation of the Weber illusion. Now the question is whether such fibers are found in man. I give that question to Dr. Johansson. Thus, far, you have not looked for them, have you?

DR. JOHANSSON: Temperature effects on the mechanoreceptive fibers? No, we have not looked for it.

DR. HENSEL: We found them in our first experiments done together with Boman (Hensel and Boman, 1960). We found mechanosensitive fibers responding to mechanical stimulation and cooling, and more recently we have found, in the group of SA II fibers, about 30 per cent sensitive to mechanical stimulation as well as to cooling. This finding has not been published yet, but I think, in humans, there are quite a few fibers that fit these requirements. Still, the question remains, "What about the warm side?" I have no explanation for that.

DR. IGGO: So far as the SA mechanoreceptors are concerned, there are two effects I think you need to bear in mind. One is that many of them, and probably in the right circumstances, all of them will be excited when the skin is cooled. But they also show a static thermal sensitivity. The peak sensitivity varies among the different fibers, in the range $30°$ to $40°C$. I think that you need to be careful, in psychophysical testing, to make sure that you bear in mind these two possibilities, because whenever you place a cold object on the skin, you will certainly get excitation of the mechanoreceptors by the falling temperature of the skin together with that of the mechanical stimulus. However, if you leave the object on the skin, then you will have the static component coming in, and there one finds that the receptors cease to respond at temperatures down below $20°C$. and also cease to respond at temperatures up above $40°$ to $45°C$., or so. This varies according to the receptors.

DR. VERRILLO: Yes, but I think this adds motivation, actually, for looking at the time course of the thermal intensification, which is a variable that we want to get at soon. I think that we also want to look at some other body regions, because the difference between the forehead and the forearm suggests that you might possibly find even bigger differences between other regions.

DR. TOREBJORK: I will describe an experiment which I think is of

relevance in this context. If you put a piece of thin brass plate
on the dorsum of the hand and record from the radial nerve, you
often find spontaneous activity going on in the SA II receptors.
If you then put on a few drops of ether, cooling the metal plate,
this activity will increase and the blind-folded subject will say,
"Now you have increased the weight on the hand." Then, if you just
breathe on the plate, increasing the temperature, the spontaneously
occuring activity ceases completely, and the subject will tell
you that you have taken the plate away. So there seems to be a
correlation between the activities in these receptors and the
perceptions which I have described.

DR. ZOTTERMAN: I also recall some data which could explain it, if
the conditions are the same in man as in cat. It deals with the
persisting cold sensation. If you press a cold object against the
skin and then take it off, after a second or two there is a cold
sensation when the skin is warming up. Thus, we have explanations
for both Weber's illusion and the phenomenon of the persisting
cool sensation.

DR. STARR: The cooling of the skin obviously has an effect on the
receptors, but there is another problem that cooling slows nerve
conduction velocities in the skin and I have always wondered how
one would handle this, because that would theoretically mean decreased efficiency of nervous activity and, at least in this
country, we think, the faster you go, the better you are.

DR. IGGO: The effect of cold on nerve conduction is very real.
If you cool the nerve you will eventually block it. To block the
myelinated fibers, they have to be cooled down, in the cat saphenous
nerve, to about $7.4^{\circ}C$. which is, despite the $0^{\circ}Cs$ on the figures,
a good deal colder than the skin ever got in Dr. Steven's experiments. Long before you get to such low temperatures, conduction
in the nerve is affected. Even at temperatures as high as $20^{\circ}C$,
at high discharge rates, the nerve will be blocked. So what
happens is that as the nerve becomes colder, the heavy weights
ought to feel lighter. I would like to ask our speaker if he has
ever observed that phenomenon, that is, if the heavy weights become
lighter when you have low temperatures?

DR. STEVENS: Never. No.

DR. IGGO: One would expect, in the slow adapting fibers anyway,
that there would be a halving of the number of impulses going
through the nerve, or a quartering, or so on. However, the nerve
itself has not been cooled, and I would suggest to Dr. Stevens
that he would now do other experiments in which he cools the nerve
and leaves the skin alone.

DR. POULOS: In agreement with Dr. Iggo's comment, the difference
one sees in the monkey trigeminal system between purely thermal
receptors and those that also respond to mechanical stimuli is that
the thermal will give a brief dynamic response to rapid cooling,
say from 35° to 15°C and then they shut off, and go completely
silent. The units that respond to both thermal and mechanical
stimulation will give a dynamic response and very often will
maintain ongoing activity at 15°C. However, if one attempts to
stimulate them mechanically, one does not elicit a dynamic response to a mechanical stimulus until the skin is warmed up.

DR. CRAIG: Could you differentiate between cooling the skin or
warming the skin and leaving the cylinder at the same temperature.

DR. STEVENS: We could differentiate that, and that is one of the
things that we plan to do.

DR. CRAIG: Would such a procedure get at some of the questions
of nerve block that have been raised?

DR. STEVENS: Yes, I think it will.

DR. IGGO: I would like to ask you to comment on a possible role
of the thermoreceptors in the effects that you have been describing. Do you think they have anything to do with this?

DR. STEVENS: I did at first, I thought this was probably a
central kind of summing between thermal nerve inputs and mechanical inputs. But when we found nothing like that for the forehead, we turned toward a peripheral explanation. When we found
a difference between the forehead and the forearm, we were even
more convinced the effect was peripheral. Of course, we cannot
really rule out a possibility of central summation.

DR. KENSHALO: Would you comment on the relationship between
temperature and the high frequency portion of your vibratory
threshold curve? Why are the Pacinian corpuscles effected and the
other ones are not?

DR. GREEN: I would like to be able to answer that. I think
actually there are people here that could answer it better than I,
except that I was aware that the Pacinian corpuscles show a pretty
strong temperature effect over the range of temperatures that I
measured. I believe Sato (1961) made the original measurements
on its change in sensitivity with changes in temperature. As Dr.
Stevens mentioned, the fact that the effect is frequency dependent
does seem to suggest that it is the receptor that is being affected and not the skin. However, if you have two different

systems, one spatially summating and one not, then if there are physical differences, say vasodilation or constriction, you might expect those physical differences to effect sensitivity in the high frequency summating range and perhaps not effect the low frequency non-summating range.

DR. JOHANSSON: When one compares the Meissner (non-Pacinian system) and Pacinian corpuscles, one should have in mind that the Pacinian corpuscles are located much deeper so the direct effect of cooling on the receptor may come first to the Meissner corpuscle as they are located more superficially.

REFERENCES

Hensel, H. & Boman, K. K. A.   Afferent impulses in cutaneous sensory nerves in human subject. Journal of Neurophysiology, 1960, 23, 564-578.

Sato, M.   Response of Pacinian corpuscles to sinusoidal vibration. Journal of Physiology, 1961, 159, 391-409.

THERMO-TACTILE INTERACTIONS: EFFECTS OF TOUCH ON THERMAL LOCALIZATION

Barry G. Green

Yale University and The John B. Pierce Foundation

Laboratory, New Haven, Connecticut

It has long been known that spatial discrimination is much better in the tactile sense than in the thermal senses (Pritchard, 1931). Results like those of Cain (1973), who discovered that 20 percent of the time subjects fail to distinguish between radiant heat stimulation of the stomach and back, teach us that the thermal senses do not function as spatially discriminative senses. There is little reason they should: thermal stimulation commonly affects large areas of the body, as in the case of radiant or convective heating and cooling. When thermal stimulation is discrete, as in the case of conductive heating and cooling, the accompanying tactile stimulation supplies an accurate cue to locus. But there appears to be more to the perception of combined thermo-tactile stimulation than a simple spatial coincidence of the two sensations. The diffuse nature of thermal sensation prevents exact spatial coincidence, yet we routinely perceive thermal sensations as limited to the area of mechanical stimulation. The phenomenon described here, in which a tactile stimulus adopts the thermal quality of an adjacent conductive thermal stimulus, reveals a mechanism whereby relatively diffuse thermal sensations combine with tactile sensations to form discrete and unitary perceptions.

Thermal Referral With Three Stimulators

Referral of thermal sensations to the site of tactile stimulation was discovered outside of the laboratory in a simple experiment: Two pennies were tossed in a freezer to cool while a third, thermally neutral penny was held in the hand. After a minute or so the two cold pennies were removed from the freezer and placed on a table, and the neutral penny placed between. Touching

the three coins simultaneously with the first three fingers of the
hand gave a startling result: All three coins felt cold! Additional informal tests affirmed the validity of the phenomenon,
and led to a series of formal experiments in the laboratory.

     Figure 1 shows the results of the laboratory version of the
"three-penny experiment" (Green, 1977). Instead of pennies,
Peltier devices served as stimulators, and subjects reported perceived magnitudes of thermal sensations at the center stimulator
when (a) the center stimulator was warmed or cooled directly and
the outer stimulators held neutral (filled circles), or (b) when
the center stimulator was held neutral and only the outer stimulators were warmed or cooled (open circles). Surprisingly, the
perceived magnitude of the thermal sensation at the center stimulator was the same in both conditions. If the center stimulator
is itself neutral but adjacent fingers touch warm or cool stimulators, the center stimulator appears as warm or cool as when
its temperature actually changes.

     This phenomenon has been called "thermal referral" because
thermal sensations "refer" to the site of tactile sensation in a
way reminiscent of the way visceral pain seems to refer to

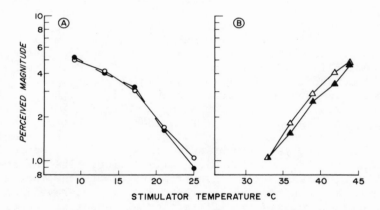

Fig. 1.   Part A shows the perceived magnitude of cold sensation at
          the middle finger as a function of stimulator temperature,
          with the temperature of the center stimulator alone varied
          (filled circles) or with the temperatures of the outer
          stimulators varied and the center stimulator held at 30°
          (open circles). Part B shows the perceived magnitude of
          warmth sensation at the middle finger as a function of
          stimulator temperature, with the temperature of the center
          stimulator alone varied (filled triangles) or with the
          temperature of the outer stimulators varied and the center
          stimulator held at 30°C (open triangles) (Green, 1977).
          1977).

superficial areas of the abdomen. One notable difference in the two types of referral is that thermal referral occurs without significant alteration of the spatial or intensive properties of the thermal sensation at the veridical site.[1]

Proof that referral requires the presence of parallel tactile input lies in the observation that the middle finger remains thermally neutral if held just above the center stimulator. Once in contact, the surface of the stimulator appears to warm-up or cool-down depending on the temperature of the outer stimulators. More convincing evidence of tactile involvement comes from the following tests: slow submersion of three fingers in three cups of water (the outer fingers in warm or cold water, the middle finger in neutral water) fails to produce referral. However, wiggling the fingers, which heightens tactile stimulation, sometimes produces a sensation of warmth or cold at the middle finger. Better still, placing a tight-fitting surgical glove on the hand and again submerging the fingers produces a clear sensation of warmth or cold at the middle finger. The thermal sensation actually creeps above the water-line and into the hand, presumably because of the strong tactile stimulus the glove produces throughout the hand.

Enhancement, Domination, and Synthetic Heat

Thermal referral also occurs when the center stimulator is itself heated or cooled along with the outer stimulators. Figure 2 shows that when the outer stimulators are held at a warm or cool temperature, and the center stimulator is varied in temperature, the center stimulator appears warmer or cooler than when it is heated or cooled alone. The presence of adjacent thermal stimulation enhances the perception of warmth or cold at a nearby site.

But what happens when bracketing and middle stimulators are heated or cooled in opposition to one another? Figure 3 gives the answer. The open circles on the left and the open triangles on the right replicate the results of Fig. 2, where outer and center temperatures were both warm or cold. The open triangles on the left and open circles on the right show what happens when thermal qualities oppose one another. With a cool center stimulator and warm outer stimulators, the perceived magnitude at the center

---

[1]An experiment, nearly complete at this writing, indicates that thermal referral causes almost no alteration in the thermal sensation at the veridical site. Specifically, the perceived magnitude of thermal sensation produced by warming the index finger directly remained largely unchanged when the second finger touched a neutral stimulator, which induced referral.

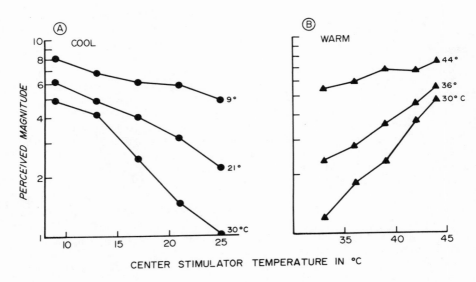

Fig. 2. Perceived magnitude of cold (A) or warmth (B) at the
middle finger as a function of center stimulator temperature. The parameter is the temperature of the outer stimulators (Green, 1977).

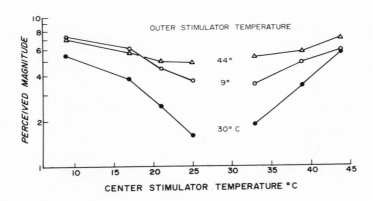

Fig. 3. Perceived magnitude of the thermal sensation at the middle
finger as a function of center stimulator temperature.
The parameter is the temperature of the outer stimulators.
The open circles on the right and the triangles on the
left represent conditions in which the quality of the
thermal sensations aroused by the center and outer stimulators differed (Green, 1977).

stimulator is once again enhanced. Enhancement of cold sensation by adjacent warm sensations is so great that with center stimulator temperatures of 25° and 21°C, warm outer stimulators contribute more to the center stimulator than do cold outer stimulators. Enhancement also occurs with a warm center and cold outer stimulators, but to a lesser degree.[2]

When enhancement occurs between stimulators of opposite thermal quality, what thermal quality is felt at the center stimulator? To answer this question, subjects were instructed to report on each trial whether the center stimulator felt very cold, cold, cool, warm, very warm, or hot. The results of this task appear in Fig. 4. The squares in both A and B illustrate the percent of warm and cool judgments (collapsed across the three subcategories for the two qualities) as a function of center stimulator temperature when the outer stimulators were neutral. The circles show what happened when (A) the outer stimulators were at 44°C, or when (B) the outer stimulators were at 9°C. In both cases, even extremely warm and extremely cold center temperatures resulted in "incorrect" judgments. That is, the thermal quality of the outer stimulators often dominated judgement of the thermal quality of the center stimulator.

On some trials when warm outer stimulators opposed a cool center stimulator, subjects reported sensations indicative of the perception of "synthetic heat." The phenomenon of synthetic heat was discovered in the 19th century (Alrutz, 1898), but has received scant attention since except by the early introspectionists (e.g., Burnett and Dallenbach, 1928). Typically produced by spatial alternation of warm and cool stimuli on the skin, synthetic heat is perhaps best explained as the result of simultaneous activity in warm and cold fibers on adjacent areas of skin (Alrutz, 1898). The logic is that under conditions of extreme warmth, cold fibers often fire paradoxically (Dodt and Zotterman, 1952), thus sending the CNS a mix of warm- and cold-fiber activity that somehow signals heat. This seemingly parsimonious explanation should be accepted with caution, however, since more recent findings indicate that cold fibers may fire paradoxically only at temperatures of 50°C or higher, temperatures well above those necessary for the perception of heat (Long, 1977).

To get a better idea of the frequency of occurrence of synthetic heat in the referral paradigm, the frequency of very warm or hot judgments was plotted as a function of center stimulator temperature. Figure 5A shows that under the conditions of the

---

[2]Warm refers more effectively to the site of cold stimulation than does cold to the site of warm stimulation, even though 9°C produce similar perceived magnitudes (Fig. 1).

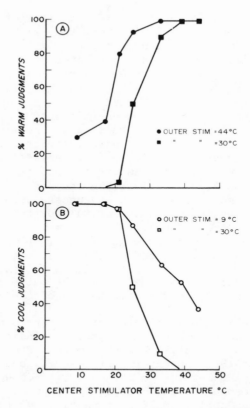

Fig. 4.   The percent warm judgments (A) and percent cool judgments
          (B) as a function of center stimulator temperature. The
          parameter is the temperature of the outer stimulors (Green,
          1977).

experiment, perceptions of heat seem to occur most often when outer
stimulators reach 44°C and the inner stimulator temperature falls
to 21°C. Puzzling, however, is Fig. 5B, where a similar peak in
judgments of extreme cold occurs with an outer temperature of 9°C
and a center temperature of 39°C. The nonmonotonic nature of the
functions in Fig. 5 argues against the idea that simple dominance
of thermal quality occurred. Dominance should vary monotonically
with the difference between center and outer temperatures, as in
Fig. 2. It is possible, however, that the peak in cold judgments
reflects "synthetic cold," a sensation characterized by qualities
of pricking or burning mingled with cold. Also, cold is often the
first thermal sensation perceived in a synthetic heat experiment
(Burnett and Dallenbach, 1927), and the relatively brief (3 sec)
contact allowed in these experiments may have favored judgments of

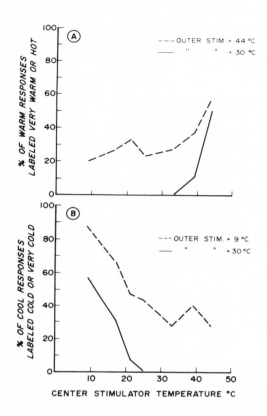

Fig. 5.   The percent of warm responses labeled very warm or hot (A)
         and the percent of cool responses labeled cold or very
         cold (B), as a function of center stimulator temperature.
         The dashed lines show what results when the outer stimu-
         lators are held at 44°C (A) or 9°C. The solid lines were
         obtained with the outer stimulators held at 30°C (Green)

cold. Germane, too, to the peak in cold judgments is the observation that subjects never abruptly removed their fingers from the
stimulator when the center stimulators was warm and the outer
stimulators cold, as they sometimes did when the center stimulator
was cold and the outer stimulators warm.

     Referral with Two Stimulators

     Soon after work on referral began it was discovered that
thermal sensations sometimes refer between just two stimulators
when one is warmed or cooled and the other neural. An earlier

attempt to define the spatial limits of referral with three stimulators failed when referral remained robust over the length of the
forearm. The discovery of referral between two stimulators offered
a more promising approach to the problem.

    Returning to the forearm, referral of both warmth and cold was
measured at four stimulator separations using two procedures. One
procedure, which required subjects to judge the ratio of thermal
sensations between stimulators, was expected to bias subjects toward reporting more referral by heightening the expectation of
sensation at both stimulators. The second procedure, which required subjects to report the perceived magnitude of thermal sensations at the two sites independently, was expected to produce
less referral by encouraging independent assessment of sensation
at the two stimulators. Thus the questions asked in this experiment were, (a) How much is referral affected by task, and (b) Do
warmth and cold refer equally as the distance between stimulators
increases?

    Figure 6 answers both questions. First, task does affect re-
ports of sensation at the neutral stimulator. As expected, the
ratio estimation procedure produces more referral than the magnitude estimation procedure. Hence when referral is weak, response
bias becomes a factor. But more importantly, at all separations
warmth refers more strongly to a tactile stimulus than does cold,
and the rate of decline in referral over distance is unaffected by
task. Note that referral remains significant for warmth when
stimulators are separated by 16 cm. Thus two-stimulator referral
reveals a difference between warmth and cold that remained hidden
in the abundance of referral produced with three stimulators.

    Or are the fingers and arm simply different? To check this
possibility referral was tried again on the hand, this time with
two stimulators. Provisions were made to test referral between
finger pairs and across the four fingers. In addition, preliminary
observations indicated that the direction of referral mattered,
(i.e., toward or away from the index finger) so referral was tested
in both directions. Figures 7 and 8 illustrate the results for
warmth and cold. Three points emerge from the data: (a) Referral
for warmth exceeds that for cold, in agreement with data from the
arm, and also in agreement with data recently collected in this
laboratory showing cold to be better discriminated spatially than
warmth[3]; (b) The magnitude of referral depends on direction. Referral occurs more readily in the direction away from the index
finger (e.g., when finger 2 is warmed and finger 3 is neutral).
(c) The spatial pattern of referral differs between thermal modalities, suggesting different innervation patterns exist for warmth
and cold either peripherally, centrally, or in both places.
Clearly, there is more to referral than initial experiments with
three stimulators indicated.

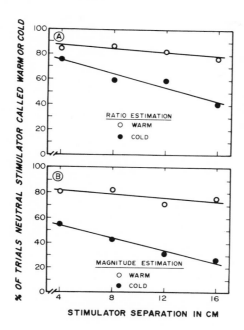

Fig. 6.   The percent of trials the neutral stimulator was called
warm (filled circles) or cold (unfilled circles) as a
function of stimulator separation. Data in (A) come from
the ratio estimation task, and data in (B) come from the
magnitude estimation task.

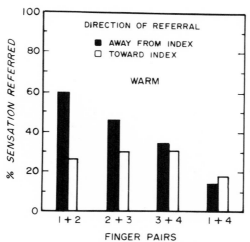

Fig. 7.   Percent of warmth sensation referred to neutral stimulator
for four finger pairs in two directions. One-hundred percent referral means the neutral stimulator feels equal in
warmth to the warmed stimulator.

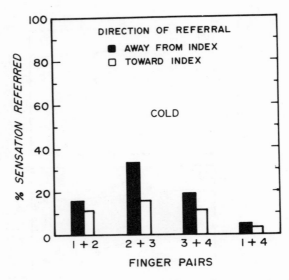

Fig. 8.   Percent of cold sensation referred to neutral stimulator
         for four finger pairs in two directions.

DISCUSSION

     That a tactile stimulus adopts thermal sensations from ad-
jacent conductive thermal stimuli reveals that the central nervous
system focuses thermal sensations at the site of tactile stimulation.   Thus referral stands as a unique example of a multimodal
interaction that binds thermal and tactile sensations together into
cohesive percepts. By so doing, thermal sensation may become more
an attribute of the object than an attribute of the skin. One can
even think of referral as a means of "externalizing" thermal sensation: Without tactile stimulation (as for example during radiant
warming or cooling) the perception is simply one of warm or cold
skin; with tactile stimulation the perception is more one of warm
or cold object. Whereas tactile sensation usually seems external
in origin, and pain sensation usually superficial or internal in
origin, the apparent locus of thermal sensations may depend on the
presence or absence of tactile stimulation.

_____

     [3]Tactile cues to thermal locus are eliminated by resting the
arm on a flat surface through which thermal stimulators contact the
skin. Requiring subjects to report which of two stimulators is
warmed or cooled results in significantly better performance for
cold compared to warm stimuli (a difference in error rates of as
much as 4-to-1).

The mechanism that underlies referral also has consequences for the perception of cutaneous qualities. Referral means that information about quality can be integrated across nerve fibers. Synthetic heat is a case in point, where referral of warmth to the site of cooling produces a sensation of heat with qualities both similar to and different from its thermal and tactile elements. Thus we have a system wherein the stimulus selectively afforded by different modalities in the periphery combines centrally to produce rich perceptions without loss of information. One could argue that information is actually gained by linking thermal sensations with tactile stimulation, in that ambiguity about the source of thermal stimulation is reduced.

The neurophysiological basis for referral escapes easy explanation. That it is a central effect is apparent from the presence of referral across fingers, along the length of the forearm, and even across the midline of the abdomen (all readily observable with two or three pennies). The peculiar effects of the direction and pattern of referral on the hand goes unexplained by peripheral innervation. If communality of peripheral innervation were crucial, referral on the hand would reach a maximum for both warmth and cold between fingers 1 and 2 (which share the median nerve), and would show directional symmetry. Referral does reach a peak for warmth between fingers 1 and 2, but not for cold (Fig. 8), and the requirement of directional symmetry fails in both modalities.

Thus we are faced with a central effect that escapes easy physiological analysis but appeals well to functional necessity and convenience. What at first glance seems simply an anomaly of thermal localization, may upon closer examination turn out to be the manifestation of a mechanism that sharpens and unifies the perception of cutaneous stimuli.

SUMMARY

A thermo-tactile interaction is described in which thermal sensations "refer" to the site of nearby tactile stimulation. Referral of thermal sensations was studied when a tactile stimulus adjacent to a thermal stimulus: (a) was thermally neutral; (b) had the same thermal quality as the inducing stimulus, in which case its perceived magnitude was enhanced; (c) had the opposite thermal quality to the inducing stimulus, in which case the inducing quality either dominated the quality of the adjacent stimulus, or synthetic heat was produced. Referral between just two loci reveals that warmth refers more readily to a tactile stimulus than does cold. The neurophysiological basis of the effect is unknown but probably resides centrally. It is suggested that from a functional standpoint referral acts to combine thermal and tactile sensations into unitary percepts.

ACKNOWLEDGEMENTS

This work was supported in part by grants from the National Institute of Health (ES-00123-08) and the National Science Foundation (BNS76-24341).

REFERENCES

Alrutz, S. On the temperature senses: II. The sensation 'hot.' Mind, 1898, 2 ser., 7, 140-144.

Burnett, N. C., & Dallenbach, K. M. The experience of heat. American Journal of Psychology, 1927, 38, 418-431.

Burnett, N. C., & Dallenbach, K. M. Heat intensity. American Journal of Psychology, 1928, 40, 484-494.

Cain, W. S. Spatial discrimination of cutaneous warmth. American Journal of Psychology, 1973, 86, 169-181.

Dodt, E., & Zotterman, Y. The discharge of specific cold fibers at high temperatures (the paradoxical cold). Acta Physiologica Scandinavica, 1952, 26, 358-365.

Green, B. G. Localization of thermal sensation: An illusion and synthetic heat. Perception and Psychophysics, 1977, 22, 331-337.

Long, R. R. Sensivitity of cutaneous cold fibers to noxious heat: Paradoxical cold discharge. Journal of Neurophysiology, 1977, 40, 489-502.

Pritchard, E. A. B. Cutaneous tactile localization. Brain, 1931, 54, 350-371.

DISCUSSION

DR. VERRILLO: I notice that most of your experiments on the hand were mediolateral and on the forearm were proximodistal. Have you tried mediolateral placements on the forearm?

DR. GREEN: Yes, I have, informally. I did find that I got referral that way. It is difficult to tell whether or not I got more referral up and down the arm than across, which may be the case. When you happen upon this kind of thing it is very difficult to decide what to do next. I have to plead guilty of looking for the big effects at this point.

DR. GESCHEIDER: If it is true, as you suggested, that the tactile system is actually helping the temperature system in spatial acuity, that seems to imply that perhaps textual differences in terms of touch would be important in the degree to which you would be able to benefit by this phenomenon, and I was wondering if you had done any experiments on varying textual difference between the test stimulus and the inducing stimuli. If so did you find any kind of improvement or disruption of the effect if the differences in texture were really great, such as differences in sandpaper grade or perhaps differences in vibration frequency? It might be interesting to try very low frequency vibration and very high frequency vibration to see if you could disrupt the effect in that way.

DR. GREEN: Yes, I think that is an excellent suggestion. I have thought about the vibration experiment, but that is a little way down the line, I think. Texture is very important. I have, looked at gross differences in texture, for example, between metal objects and a cloth object and found that I cannot really perceive the cloth object to get cool, whereas the metal object does very readily. It becomes complicated, however; for example the demonstration I mentioned earlier, about sticking your two outer fingers in cups of water and then touching the middle to a metal object still allows referral. In that case, one seems to have almost no tactile sensation referring to a very profound tactile sensation. Incidentally, you can get synthetic heat that way, as well.

DR. VERRILLO: Along the same point, your demonstration with a glove would suggest that perhaps there is an interaction with slowly adapting mechanoreceptors. I do not know what these polymodal fibers that respond to both mechanical and thermal stimulation contribute. On the mechanical side, are they slowly adapting fibers?

DR. IGGO: They are.

DR. HENSEL: I have no answer to that but I would like to raise
another question. Did you also find any direct interferences
between mechanical stimulation and thermal sensation? For
example, was the thermal sensation dependent on the pressure on the
skin?

DR. GREEN: On the intensity?

DR. HENSEL: Yes, this was my first question. Secondly, I would
like to make a comment; namely, that the main biological significance of thermal reception, in my opinion, is temperature re-
gulation and that spatial discrimination is relatively unimportant for the temperature sense. I think there are only exceptional
biological situations where it might be important to precisely
localize the thermal stimulus.

DR. GREEN: I agree with that comment. There really is no need
for good spatial discrimination of warmth and cold, except perhaps,
when you come in contact with an object. Then you have the tactile
sense to tell you where things are. With respect to your first
question, I did some pilot work on that very point, whether or not
referral would increase with increased pressure on the center
simulator, I used weights placed on the arm. I did not complete
that experiment for several reasons, but mainly because the data
was too noisy. Subjects had difficulty discriminating the center
weight from the end weights when I placed 3 weights on their arm.
If there is an effect, it is not very large.

DR. LEDERMAN: I was interested in George's (Gescheider) comment on
the relationship between texture and the temperature sense. There
is an unpublished experiment that Bob Gibson mentioned to me a
number of years back in which he and a student ran an experiment
where they were feeling a series of grids - ruled lines, and both
the hand and the plate were presented either at a neutral temperature, or raised $10^\circ C$ above neutral temperature, or the hand and
the plate were both lowered $10^\circ C$. What he found was that the
texture, the smoothness, increased for the cold temperature. This
relates also to your work, as well as, Joe's (Stevens). The surfaces
felt smoother when the hand and the surfaces were cold. The texture felt about the same, from what he told me, if they were neutral
or warmer temperatures. So I was also wondering, since you find
again at a higher nervous system level, this interrelationship
between texture and temperature, whether you could enhance or possibly suppress the kind of effect that you're talking about by
introducing a textural component?

DR. GREEN: I will just say only that this potential effect does
deserve further investigation. The pilot work I mentioned suggests

that texture makes a difference.

DR. IGGO: Your effects clearly cannot be related to the spatial characteristics of the receptive fields of the primary afferent fibers, since these in both cold and warm receptors, are known to be very small. But, if one moves farther up the sensory pathway to the dorsal horn, first, the dorsal horn neurons that respond specifically to temperature changes are insensitive to any mechanical input from the fast mechanoreceptors. It is quite clear, I think, that the interactions that you are finding cannot be related to effects at that early part of the sensory pathway for cold and warmth. Secondly: the receptive fields for the dorsal horn neurons responding to cooling the skin, driven by the cold receptors presumably, are very much larger than the receptor fields for the primary afferent fibers. They may cover, in the case of the monkey, perhaps one-quarter of the hand. It is clear that the spatial discrimination available for cold and for warmth, is very poor when you consider the first stage in the sensory pathway. Perhaps your interactions, which clearly cannot be occurring in that early stage in the cold pathway, must be occurring farther up, because the dorsal horn neurons respond specifically to cooling the skin. Some of them at least are projecting directly into the crossed lateral pathway (anterolateral). This information is being preserved, uncontaminated by any mechanical input, until it gets to the thalamus.

DR. GREEN: This has stirred a memory of my own that relates to what Dr. Stevens talked about earlier and also perhaps as to why referral does not occur quite as much for cold as it does for warmth and why cold stimuli may be better localized. That is, if there are so many mechanoreceptors that are stimulated by cooling the skin, then in effect you may never get a "pure cold stimulus." Whenever you cool the skin, to any significant degree, you have a parallel tactile input as well. In a sense, you may have referral going on whenever you cool the skin to the extent that both thermal and tactile information is coming in; that presupposes that the mechano-receptors are signalling touch when they are being cooled and not cold.

DR. ZOTTERMAN: Dr. Hensel and I have discussed that these fibers that respond to both mechanical stimulation and cooling must mediate tactile sensations. You cannot arouse a cool sensation by mechanical stimulation of the skin with a thermally neutral probe. For that reason we believe that these fibers never mediate sensations of cool, in itself, when they are stimulated.

DR. JARVILEHTO: In this experiment where you have hot outer stimuli and a cold inner stimulus, have you tried a temporal separation between the two stimuli so that you first heat and then cool. Do you get a heat sensation then?

DR. GREEN: If you put your fingers down on the warm stimulators first and let them warm up, then touch the cold stimulus you do get a heat sensation. However, if you put the finger down on the cold one first then touch the outer warm ones, it is ambiguous because you know it is cold.

DR. JÄRVILEHTO: I ask this because in the experiments which I am going to report in the afternoon, we have studied this paradoxical heat which occurs when cooling. We get it very clearly when we first heat the skin and then cool the same place. We experience a very clear heat sensation when cooling.

DR. LINDBLOOM: Do you think that is actually the same phenomenon?

DR. JÄRVILEHTO: Yes, because we have thought that the simplest explanation for this heat sensation would be some type of facilitation of some peripheral receptors. But what you have shown, suggest that there are some central interactions.

DR. GREEN: Right, the classic explanation of synthetic heat is that it results from activity in both cold fibers and warm fibers, mixing centrally and giving you a sensation of heat. That is based on the assumption that you feel heat when you raise skin temperature and begin to fire cold fibers paradoxically, so that the normal sensation of heat involves input from both warm and cold fibers. It seems though that recent data indicates that you do not get this paradoxical firing until you reach $50^\circ C$, or above. If you do not get paradoxical activity in cold fibers until you clearly get into the pain range, then I do not know if that explanation is valid.

DR. STEVENS: My question was prompted by the remark that Dr. Iggo made a few minutes ago. We have studied the property of spatial summation a great deal in our laboratory. It has also been studied here extensively by Dr. Kenshalo and one of his students here, Andrew Rożsa. It always seemed to me that the lavish spatial summation that you get had something to do with the large receptive fields of the central cells that you record from. These receptive fields measured by (Hellon & Mitchell, 1975) are not only large but they even are bilateral and all of us have found that summation moves freely across the mid-line and dermatone boundaries, in general. My question may be a bit metaphysical in nature. It is this; why did nature design a peripheral nervous system that would take all the information about tiny spots all the way up into the core of the brain and then throw it away by funneling it into a few cells?

DR. IGGO: I think the problem is, to start with, all this marvelous information of little spots out in the periphery and all the rest of it, appeared to have been thrown away. In the early experiments it was missing, but there is now more information that some of it, at least, is being preserved. There is no doubt that a good deal of convergence is occurring. The thermosensory pathway is so difficult to work on, and we have got such a small yield of units that we may be jumping to the wrong conclusion. The available evidence indicates that for the cold system the spatial information certainly has been thrown away, but in the mechanoceptive system and the nociceptive system, there certainly is preservation, particularly if you move down to the spinal cord, the receptive fields of the dorsal horn and of the dorsal column nuclei cells can be quite small. Maybe nature says a little redundancy is required because, after all, as we get older we have just been hearing that we lose 1 per cent of our myelinated fibers each year. I gather you have got to have an awful lot to start with in order to have enough left at the end.

DR. POULOS: In the trigeminal system, where perhaps things are a bit more discreet, at the level of the spinal nucleus of V and thalamus, we have never seen receptive fields that cross the midline. In a sense they are large, but are maintained quite discreetly in the cold system. My question is whether your referral occurs across the midline. It would be interesting to look into whether differences occur at the spinal level and in the face, where we know there is a clear ipsilateral and contralateral input.

DR. GREEN: I have not done any formal experiments with the bilaterality question. Referral can be produced with pennies across the forehead. I have gotten it with just two pennies or stimulators, across the midline on the stomach. However, you don't get it from one hand to the other. I am sure it does break down as the distance between the stimulators is increased.

DR. KENSHALO: With regard to the paradoxical stimulation of cold fibers, we found approximately 30 per cent of a small population of cold fibers that could be fired paradoxically by warming from 45° to 50°C. Long (1973) seems to think that this is a function of body core temperature and he has reported some paradoxical discharges at fairly low intensities of warming.

DR. GREEN: It was Long I was thinking of when I said that the more recent data had indicated that paradoxical firing started at higher temperatures. My recollection was that it was around 50°C.

DR. IGGO: This is again relating to the question of the paradoxical

discharge of cold fibers. I have been doing some experiments on
monkey cold receptors in Delhi and was aware of Long's results
and very puzzled by them because he was appearing to suggest that
there was some kind of effect, perhaps coming out from the CNS, to
alter the sensitivity of the receptors. In fact, what we have been
doing is to establish that the cold fibers are very dependent on
the skin being supplied with plenty of oxygenated blood. If the
flow of oxygenated blood is interrupted by giving the monkey low
oxygen gas mixtures nitrogen to breathe, then the behavior of the
cold receptors changes quite substantially and they become a good
deal less sensitive. The group discharge, for example, may dis-
appear. The effect can even be found when cutting off the blood
flow, by pressing on the skin. This kind of effect was recorded
earlier by Dr. Hensel. There is no doubt that the cold receptors,
at least, do seem to be rather dependent on having plenty of
oxygen in the blood stream. We were starting to look at the effect on paradoxical discharge but did not quite get there, because
of apparatus limitations. I suspect also, in reading Long's
paper, that the paradoxical discharge which he said is dependent
on body core temperature is actually dependent on the flow
through the skin of plenty of oxygenated blood. The paradoxical
effect is more marked when the blood flow is best.

DR. HENSEL: I would like to add that the sensitivity to oxygen
lack is so high that sometimes even the pressure of the thermode is
sufficient to change the discharge of the cold receptors.

REFERENCES

Hellon, R. F. & Mitchell, D. Convergence in a thermal afferent
        pathway in the rat. Journal of Physiology, 1975, 248, 359-
        376.
Long, R. R. Cold fiber heat sensitivity: dependency of 'paradox-
        ical' discharge on body temperature. Brain Research, 1973,
        63, 389-392.

THE NEURAL BASIS OF THE SENSORY QUALITY OF WARMTH

F. Konietzny and H. Hensel

Institute of Physiology, University of Marburg

3550 Marburg/Lahn, Germany

Our knowledge about temperature sensation is mainly based upon two experimental approaches which differ remarkably in aim and scope. First, the relationship between temperature sensation and thermal stimuli was investigated by using psychophysical ("phenophysical") methods (Kenshalo, 1970; Marks and Stevens, 1968; Stevens and Stevens, 1960; Stevens and Marks, 1967, 1971; Vendrik, 1970). Second, the neural responses to thermal stimuli in infra-human species (cats, monkeys) were compared to the sensations evoked in man by identical stimuli, thus, implying that each sensory modality in each species is mediated by the same set of sensory receptors (Järvilehto, 1973; Johnson, Darian-Smith, and LaMotte, 1973; Darian-Smith, Johnson, and LaMotte, 1975; Kenshalo, 1976; Molinari and Kenshalo, 1977; LaMotte and Campbell, 1978).

At the present time, only a few direct measurements of afferent impulses from cutaneous thermoreceptors in man are available. In conscious human subjects, Hensel and Boman (1960) first recorded afferent impulses from specific cold fibers from the superficial branch of the radial nerve. Afferent activity of specific warm units from human skin nerves was recently correlated with the conscious temperature sensation (Torebjörk, 1974; Hensel, 1976; Konietzny and Hensel, 1975; Konietzny and Hensel, 1977b, 1978; Hallin and Torebjörk, 1977) using the technique of microneurography pioneered in humans by Hagbarth and Vallbo (1967).

According to our present knowledge, temperature sensation is related to peripheral thermoreceptor activity and the sensory qualities of cold and warmth can probably be ascribed to a dual set of receptors sensitive either to cooling or to warming. This assumption is based on human sensory physiology, in particular on the discovery of separate "cold" and "warm" spots in the skin from which natural or electrical stimuli elicited cold or warm sensations (Blix, 1882), and on recent investigations in which a selective elimination of either cold or warm sensation was achieved by selective blocking of myelinated or unmyelinated cutaneous nerve fibers in humans (Torebjörk and Hallin, 1972; Fruhstorfer, Zenz, Nolte, and Hensel, 1974). However, whether this dual receptor theory can fully explain the nature of the sensory quality of "heat" as distinct from the quality of warmth has to be examined.

The present study had two main goals: The first was to make a quantitative analysis of the dynamic and steady-state properties of single specific warm units in humans. The second goal was to determine which types of primary neural afferents play a suffi-cient role in mediating the sensations of warmth and "heat".

METHODS

Single afferent units were studied with HOSTAFLON TF^R coated tungsten microelectrodes (Konietzny and Hensel, 1974) percutaneously inserted in the superficial branch of the human radial nerve about 2 cm proximal to the wrist. Subjects were 28 paid volunteers, 19 females and 9 males, aged between 20 and 31 years.

The neural acitvity was amplified with a conventional AC-coupled amplifier, audio-visually monitored and stored on analog magnetic tape along with the electrical analog of the thermal stim-uli. Each receptive field was mapped with different mechanical stimulators, a heat radiator and several water perfused copper thermodes described in previous publications (Konietzny and Hensel, 1977a,b).

The quantitative response of each receptor to various temper-atures was then studied with a thermal stimulator operating on the Peltier principle (Kenshalo, 1963). A thermistor attached to the 1 cm^2 stimulating surface measured the temperature of the thermode-skin interface and provided feedback to a current controller which maintained the stimulator at any predetermined temperature level between 5° and 45°C. Temperature changes in either the cool or warm direction could be produced at rates up to 1.5°/sec.

The axonal conduction velocities of identified units were de-termined by combined electrical and natural stimuli using a compact time presentation of the induced nerve responses (Torebjörk and Hallin, 1974, a,b). The environmental temperature was kept at approximately 23°C.

RESULTS

General Characteristics of Neural Afferents Responding to Thermal
Stimulation of the Skin.

The receptors described in this paper were on the hairy skin
of the human hand. A total of 43 units were isolated from the
superficial branch of the radial nerve and classified according to
conduction velocity, receptive field size and in relation to their
"sensory" and "biophysical" specificity (Hensel, 1973b). Sixteen
units were classified as Type II slowly adapting mechanoreceptors
(Chambers, Andres, Düring, and Iggo, 1972). These units were
spontaneously active in the absence of any stimulus showing a
highly regular discharge of about 10 ± 3.2 imp/sec (SD). Five
units of this sample, i.e., 31 percent were extraordinarily sensitive to cooling of their receptive field. They were excited by
a fall in temperature and the resting discharge was temporarily
depressed when the skin temperature rose. Figure 1 shows the
change in neural activity to cooling the receptive field of a Type
II slowly adapting mechanoreceptor from human hairy skin. A maximum steady-state frequency of discharge of about 6 imp/sec occurred
at a skin temperature between 25° and 30°C. At about 20° to 17°C
the regular discharge ceased and bursts of impulses appeared.

Twenty-two fibers could be identified as warm units. Of
these, 15 had satisfactory signal-to-noise ratios and were held
sufficiently long to record their static and dynamic responses to
intensity-rate series of temperature changes from adapting temperatures between 27° and 49°C. Ten units of this sample were
spontaneously active at skin temperatures between 30.4° and 33.6°C.
(low-threshold units), whereas 5 units started discharging tempera-

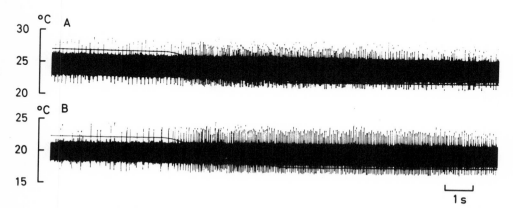

Fig. 1.   Dynamic discharge of a Type II slowly adapting mechano-
          receptor from human hairy skin when cooling the receptive
          field from 27° to 22°C to 17°C (B).

tures of about 35° to 38°C (high-threshold units). Both groups of units were insensitive to mechanical stimuli such as touch, lateral stretching of the skin, vibration or pricking the skin. The receptive fields of the warm units were spot-like areas of about 1 mm². Conduction velocity measurements carried out on 5 units were found to vary between 0.5 and 1.0 m/sec (mean: 0.72 m/sec), indicating that these units were predominantly innervated by C fibers.

Four units showed a response characteristic similar to those of "polymodal nociceptors" (Bessou and Perl, 1969). The units were not spontaneously active and were excited by heating the skin up to the noxious temperature level and by strong mechanical stimuli, e.g., pin-prick or squeezing the skin with small forceps. The threshold of discharge, i.e., the skin temperature at which the first spike appeared in these units, ranged from 40° to 43°C. The receptive fields were round or elliptic areas ranging from 1 to 14 mm² in size. Conduction velocities determined in 3 units were in the range for unmyelinated C fibers (mean: 1.3 m/sec; SD: 0.5 m/sec). One unit showed a response characteristic of a specific cold receptor (Hensel, 1973a).

Steady-state Response of Warn Units to Temperature Stimuli

Specific warm receptors identified in our studies showed a more or less regular static discharge at constant skin termperatures between 30° and 46°C. The individual steady-state frequencies of 6 specific warm units from human hairy skin as a function of the adapting temperature as shown in Fig. 2.

They were not a uniformly sensitive group but there seem to be two major groups similar to those described by Hensel and Iggo (1971) and Sumino, Dubner and Starkman (1973) in the Rhesus monkey. A first group of receptors had threshold responses to constant temperatures at about 30° to 33°C with peak firing rates occurring between 40° and 43°C with 7 and 9 imp/sec, respectively. This group of receptors shows an approximately bell-shaped response characteristic. The second group had threshold responses between 35° and 38°C showing a monotonically increasing discharge rate to increasing temperature. Peak firing rates between 8 and 12 imp/sec occurred at or above 45°C.

Dynamic Response of Warm Units to Temperature Stimuli

In addition to their steady-state response at constant temperatures, warm receptors are characterized by their dynamic response to temperature changes. On sudden warming of the receptive field of a warm unit, the frequency of discharge rises to a maximum, whereas cooling the skin causes a transient inhibition of the discharge. As shown in Fig. 3, linear temperature changes of 1.5° C/sec, starting from adapting temperatures of 27°, 32°, 35° and 37° C caused an overshoot in the frequency of discharge depending on

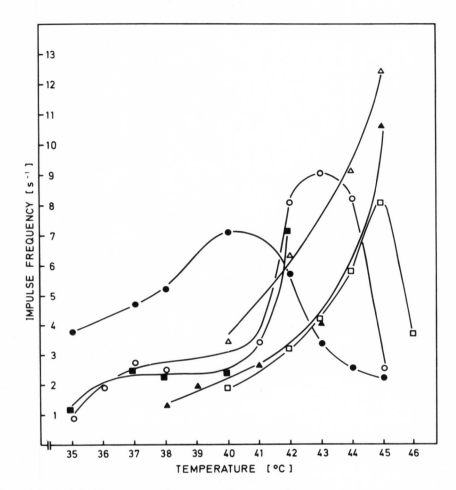

Fig. 2.   Individual steady-state frequencies as a function of the
          adapting temperature of 6 specific warm units from human
          hairy skin

the level of the adapting temperature prior to warming the skin.
When warm fibers are stimulated by a +5°C change in skin temperature
complete adaptation to a new steady-state response level requires
about 30 to 60 seconds but, as Kenshalo and Scott (1966) have
shown, complete adaptation of thermal sensations requires minutes.
A second series of experiments showed that the magnitude of the
dynamic response as seen in Fig. 4, depends on the amount of the
temperature change.   The response magnitude of the warm unit is

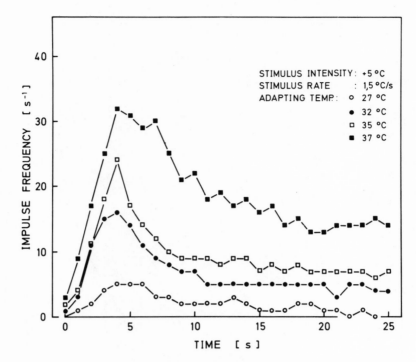

Fig. 3.   Dynamic responses of a single warm unit from hairy skin
          to warming by 5°C at a rate of 1.5°C/sec as a function
          of the temperature to which the receptive field has been
          adapted.

small to a 1°C warming step but increases markedly at higher intensities.

     When using the cumulative number of impulses that occurred
during the rising phase of the stimulus as an index of the dynamic
response magnitude, an approximately linear relationship was found

Fig. 4.   Response of a warm unit to warming the receptive field at
          a rate of 1.5°C/sec by 1, 2, 3, 4, and 5°C (from A to E,
          respectively). Adapting temperature was 32°C. Each dot
          represents the duration of the interval between two suc-
          cessive impulses expressed as instantaneous frequency
          (Sec^{-1}). The arrow on the abscissa indicates the onset
          of the thermal stimulus.

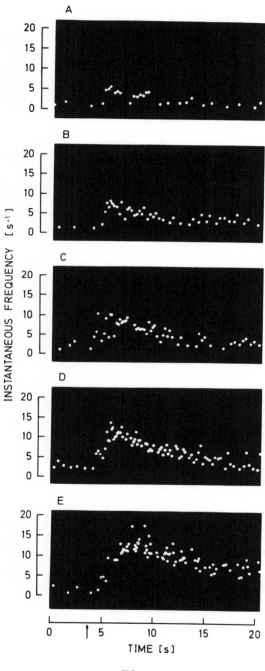

Fig. 4

between the response magnitude and the level to which the skin was
warmed. The results from this experiment for a 32° and 37°C adapting temperatures are shown in Fig. 5.

Neural Encoding of Threshold Warm Sensation

     At skin temperatures between 30° and 34°C some warm receptors
in humans are continuously active but no conscious warm sensation
is present. As proposed by Hensel (1974) the sensation begins when
relatively high number of impulses arrives in the central nervous
system within a certain period of time ("central threshold").

     When the rate of temperature change was systematically varied
at 0.5°, 1.0° and 1.5°C/sec, starting from an adapting temperature
of 32°C, we found that the threshold for the sensation of warmth

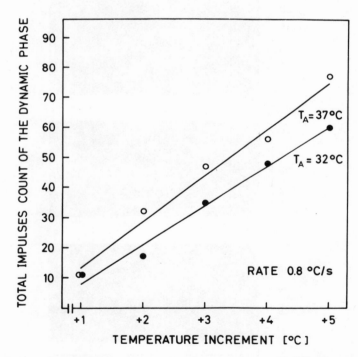

Fig. 5. Comparison between cumulative number of impulses obtained
         during the dynamic phase of response in a single human
         warm unit adapted to either 32° or 37°C as a function of
         stimulus intensity.

remained rather constant (mean: 34.6°C; SD 0.48°C). On the other hand, at slower rates of temperature change, i.e. less than 0.1°C/ sec the threshold systematically increased. The results of this experiment agree well with those reported earlier by Hensel (1950, 1952) and Kenshalo, Holmes, and Wood (1968).

The response peak frequency, the cumulative number of impulses, and the average dynamic frequency evoked during each stimulation of human warm afferents are measures that may be compared to the sensation of warmth at its absolute threshold. Afferent activity recorded in warm units when stimulated with linear rising temperature changes of 0.5° to 1.5°C/sec, starting from a constant skin temperature of 32°C, showed that both the response peak frequency and the cumulative number of impulses did not correlate well with human threshold warm sensation.

Slow rates of temperature change require longer time periods to reach the human threshold of warmth sensation and induce a larger total number of impulses during the temperature increment than do fast changes.

The peak frequencies like the cumulative number of impulses are affected more by increasing the warming rate from 0.5° to 1.5° C/sec where human sensation threshold remains unaltered. On the other hand, the average dynamic frequency provides a much better index for the human threshold warmth sensation. With a mean impulse frequency of 9 ± 0.7 imp/sec (SD) the average dynamic frequency of discharge, like the average sensation threshold of warmth, changes little across stimulation rates between 0.5° and 1.5°C/ sec.

Since no more than one warm spot was excited the threshold of conscious warm sensation ("central threshold"), as expressed by neural parameters, may be smaller than that for a cold sensation (Järvilehto, 1973).

From our observations in man it is very unlikely that slowly adapting mechanoreceptors contribute to thermal sensations. Though they show an apparently bimodal sensitivity (Chambers et al., 1972; Duclaux and Kenshalo, 1972) it appears probable that the significant function of these units is in the tactile domain.

Warm stimulation resulted in a decrease or complete suppression of the steady-state activity of Type II slowly adapting mechanoreceptors and, as former studies in humans have shown, radiant heat applied to the receptive field of Type I slowly adapting mechanoreceptors (Brown and Iggo, 1967) was ineffective in initiating activity. So far our results are similar to those of Duclaux and Kenshalo (1972) for Type I slowly adapting mechanoreceptors in the cat and monkey skin.

Receptors Responsible for Encoding of "Heat" Sensation

One of the most controversial problems in the history of sensory physiology concerns the nature of the physiological process
producing the sensation of "heat", a special sensory quality to be
distinguished from warmth.   Alrutz (1897) has proposed that the
quality of "heat" depends upon excitation of warm receptors and
simultaneously paradoxical excitation of adjacent cold receptors.
Thus "heat", he concluded is a fusion of warmth and cold.   Thunberg
(1896) argued from his observations that the quality of "heat" is
an imperfect fusion in which cold and warmth could still be separately perceived. Goldscheider (1912) on the other hand pointed
out, that in the quality of "heat" there is an additional pain component.   Herget and Hardy (1942) found, that in contrast to
Alrutz's theory, the sensation of "heat" is mediated by its own
receptor type.

When the skin temperature is slowly raised from the zone of
physiological zero (i.e., 30° to 33°C) the subjects first experience a sensation of faint warm, then distinct warm and, with a
further increase of the skin temperature, the subjects reported a
sensation of "heat" at a skin temperature of about 44 to 45°C.
When using a stimulation area of 1 cm^2, this sensation of "heat"
was reported by the subjects to be a non-painful one, except when
the skin temperature was increased beyond the 47°C temperature
level. To explain this non-painful "heat" sensation elicited by
skin temperatures just below 46°C, it would be important to know
which cutaneous afferents are predominantly activated at this
temperature range. The existence of cutaneous afferents with receptors that respond to heating the skin as well as to strong
painful mechanical stimuli has been well established in cats and
monkeys (Zotterman, 1939; Iggo, 1959; Hensel, Iggo and Witt, 1960;
Bessou and Perl, 1969; Iggo and Ogawa, 1971; Beck, Handwerker, and
Zimmermann, 1974; Croze, Duclaux, and Kenshalo, 1976; Handwerker
and Neher, 1976; LaMotte and Campbell, 1978). Units with response
characteristics similar to those of "polymodal nociceptors" were
recently observed in humans (van Hees and Gybels, 1972; Hallin and
Torebjörk, 1974; Torebjörk and Hallin, 1974a;b; Torebjörk, 1974).

In order to obtain more quantitative information about the
response properties of these units a series of controlled heating
of the skin was achieved. The dynamic sensitivity of 4 units
whose responses were similar to those of "polymodal nociceptors"
has been investigated. The experimental series consisted of heating their receptive field of 43°, 45°, 47°, and 49°C, starting from
an adapting temperature of 35°C. Three units were characterized
both by an acceleration of the total number of impulses counted in
the dynamic phase of heating up to 49°C and by the maximum frequency
of impulses. On the contrary, one unit showed a depressed response at 49°C. The results appear in Figs. 6 and 7. Comparable

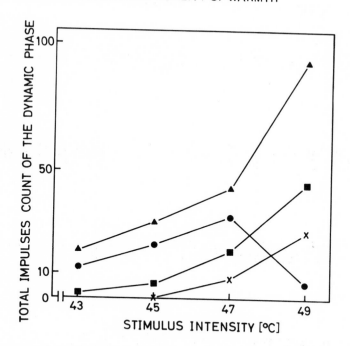

Fig. 6.   At skin temperatures of about 40° to 43°C another class
           of neural afferents was activated which exhibits a re-
           sponse characteristic similar to those of "polymodal no-
           ciceptors" (Bessou and Perl, 1969). Quantitative in-
           formation about the response properties of these units to
           a series of controlled heating of their receptive field
           was achieved.

results have been obtained in monkeys (Beitel and Dubner, 1976;
Croze et al., 1976).

     When temperature shifts into this temperature range were
applied to high-threshold warm units, their afferent discharge was
suddenly inhibited at about 46 to 47°C or, as observed in one case,
the typical pattern of discharge was bursts of impulses of high
frequency. After a sudden suppression of the response at about
47°C this unit started to discharge again irregularly at temperatures up to about 49°C. Handwerker and Neher (1976), who have
described in the cat, receptors with similar response properties,
concluded that these units transmit little quantitative information about noxious temperature levels.

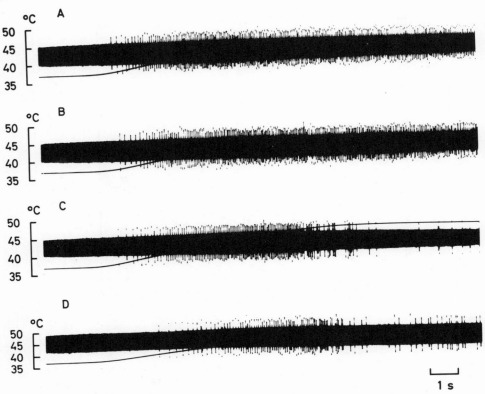

Fig. 7. The possible neural analog for the sensation of "heat" is
        described.

        From out results it seems reasonable to assume that the sen-
sation of non-painful "heat" evoked by thermal stimulation of the
human skin near 46°C is mediated predominantly by high-threshold
warm units. Units with response characteristics similar to "polymodal nociceptors" (Bessou and Perl, 1969) may participate in the
same function since they started responding in the non-noxious
range of heating (40° to 43°C), but vigorous activity was not seen
before 47° to 49°C when burning pain became the dominant sensation.

SUMMARY

1. Quantitative measurements of the steady-state and dynamic response properties of single specific warm fibers innervating human
hairy skin were carried out with tungsten microelectrodes percutaneously inserted in the superficial branch of the radial nerve.

2. Thermal sensations and the responses of primary warm and noci-ceptive fibers were compared in conscious human subjects in order to determine possible neural codes underlying the sensation of warmth and "heat".

3. Within the population of warm receptors two groups could be identified. The first group had threshold responses to constant skin temperatures of about 30°C with peak firing rates occurring at about 40° to 43°C. The second group had threshold responses between 35° and 38°C and peak firing rates occurred at or above 45°C.

4. When stimulated by a + 5°C change in temperature complete adaptation of a warm unit to a new steady-state response level required about 30 to 60 sec.

5. When the rate of temperature change was varied from 0.5° to 1.5° C/sec, starting from an adapting temperature of 32°C, the warmth threshold remained relatively constant (mean: 34.6°C; ±0.48°C SD) as does the average dynamic frequency of discharge in the single warm unit.

6. At skin temperatures of about 40° to 43°C another class of neural afferents was activated which exhibits a response character-istic similar to those of "polymodal nociceptors" (Bessou and Perl, 1969). Quantitative information about the response properties of these units to a series of controlled heating of their receptive field was achieved.

7. The possible neural analog for the sensation of "heat" is des-cribed.

ACKNOWLEDGEMENTS

This research was supported by the Deutsche Forschungsgemin-schaft.

REFERENCES

Alrutz, S. Bidrag till kännedomen om hudens kall - och varmpunkter. Upsala Läkare Förening Förhandlinger, 1897, 2, 246-263.
Beck, P. W. Handwerker, H. E., & Zimmermann, M. Nervous outflow from the cat's foot during noxious radiant heat stimulation. Brain Research, 1974, 67, 373-386.
Beitel, R. E. & Dubner, R. The response of unmyelinated (C) polymodal nociceptors to thermal stimuli applied to the mon-key's face. Journal of Neurophysiology, 1976, 39, 1160-1175.

Bessou, P. & Perl, E. R.   Response of cutaneous sensory units with unmyelinated fibers to noxious stimuli. Journal of Neurophysiology, 1969, 32, 1025-1043.

Blix, M.   Experimentaia bidrag till losning af frågan om hadnervernas specifika energi. I. Upsala Läkare Förening Forhandlinger, 1882-1883, 18, 87-102.

Brown, A. G. & Iggo, A.   A quantitative study of cutaneous receptors and afferent fibres in the cat and rabbit. Journal of Physiology (London), 1967, 193, 707-733.

Chambers, M. R., Andres, K. H., During, M. v., & Iggo, A.   The structure and function of the slowly adapting Type II mechanoreceptor in hairy skin. Quarterly Journal of Experimental Physiology, 1972, 57, 417-445.

Croze, S., Duclaux, R., & Kenshalo, D. R.   The thermal sensitivity of the polymodal nociceptors in the monkey. Journal of Physiology (London), 1976, 263, 539-562.

Darian-Smith, I., Johnson, K. O., & LaMotte, R.   Peripheral neural determinants in the sensing of changes in skin temperature. In H. H. Kornhuber (Ed.), The somatosensory system. Stuttgart: Thieme, 1975.

Duclaux, R. & Kenshalo, D. R.   The temperature sensitivity of the Type I slowly adapting mechanoreceptors in cats and monkeys. Journal of Physiology (London), 1972, 224, 647-664.

Fruhstorfer, H., Zenz, M., Nolte, H., & Hensel, H.   Dissociated loss of cold and warm sensibility during regional anaesthesia. Pflügers Archiv, 1974, 349, 73-82.

Goldscheider, A.   Über die Empfindung der Hitze. Zeitschrift für Klinische Medizin, 1912, 75, 1-14.

Hagbarth, K.E. & Vallbo, Å. B.   Mechanoreceptor activity recorded percutaneously with semi-microelectrodes in human peripheral nerves. Acta Physiologica Scandanavica, 1967, 69, 121-122.

Hallin, R. G. & Torebjörk, H. E.   Activity in unmyelinated nerve fibers in man. In J. J. Bonica (Ed.), Advances in neurology (Vol. 4). New York: Raven Press, 1974.

Hallin, R. G. & Torebjörk, H. E.   Receptors with C fibers responding specifically to warmth in human skin. Proceedings of the International Congress of Physiological Sciences, 27th, Paris, 1977, 301.

Handwerker, H. O. & Neher, K. D.   Characteristics of C-fiber receptors in the cat's foot responding to stepwise increase of skin temperature to noxious levels. Pflügers Archiv, 1976, 365, 221-229.

Hees, J. v. & Gybels, J. M.   Pain related to single afferent C-fibers from human skin. Brain Research, 1972, 48, 397-400.

Hensel, H.   Temperaturempfindung und intracutane Wärmebegwegung. Pflügers Archiv, 1950, 252, 165-215.

Hensel, H.   Physiologie der Thermoreception. Ergebnisse Physiologie, 1952, 47, 166-368.

Hensel, H. Cutaneous thermoreceptors. In A. Iggo (Ed.), Handbook of sensory physiology (Vol. 2) Somatosensory system. Berlin, New York: Springer, 1973a.

Hensel, H. Zur Elektrophysiologie der Hautsinnessysteme unter Berucksichtigung informationstheoretischer Betachtungen. Nova Acta Leopoldina N.F., 1973b, 37, 211-222.

Hensel, H. Thermoreceptors. Annual Review of Physiology, 1974, 36, 233-249.

Hensel, H. Correlations of neural activity and thermal sensation in man. In Y. Zotterman (Ed.), Sensory functions of the skin. Oxford: Pergamon Press, 1976.

Hensel, H. & Boman, K. K. A. Afferent impulses in cutaneous sensory nerves in human subjects. Journal of Neurophysiology, 1960, 23, 564-578.

Hensel, H. & Iggo, A. Analysis of cutaneous warm and cold fibers in primates. Pflügers Archiv, 1971, 329, 1-8.

Hensel, H., Iggo, A., & Witt, I. A quantitative study of sensitive cutaneous thermoreceptors with C afferent fibers. Journal of Physiology (London), 1960, 153, 113-126.

Herget, C. M. & Hardy, J. D. Temperature sensation: The spatial summation of heat. American Journal of Physiology, 1942, 135, 426-429.

Iggo, A. Cutaneous heat and cold receptors with slowly conducting (C) afferent fibers. Quarterly Journal of Experimental Physiology, 1959, 44, 362-370.

Iggo, A. & Ogawa, H. Primate cutaneous thermal nociceptors. Journal of Physiology (London), 1971, 216, 77P-78P.

Järvilehto, T. Neural coding in the temperature senses. Annales Academiae Scientiarum Fennicae; Series B, 1973, 184, 1-71.

Johnson, K. O., Darian-Smith, I., & LaMotte, R. H. Peripheral neural determinants of temperature discrimination in man: A correlative study of responses to cooling skin. Journal of Neurophysiology, 1973, 36, 347-370.

Kenshalo, D. R. Improved method for the psychophysical study of the temperature sense. Review of Scientific Instruments, 1963, 34, 883-886.

Kenshalo, D. R. Phychophysical studies of temperature sensitivity. In W. D. Neff (Ed.), Contribution to sensory physiology, (Vol. 4). New York: Academic Press, 1970.

Kenshalo, D. R. Correlation of temperature sensitivity in man and monkey, a first approximation. In Y. Zotterman (Ed.), Sensory functions of the skin. Oxford: Pergamon Press, 1976.

Kenshalo, D. R., Holmes, C. E., & Wood, P. B. Warm and cool thresholds as a function of rate of stimulus temperature change. Perception and Psychophysics, 1968, 3, 81-83.

Kenshalo, D. R. & Scott, H. H. Temporal course of thermal adaptation. Science, 1966, 151, 1095-1096.

Konietzny, F. & Hensel, H. Hostaflon TF^R coating of tungsten sensory micro-needles. Pflügers Archiv, 1974, 351, 357-360.

Konietzny, F. & Hensel, H. Warm fiber activity in human skin nerves. Pflügers Archiv, 1975, 359, 265-267.

Konietzny, F. & Hensel, H.   Response of rapidly and slowly adapting
    mechanoreceptors and vibratory sensitivity in human hairy
    skin. Pflügers Archiv, 1977a, 368, 39-44.
Konietzny, F. & Hensel, H.   The dynamic response of warm units in
    human skin nerves. Pflügers Archiv, 1977b, 370, 111-114.
Konietzny, F. & Hensel, H.   The static response of human warm re-
    ceptors. Pflügers Archiv, 1978, 373, R90.
LaMotte, R. H. & Campbell, J. N.   Comparison of responses of warm
    and nociceptive C-fiber afferents in monkey with human judge-
    ments of thermal pain. Journal of Neurophysiology, 1978, 41,
    509-528.
Marks, L. E. & Stevens, J. C.   Perceived warmth and skin tempera-
    ture as functions of the duration and level of thermal irra-
    diation. Perception and Psychophysics, 1968, 4, 220-228.
Molinari, H. H. & Kenshalo, D. R.   Effect of cooling rate on the
    dynamic response of cat cold units. Experimental Neurology,
    1977, 55, 546-555.
Stevens, J. C. & Marks, L. E,   Apparent warmth as a function of
    thermal irradiation. Perception and Psychophysics, 1967, 2,
    613-619.
Stevens, J. C. & Marks, L. E.   Spatial summation and the dynamics
    of warmth sensation. Perception and Psychophysics, 1971, 9,
    291-298.
Stevens, J. C. & Stevens, S. S.   Warmth and cold: Dynamics of
    sensory intensity. Journal of Experimental Psychology, 1960,
    60, 183-193.
Sumino, R., Dubner, R., & Starkman, S.   Responses of small myelin-
    ated warm fibers to noxious heat stimuli applied to the mon-
    key's face. Brain Research, 1973, 62, 260-263.
Thunberg, T.   Förnimmelserne vid till samma stälie lokaliserad,
    samtidigt påäende köld - och värmeretning. I. Upsala
    Läkare Förening Förhandlinger, 1896, 2, 489-495.
Torebjörk, H. E.   Afferent C units responding to mechanical, ther-
    mal, and chemical stimuli in human non-glabrous skin. Acta
    Physiologica Scandinavica, 1974, 92, 374-390.
Torebjörk, H. E. & Hallin, R. G.   Activity in C fibers correlated
    to perception in man. In C. Hirsch & Y. Zotterman (Eds.),
    Cervical pain. Oxford: Pergamon Press, 1972.
Torebjörk, H. E. & Hallin, R. G.   Responses in human A and C fibers
    to repeated electrical intradermal stimulation. Journal of
    Neurology, Neurosurgery and Psychiatry, 1974a, 37, 653-664.
Torebjörk, H. E. & Hallin, R. G.   Identification of afferent C units
    in intact human skin nerves. Brain Research, 1974b, 67, 387-
    404.
Vendrik, A. J. H.   Psychophysics of the thermal sensory system and
    statistical detection theory. In J. D. Hardy, A. P. Gagge,
    & J. A. J. Stolwijk. Physiological and behavioral tempera-
    ture regulation. Springfield: Ill: Thomas, 1970.
Zotterman, Y.   Touch, pain and tickling: An electrophysiological
    investigation on cutaneous sensory nerves. Journal of Phy-
    siology (London), 1939, 95, 1-28.

DISCUSSION

DR. DUCLAUX: I have two questions. First, do you have any explanations for the fact that some SA II receptors do not respond
to cooling? The second question is: You show a relationship
during the dynamic change in temperature between the number of
spikes and the temperature change. Are you suggesting that the
central nervous system is using this as a code of the dynamic
change?

DR. KONIETZNY: The first question is I think very difficult. I
have seen recordings of receptors that I thought were depressed in
activity when warming their receptive fields and we have seen that
some populations were excited when the temperature falls. We do
not know what the reason for this could be. We have started to
build a new experimental setup in order to establish whether these
cold sensitive SA II receptors have a functional property in terms
of singalling cold sensation, as we have discussed this morning.
We are collaborating with Professor Andres at Bochum and we are
going to investigate the relationships between the electrophysiological response, the sensation of the subject, and the
anatomical structure of this type of receptor. Perhaps, we can
find something that may be due to the cold activity.

DR. DUCLAUX: Are you suggesting that the central nervous system
is using this as a signal to judge the amount of temperature change?

DR. KONIETZNY: I think the sensation magnitude might be encoded
by the number of spikes during the temperature change.

DR. IGGO: I would like to express a certain amount of disappointment. You are presenting results that I presume are from non-
myelinated afferent fibers and nobody seems to be excited. It
seems to me to be quite a remarkable technical achievement that we
can now sit around in a room like this and quietly and calmly
accept the fact that it is possible to record from human C-fibers.
It is encouraging to see that their responses are rather similar to
those in subhuman animals. But I would like to ask you why you
have so few cold fibers?

DR. KONIETZNY: It might be that the warm receptors I have shown
were unmyelinated and, one knows from other experiments, that cold
fibers were also unmyelinated. One should expect to find these as
well in the same population, but it depends on the point of view
when one starts an experiment. When we started the experiment with
the rapidly adapting mechanoreceptors we concentrated only on this
fiber type. This might be the reason that we have found very few
(2) cold receptors, at least. Perhaps, in the future when we
intend to find cold receptors we will.

DR. IGGO: But, my point is that in subhuman primates there are
non-myelinated cold fibers. However, at least half the population
of the myelinated axons in a peripheral human nerve are below about
5 μm in diameter. They have conduction velocities from say 30 m/
sec down to 5 m/sec. We know from the monkey experiments that
there are a very large numbers of cold afferent units that have
conduction velocities with a peak around about 9 msec, indicating
that they are about 2 μm in diameter, and, hence, are myelinated
fibers. It is very surprising that, working in Dr. Hensel's
laboratory, you should fail to find any cold fibers. It is quite
likely looking at your records, that the cold fibers that you have
shown us actually had non-myelinated axons. We still have this
awkard problem of why this marvelous new technique should be able
to record from the large myelinated afferent fibers and from non-
myelinated afferent fibers, yet seems to miss all the smaller
myelinated fibers. This is really what puzzles me. Is there
something about the technique that could account for this? After
all, the unit that you showed did not have the characteristic
well-marked grouping of impulses that one sees in the subhuman
cold fibers. It could be, of course, as Dr. Hensel showed with
Dr. Boman, a long time ago, that perhaps man is really different
from the monkey after all.

DR. KONIETZNY: Well, I can only guess based on the results of the
warm units. We have found that they tend to lie in small bundles,
close together. I have often found that when I isolated one warm
fiber and I penetrated deeper within this bundle, I found more
than one lying close together. That might be the reason for this.

DR. JÄRVILEHTO: I just wanted to confirm what Dr. Konietzny said.
It depends somewhat on what one looks for in the nerve. We had
the same experience also, in that when we found our first cold
fiber, then we found the second. Most people who have worked in
cats, see that the fibers seem to be organized in certain bundles.

DR. IGGO: But still half the myelinated axons are less than 5 μm
in diameter yet there are so few recordings from them.

DR. HENSEL: There is no really satisfactory explanation yet as to
why you get so few cold fibers with the microelectrodes. I often
wonder if I should not return to our old technique of nerve dissection in human subjects to get more insight into the discharge
of the cold fibers. One possible explanation might be that they
are concentrated in certain bundles. This is the case in the
warm fibers of humans and in the monkey the warm fibers also seem
to be concentrated. Once you happen to have a preparation with one
fiber, there might be several more warm fibers. This is just
speculation, of course, and I have no satisfactory answer yet about
these strange results.

DR. PERL: We used quite a different microelectrode technique in animals, and our experimental protocols show that one day several cold fibers would be found and then ten experiments later another would finally appear. Yet about the same number of elements were sampled each time. We have always suspected, without a shred of proof, that there is a sort of congregation of elements within the peripheral nerve bundles or the dorsal roots. There does seem to be some peculiarity in the distribution of elements within a given bundle. In our dissection experiments, a number of peripheral nerves also evidenced a congregation of cold fibers in the C-fiber range. There was a definite tendency for the elements to appear together. I suspect that is at least part of the explanation.

When Professor Iggo stood up a moment ago, I thought he was going to bring up something else, because the initial question was related to the SA II mechanoreceptor fiber and temperature. It seems to me that we ought to consider his view of some time ago. He seemed to have retired the issue of such mechanoreceptors having a role in temperature sensibility, for several reasons: their responses to maintained temperature are notably poor, on the average; their responses are more phasic than seems appropriate for temperature sensibility, as Dr. Konietzny just mentioned; and many do not respond to thermal stimuli, even with rather dramatic shifts in temperature. If they do respond, it is very weakly, though an exceptional few respond vigorously. I believe that was the same way they were first described by Witt and Hensel in 1959 .

DR. IGGO: The fact that you get 1/3 of your SA II population to respond to temperature change probably has the explanation that I seem to remember giving at a symposium in Utah in 1960. The question was raised about the effect of temperature on some cut- aneous receptors. The explanation seemed to me to lie in the accessibility of the receptor to the temperature change. If you have an SA I receptor, where the terminals are very close to the surface of the skin, within 40 to 50 µm, then the temperature change applied on the surface will reach these terminals very quickly. On the other hand, when you are dealing with the SA II receptors, and particularly in human skin where you have a much greater depth of tissue, the temperature change may not actually penetrate so readily to these tissues, particularly, if you have a conscious human subject who has a good blood flow through the skin that is resisting the temperature change that you impose. So I suspect that this, in part, may underlie the fact that some of these receptors fail to react to the temperature change. But, as I said here in 1966, the SA II are spurious thermoreceptors.

REFERENCES

Witt, I., & Hensel, H. Äfferente Impulse aus der Extremitätenhaut der Katze bei thermischer und mechanischer Reizung. Pflügers Archiv, 1959, 268, 582-596.

PROBLEMS OF CORRELATING CUTANEOUS SENSATION WITH NEURAL EVENTS IN MAN

Herbert Hensel and Frithjof Konietzny

Institute of Physiology, University of Marburg

3550 Marburg, Germany

Modern sensory physiology includes various experimental approaches that can be symbolized by a triadic relationship (Fig. 1): 1. The phenomenological analysis of sensory phenomena (P). These objects are non-conceptual parts of experience constituted by the method of analytical reduction. 2. The measurement of the so-called stimuli (S), e.g., physical events. 3. The investigation of neural events (N) in the sensory channels, mainly by electrophysiological methods. In a wider sense, physiological and behavioral methods belong to this category as well.

The correlation between P-S is investigated by what is called in classical terms "psychophysics". This term reflects the Galilean-Cartesian dichotomy between subject and object, postulating that sensory phenomena are purely subjective - a view that is obsolete in modern sensory science. Therefore I prefer the more adequate term "phenophysics". The relationship P-N is investigated by phenophysiology ("psychophysiology") and S-N by the so-called objective sensory physiology. The latter does not include any immediate sensation but deals with conceptual objects of positive sciences, such as physics or physiology.

A direct comparison of the total triadic relationship between sensory phenomenon, physical stimulus and neural event has become possible when recordings from human cutaneous nerve fibers were achieved, either by nerve dissection (Hensel and Boman, 1960) or by microelectrodes (Hagbarth and Vallbo, 1967; Knutsson and Widén, 1967). More recently this technique has been improved in several respects (Konietzny and Hensel, 1974).

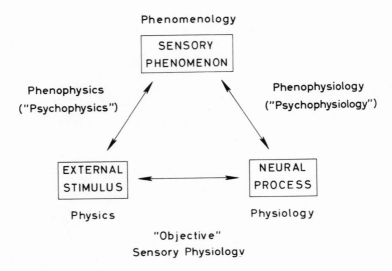

Fig. 1.   Relationship between sensory phenomenon, physical stimulus
          and neural event.

Since cutaneous nerves consist of fibers of various size and
functional significance, it is difficult to decide whether the
neuronographic recordings give a true picture of the neural activity involved in a particular cutaneous sensation (cf. Järvilehto,
1977). When recording from a whole nerve or a larger fascicle, no
detailed information of the ongoing activity can be obtained; in
particular, action potentials from small fibers may be masked by
potentials from larger ones.

On the other hand, when recording from single fibers, one has
to rely on statistical samples of fiber populations that can be
biased by preparation and recording techniques. Even when using
spot-like stimuli confined to the receptive field of a single fiber,
additional fibers may be involved in sensation, particularly in the
range of higher intensities. However, in spite of these difficulties, considerable progress has been made during the last decade.

While the specificity of cutaneous receptors was originally defined in terms of "phenomenal" specificity, as established by phenophysical experiments, neuronographic recording from single units
has made it possible to investigate also the question of "biophysical" specificity as defined by the response of cutaneous units
to various qualities of stimuli (Fig. 2).

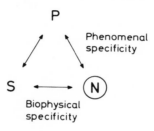

Fig. 2. Concepts of specificity. P are sensory phenomena, S external stimuli, and N neural processes.

Although both concepts of specificity are closely related, they are not identical, the criterion being the quality of a sensory phenomenon (P) in the first case and the quality of a physical stimulus (S) in the second case. Since the basic units of physics are arbitrarily defined without regard to immediate sensory qualities, it is not surprising that both definitions of specificity may differ considerably. A clear distinction between both concepts is necessary, in particular when a receptor responds to more than one kind of physical stimulus. For example, certain cutaneous receptors are excited both by mechanical stimulation and by cooling. Thus they are bimodal receptors with regard to the physical stimulus, but they may be unimodal in terms of the quality of sensation.

A number of cutaneous receptors in man are specific in the phenomenal as well as in the biophysical sense. This holds for various types of mechanosensitive units, such as hair follicles (Hensel and Boman, 1960), RA and PC units (Knibestöl, 1973, 1975; Johansson, 1976; Järvilehto, 1977; Konietzny and Hensel, 1977b) and SA 1-units (Knibestöl and Vallbo, 1976). Furthermore, specific cold and warm fibers are now well established (Hensel and Boman, 1960; Konietzny and Hensel, 1975, 1977a).

On the other hand, numerous nonmyelinated units have been found that respond to more intense mechanical stimuli, heat and chemical irritants (van Hees and Gybels, 1972; Torebjörk, 1974; Torebjörk and Hallin, 1976; van Hess, 1976) and thus classified as "multimodal receptors". From phenophysical experiments it is concluded that these units mediate pain and possibly itch. An unsolved problem is the neural correlate of "heat" and heat pain. Are there specific fibers mediating these sensory qualities, or is the neural correlate an across-fiber pattern of various types of receptors? Besides the "multimodal nociceptors" excited by heat, afferent fibers have recently been found in human skin that respond specifically to heating in the temperature range correlated with the sensation of "heat" (Konietzny and Hensel, this Symposium).

A bimodal response to cutaneous stimulation is found in certain SA II receptors. About one third of this group in humans is excited by pressure as well as by cooling the skin (Hensel and Boman, 1969; Konietzny and Hensel, unpublished). Although the sensory qualities mediated by the bimodal SA 2 receptors are not yet known, we may assume that they are pressure rather than cold sensations.

It may be mentioned that so far no identification of any cutaneous receptor in humans has been achieved by direct combination of phenophysical, neurological and electron microscopical methods.

Which number or frequency of impulses from the periphery corresponds to a conscious threshold sensation? The general assumption is that sensory channels are noisy systems and that a larger number of afferent impulses is the necessary condition for a threshold sensation. The signal detection theory considers this as a statistical problem of the signal-to-noise-ratio.

This general view should be revised because there is strong evidence now for the hypothesis (Hensel and Boman, 1960) that a single mechanosensitive fiber may be correlated with a conscious threshold sensation, as shown by the coincidence of single fiber impulses from mechanoreceptors in the human finger and reported sensations (Vallbo and Johansson, 1976). On the other hand, a certain level of activity in slowly adapting mechanoreceptors, cold and warm receptors may occur at subconscious levels. For a single warm receptor, about 10 impulses/sec are the correlate of a conscious warm threshold (Konietzny and Hensel, this Symposium), while the neural correlate of conscious cold sensations, as concluded from comparisons between cat and man, may be in the order of 80 impulses/sec when stimulating a single cold spot (Järvilehto, 1973).

Direct comparisons between vibratory sensations and the activity of single RA receptors have been made during vibratory stimulations of the skin (Konietzny & Hensel, 1977b). The thresholds of "flutter" sensations in the low frequency range corresponded with the tuning curves (threshold of 1 impulse in a single fiber per cycle of vibration) of RA receptors, the optima being between 20 and 40 Hz, whereas the thresholds for vibratory sensations decreased with frequency towards the range about 100 Hz (Fig. 3). The vibratory thresholds in this range were much lower than the thresholds of the RA fibers, so that this group can be excluded as the correlate of vibratory sensations at higher frequencies. In this range the sensations of vibration may be conveyed mainly by PC-fibers with tuning optima above 100 Hz (Järvilehto, Hämäläinen and Laurinen, 1976).

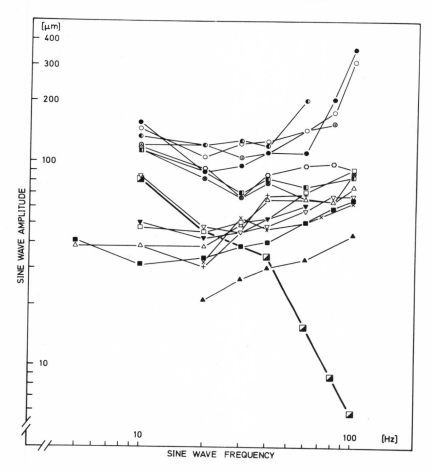

Fig. 3.   Tuning curves of various RA fibers from the human hand
          and average threshold of vibratory sensation (heavy line)
          from the same receptive field. From Konietzny and Hensel
          (unpublished).

     Particularly interesting is the relationship of neural events
and phenomenal magnitude of sensation. As far as temperature sensation is concerned, there is an almost linear correlation between
the magnitude of warming the skin and the overshoot in impulse
frequency of single warm fibers (Fig. 4), while the phenomenal
magnitude of warmth was found to be a power function of the magnitude of warming area (3.7 to 200 cm^2) and body region. The
exponent increased with decreasing stimulus area (Stevens, Marks
and Simonson, 1974).

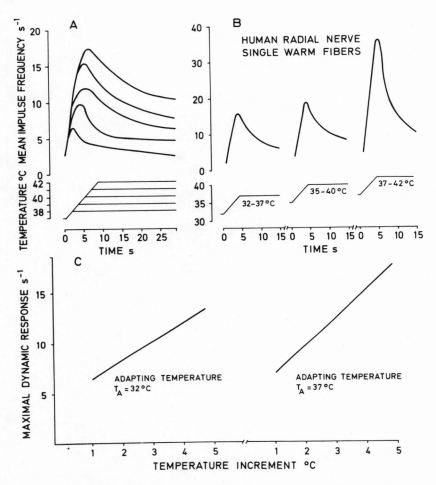

Fig. 4.   A: Average impulse frequencies of a single warm unit from
hairy skin when applying linear temperature changes of
constant rate (dT/dt = 0.8°C/s) and various magnitude
(ΔT = 1, 2, 3, 4, and 5°C). Adapting temperature T_A =
37°C.
B: Impulse frequencies of a single warm unit and skin
temperature when applying linear temperature changes of
constant rate (dT/dt = 1.5°C/s) and equal magnitude (ΔT =
+5°C). Adapting temperature T_A = 32, 35, 37°C.
C: Maximal dynamic response of the same unit as shown in
A. Adapting temperature T_A = 32 and 37°C. From Konietzny
and Hensel (1977a).

Recently we have studied the sustained temperature sensations when applying constant temperatures to the hand (Beste and Hensel, 1977; Beste, 1977). More quantitative data on human cold receptor activity are needed for a satisfactory correlation, but the results in monkeys (Dykes, 1975) show that in the lower temperature range neither the average frequency of the static discharge of a cold receptor population nor the parameters of the burst discharge can account for the curve of static cold sensation (Fig. 5 and 6). For example, the phenomenal static differential sensitivity at 25°C is zero, whereas the differential sensitivity of burst parameters is positive. Furthermore, at 16°C the phenomenal differential sensitivity is positive, that of the average discharge negative, and

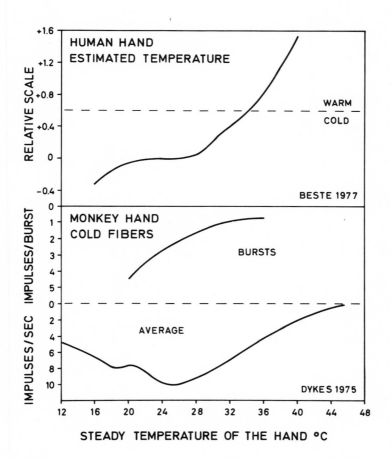

Fig. 5.   Estimated steady temperature of the hand in man, impulses/
           burst of the burst discharge and average frequency of a
           population of cold fibers in the hand of monkeys as
           function of steady skin temperature.

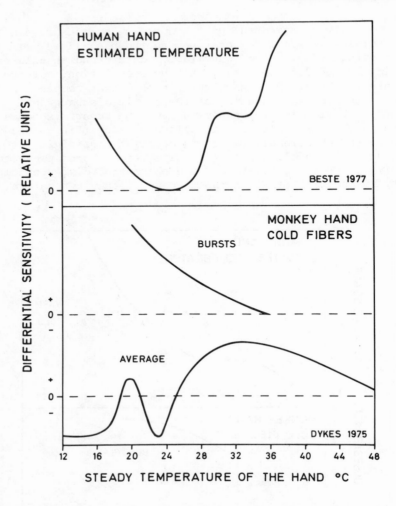

Fig. 6. Static differential sensitivity of estimated temperature
of the hand in man, burst parameters and average frequency of a population of cold fibers in the hand of
monkeys as function of steady skin temperature.

there is no regular burst discharge at this temperature. An additional argument against the significance of the burst parameters
for static cold sensations in the low temperature range is the fact
that these parameters are not conveyed to the second order neuron
(Dostrovsky and Hellon, 1978). Possibly the neural correlate of
static cold sensations at low temperatures may be an across-fiber
pattern rather than an average frequency (Hensel, 1976).

In Fig. 7 the neural activity of single RA and SA units (Gybels and van Hees, 1972) and of single SA I units (Knibestöl and Vallbo, 1976) is correlated with the estimated magnitude of sensation in a double logarithmic plot. For one series of experiments the results can be described by a power function with an exponent of 1.0, indicating a linear relationship between neural response and phenomenal magnitude, whereas the correlation in the other series does not follow a power function or at least a power function with a much higher exponent.

However, there are some general problems that should be considered in connection with such correlations:

1. It cannot be excluded that with increasing intensity additional receptors may be excited that contribute to the magnitude of sensation but do not show in the single fiber record.

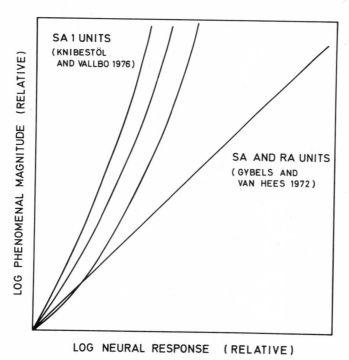

Fig. 7.   Correlation between neural response and phenomenal magnitude for various mechanosensitive fibers in human skin.

2.   In contrast to objects of classical physics, sensory objects are not independent of observation, underlying unpredictable changes with the observer's intention. Therefore the correlation between neural response and phenomenal magnitude may vary in one and the same subject as well as between different subjects.

3.   The construction of sensory power functions is based on the assumption that the scale of phenomenal magnitude is a rational scale (Stevens, 1970). This is a postulate rather than an empirical fact. As Russell (1920) said, "The method of postulating what we want has many advantages. They are the same as the advantage of theft over honest toil". If the structure of estimated magnitude were represented by a rational scale, it should follow the axioms of multiplication, with commutativity, associativity and distributivity:

$$ab = ba \qquad \text{commutativity}$$
$$m(na) = (mn)a \qquad \text{associativity}$$
$$ma+mb = m(a+b) \qquad \text{distributivity}$$
$$(m+n)a = ma+na$$

To my knowledge, this has not yet been tested experimentally. Therefore the question of phenomenal magnitude and its neural correlates needs further research both from the aspect of phenomenology and neurophysiology.

SUMMARY

By recording afferents from human cutaneous nerves, the triadic relationships between sensory phenomenon, neural event and physical stimulus can be directly investigated. As cutaneous nerves consist of fibers with various properties, only single fiber analysis can give detailed information. However, the differentiation of single fiber populations may be biased by preparation and recording techniques.

Certain mechanosensitive, warm sensitive and cold sensitive fibers in man are phenomenally and biophysically specific, while the function of cold-sensitive SA receptors and the neural correlate of heat sensation, heat and cold pain and other nociceptive sensations need still to be clarified.

The neural correlates of threshold sensations may be a single impulse in a single mechanosensitive fiber, a few impulses/sec for a single warm fiber and about 80 impulses/sec for a cold fiber. Flutter sensations in the low frequency range are mediated by RA receptors and vibratory sensations preferably by PC units. No satisfactory neural correlate is known for the static thermal sensation.

The question of phenomenal magnitude of intensity and its neural correlate needs further research both from phenomenological and neurophysiological aspects. As yet the structure of phenomenal intensity scales is not clear since these scales are based on postulates that are not experimentally verified.

ACKNOWLEDGEMENTS

Supported by the Deutsche Forschungsgemeinschaft

REFERENCES

Beste, R. Perzeption statischer thermischer Reize beim Menschen. Inaug.-Diss. Marburg, 1977.

Beste, R., & Hensel, H. Subjective estimation of static temperature at the palm in humans. Pflügers Archiv, 1977, 368, Suppl., R47.

Dostrovsky, J. O., & Hellon, R. F. The representation of facial temperature in the caudal trigeminal nucleus of the cat. Journal of Physiology (London), 1978, 277, 29-47.

Dykes, R. W. Coding of steady and transient temperatures by cutaneous 'cold' fibers serving the hand of monkeys. Brain Research, 1975, 98, 485-500.

Gybels, J., & Hees, J. van. Unit activity from mechanoreceptors in human peripheral nerve during intensity discrimination of touch. In G.G. Somjen (Ed.) Neurophysiology studied in man. Intern. Congr. Series, No. 253. Amsterdam: Excerpta Med., 1972.

Hagbarth, K.-E., & Vallbo, A. B. Mechanoreceptor activity recorded percutaneously with semi-microelectrodes in human peripheral nerves. Acta Physiologica Scandinavica, 1967, 69, 121-122.

Hees, J. van. Single afferent C fiber activity in the human nerve during painful and non-painful skin stimulation with radiant heat. In Y. Zotterman (Ed.), Sensory functions of the skin in primates (Vol.27). Oxford: Pergamon Press, 1976.

Hees, J. van., & Gybels, J. M. Pain related to single afferent C fibers from human skin. Brain Research, 1972, 48, 397-400.

Hensel, H. Correlations of neural activity and thermal sensation in man. In Y. Zotterman (Ed.), Sensory functions of the skin in primates (Vol.27). Oxford: Pergamon Press, 1976.

Hensel, H., & Boman, K.K.A. Afferent impulses in cutaneous sensory nerves in human subjects. Journal of Neurophysiology, 1960, 23, 564-578.

Järvilehto, T. Neural coding in the temperature sense. Human reactions to temperature changes as compared with activity in single peripheral cold fibers in the cat. Annales Academiae Scientiarum Fennicae; Series B, 1973, 184, 1-71.

Järvilehto, T. Neural basis of cutaneous sensations analyzed by microelectrode measurements from human peripheral nerves--a review. Scandinavian Journal of Psychology, 1977, 18, 348-359.

Järvilehto, T., Hämäläinen, H., & Laurinen, P.   Characteristics of
    single mechanoreceptive fibres innervating hairy skin of the
    human hand. Experimental Brain Research, 1976, 25, 45-61.
Johansson, R. S.   Receptive field sensitivity profile of mechano-
    sensitive units innervating the glabrous skin of the human
    hand. Brain Research, 1976, 104, 330-334.
Knibestöl, M.   Stimulus-response functions of rapidly adapting
    mechanoreceptors in the human glabrous skin area. Journal of
    Physiology (London), 1973, 232, 427-452.
Knibestöl, M.   Stimulus-response functions of slowly adapting
    mechanoreceptors in the human glabrous skin area. Journal of
    Physiology (London), 1975, 245, 63-80.
Knibestöl, M., & Vallbo, A. B.   Stimulus-response functions of
    primary afferents and psychophysical intensity estimation on
    mechanical skin stimulation in the human hand. In Y. Zotterman
    (Ed.), Sensory functions of the skin in primates (Vol.27).
    Oxford: Pergamon Press, 1976.
Knutsson, E., & Widén, L.   Impulses from single nerve fibers in man
    using microelectrodes. Nature, 1967, 213, 606-607.
Konietzny, F., & Hensel, H. Hostaflon TF coating of tungsten sen-
    sory microneedles. Pflügers Archiv, 1974, 351, 357-360.
Konietzny, F., & Hensel, H.   Warm fiber activity in human skin
    nerves. Pflügers Archiv, 1975, 359, 265-267.
Konietzny, F., & Hensel, H.   The dynamic response of warm units in
    human skin nerves. Pflügers Archiv, 1977a, 370, 111-114.
Konietzny, F., & Hensel, H.   Response of rapidly and slowly adapting
    mechanoreceptors and vibratory sensitivity in human hairy skin.
    Pflügers Archiv, 1977b, 368, 39-44.
Russell, B.   Introduction to mathematical philosophy, 2nd ed.
    New York: Macmillan, 1920.
Stevens, J. C., Marks, L. E., & Simonson, D. C.   Regional sensiti-
    vity and spatial summation in the warmth sense. Physiology
    and Behavior, 1974, 13, 825-836.
Stevens, S. S.   Neural events and the psychophysical law. Power
    functions like those that govern subjective magnitude show
    themselves in neuroelectric effects. Science, 1970, 170,
    1043-1050.
Torebjörk, H. E.   Afferent C units responding to mechanical, thermal
    and chemical stimuli in human non-glabrous skin. Acta Physio-
    logica Scandinavica, 1974, 92, 374-390.
Torebjörk, H. E., & Hallin, R. G.   Skin receptors supplied by un-
    myelinated (C) fibers in man. In Y. Zotterman (Ed.), Sensory
    functions of the skin in primates (Vol.27). Oxford: Pergamon
    Press, 1976.
Vallbo, A. B., & Johansson, R.   Skin mechanoreceptors in the human
    hand: Neural and psychophysical thresholds. In Y. Zotterman
    (Ed.), Sensory functions of the skin in primates (Vol.27).
    Oxford: Pergamon Press, 1976.

DISCUSSION

DR. ZOTTERMAN: Well, Herbert, first of all in your Fig. 5, you must understand that the subject has warm and cold fibers and these warm fibers act antagonistically to the cold ones so there must be a discrepancy.

DR. HENSEL: Yes, but I refer to this part of the curve (points to the left half of the figure) where only cold fibers are active. I want to discuss warm fibers, but as you see here, this is just the range of skin temperatures where practically no warm fibers are active, and this is just the range where you have the biggest discrepancy between sensation and any known peripheral neural activity.

DR. ZOTTERMAN: Yes, but when you consider taste, there we found that the relation between the summated electrical response and the stimulus strength in the human chorda tympany nerve always has the same function; that of the perceptual response. How could it be otherwise? If this information comes into the brain it must be so.

DR. LaMOTTE: I was wondering if you know of the unmyelinated and thinly myelinated fibers that a fellow named Georgopoulos (1977) described recently in the monkey that showed a nearly linear increase in the number of impulses evoked with increases in cooling over the range of 30° to 15°C, which is as low as he could go. They might contribute to cold sensation.

DR. HENSEL: Yes, and I think in this context one should also mention another finding that the population of cold fibers, for example in the cat's nose, seem to be distributed very inhomogeniously. There seem to be different subpopulations of cold fibers and it might be possible that the intensity of cold sensation, and perhaps the quality has something to do with different populations. One interesting point was that practically all subjects reported, not only a change in the intensity in the lower temperature range, but also a change in quality. That means that the cold sensations became relatively sharp or ice-cold, almost painful. It might be that the scale of cold temperatures is not only a matter of intensity but perhaps also of quality. Unfortunately, in human subjects, we have too little information about that as yet. At least from the cat one can conclude that there must be different populations of cold fibers. The distribution is not random.

DR. JOHANSSON: There was one thing I recalled when you discussed the problem of coding in the cold fiber population. You are referring to units, I suppose, just units which have receptive fields located under the stimulus probe. However, there should be a number of cold units stimulated by the temperature gradient with the distance from the probe. Units under the probe would respond a certain amount, but the unit located close to the probe, but not under it, may have less cold stimulation and would respond; to that amount, and so on. You would then have a continuous distribution of unit responses and this will follow the decrease and increase in the temperature of the probe.

DR. HENSEL: In the experiments on human static cold sensation, we had a large thermode covering the whole palm of the hand, so it is not a matter of a gradient. Also we waited until the whole temperature was absolutely constant, as I said for at least half an hour, but of course you could be right if you use a smaller stimulator. In the other experiments we even put the whole hand into constant temperature water bath, so there is no local temperature gradient from the center to adjacent cold receptors, or didn't I understand you correctly?

DR. JOHANSSON: You will always have a gradient, and the larger the stimulus area, the larger is the edge around the area and the larger is the unit population within this gradient.

DR. HENSEL: Yes, that's why by putting the hand into water, you have only a gradient at the wrist, but the temperature sensation comes very distinctly from the hand. I do not think it's a matter of the few cold receptors around the wrist.

DR. FRANZÉN: I have a couple of comments. First, as to the correlation between neural discharge on the detection threshold; we have run a lot of experiments on the primary cortical potential in humans evoked by tactile stimuli applied to the pad of the finger tip. We also obtained magnitude estimations to the same stimuli in the same subjects at the same time. When we plotted the estimates as a function of the peak to peak value of the primary component in microvolts, we always got a negative intercept so when the sensation was zero, there is a response in the cortex (Franzén, 1970). This was for touch. I will present data later for the visual system, where we looked at the contrast response, in humans, to gratings. The relationship was the same, again we got a negative intercept of the same sort. These results are very consistent with one another, and it obviously points to the conclusion that there is some activity in the brain in response to a stimulus although you may not experience any sensation. So, that means there must be more than one spike from the periphery.

To answer you second question, I agree there is a lot to be done with respect to methodology in psychophysics, and especially when we are dealing with correlations. Here, you have put your finger on a sensitive point and that is whether we are dealing with a ratio scale in our estimates. Is there any real indication of having ratio data? I have one example, and will go back to my touch data where I stimulated the index and middle fingers. I can stimulate them at the same time or I can stimulate only one. The input there is 2 to 1. Then I ask the subject to estimate how much of an increment they left when I go from one finger to two (Franzén, 1969; Franzén and Offenloch, 1969). The subjective response for two fingers over one was the square root of two.

I have data of magnitude from estimates of warm sensations starting from an adapting temperature of 40°C and you stimulate from 40° to 47°C. You find the slope between 40° and 43°C is about 1, but then it goes up steeply. At this point, the subject says that it begins to become hot or painful. Of course, 47°C is painful they say, "it's burning, take it away." So it is interesting that here you see power transformation as though another system is brought in, like the C-fibers and the Aδ fibers.

DR. STEVENS: I think I should have an opportunity here. The 1960 study referred to was the first scaling study of temperature using magnitude estimation and, as you say, we got an exponent of about 1.6 for warm and about 1 for cold. Very modestly at the end of that first foray into the temperature field Smitty Stevens and I said, "You know, this is only one condition of stimulation, (little temperature contactors, about 3 cm^2, and one of the things that might matter is size." So we set out since then, at the Pierce foundation, to explore the role of the size of the field for warmth, and it turns out that there is no one power function for warmth, but a whole family of functions, whose constants depend on the area of the stimulator. These incorporate the laws of spatial summation governing warmth. The functions converge and in all cases the point of convergence turns out to be the threshold of thermal pain where there is no spatial summation. I would just like to add that even if these are not rational scales they are clearly different for different areas. The point being that I do not think we can explain the growth rate of warmth solely in peripheral terms, because we must take into account complex central interactions. Now in the case for cold, which we have only recently looked at, and which has also been looked at in Dr. Kenshalo's laboratory, the exponent is constant and the intercept of the function varies, depending on the area; the bigger the area, the colder the sensation, but the growth rate seems to be the same. Again, whether these are ratio scales or not, they are the same, in contrast to warmth.

DR. HENSEL: I agree completely with you and, in particular, I think it is very important to always mention the particular conditions under which you are using such scales. Of course, it

is not possible to compare one condition directly with another.
There is one interesting thing. We did some recent experiments
to investigate the influence of the general thermal state of the
body to local thresholds. We found that there is more influence
on the warm side for warm sensation than for cold sensation. This
has some resemblance to your two types of curves.

May I make a final comment to Dr. Franzén's remarks? I think
the main question now is to investigate the structure of this scale
in the purely phenomenal range. Not by comparing it with impulses
or stimuli, but the phenomenal structure. For example, you could
test the axiom of commutativity estimating, say, phenomenal
magnitude three times a given magnitude and another two times this
magnitude, and then reverse it. Take two times and then three
times and you must arrive at the same magnitude of intensity, and
so on. This sort of experiment, to my knowledge, hasn't been done
yet using the whole range of these rational axioms. I think it
would be very important to continue with these experiments in
order to find out the structure of this scale but only if the
structure on the abscissa and on the ordinate are identical
structures in the mathematical sense, you can make such a plot.

DR. POULOS: Dr. Iggo has a closing comment.

DR. IGGO: I am not closing the discussion. I am just trying to
drag you back to the real world, and away from the epiphenomenal
world. You have suggested that some of the problems in relation
to cold sensation may be related to different populations of cold
receptors responding in different ways. I really just wanted to
give you the opportunity to put into the record your own experimental experience in recording from second order or third order
cold neurons which I believe you have been doing, and whether you
have any evidence from these experiments which would support this
idea that you have separate populations of cold receptors. Unless
these separate populations of cold receptors are feeding into
different central neuronal pools, then of course, it all gets
smothered out and there is no advantage. Do you have any such
evidence from your experiments?

DR. HENSEL: No, not yet.

REFERENCES

Franzén, O. Neural activity in the somatic primary receiving area
        of the human brain and its relation to perceptual estimates.
        International conference on tactile displays at Stanford Re-
        search Institute (SRI), Menlo Park, Calif., U.S.A., April,
        1969, Special issue of the IEEE Transactions on Man-Machine
        System,. MMS-II ($\underline{I}$), 1970, 115-117.

Franzén, O. & Offenloch, K.   Perceived contrast at low spacial fre-
     quencies of frog and man: A neurophysiological study.
     Scandinavian Journal of Psychology, 10, in preparation.
Franzén, O. & Offenloch, K.   Evoked response correlates of psycho-
     physical magnitude estimates for tactile stimulation in man.
     Experimental Brain Research, 1969, 8, 1-18.
Georgopoulos, A. P.   Stimulus-response relations in high threshold
     mechano-thermal fibers innervating primate glabrous skin.
     Brain Research, 1977, 128, 547-552.
Steven, J. C. & Stevens, S. S.   Warmth and cold: Dynamics of sen-
     sory intensity. Journal of Experimental Psychology, 1960, 60,
     183-192.

TOUCH AND THERMAL SENSATIONS: PSYCHOPHYSICAL OBSERVATIONS AND UNIT ACTIVITY IN HUMAN SKIN NERVES

T. Järvilehto and H. Hämäläinen

Department of Psychology, Experimental Laboratories

University of Helsinki, Finland

The method of microelectrode recording from human peripheral nerves (Hagbarth and Vallbo, 1967) has proved to be useful in the analysis of the peripheral neural basis of the cutaneous sensations. At the present, however, the main advantage of this method - the psychophysical measurement of sensations with simultaneous electrophysiological recording - has not yet been fully exploited. Several reports on physiological characteristics of different types of human receptors located in the glabrous or hairy skin are available, but simultaneous measurement of cutaneous sensations and unit activity in skin nerves are still few (Järvilehto, 1977, for a review).

When trying to combine psychophysical analysis of cutaneous sensations with the recording of unit activity from human nerves, one of the first questions is whether such an approach offers more knowledge about the coding of cutaneous information than psychophysical work in man correlated with electrophysiological recordings in animals. In both approaches correlations between electrophysiological observations and psychophysical measurements form the basis of the conclusions about the possible coding mechanisms. It is also evident that in most experiments the sensation examined is not solely based on activity of the fiber seen by the microelectrode. Furthermore, psychophysical measurements may be contaminated by the effects of the microelectrode recording, e.g., by painful sensations caused sometimes by the electrode.

Simultaneous electrophysiological and psychophysical analysis of sensations has several advantages as compared to the use of the animal models. No assumptions on the similarity of the receptors is needed, anesthesia is not necessary, and the time relations

between peripheral spike trains and sensations may be studied.
For the successful use of the method it is, however, important that
the experiments are combined in the same laboratory so that the
stimuli used in the electrophysiological recordings are the same
as those used in the psychophysical analysis of sensations. The
coding carried out by the receptors may be uncovered only if we
know what is coded and how the sensations of the subject change
with varying stimulus parameters. Such an analysis is not usually
possible in the electrophysiological recording situation because
of the lack of time. It is also important to study, in separate
experiments, the physiological properties of human receptors to
be able to screen the possible candidates for coding of the given
sensations.

In our work we aim at combining psychophysical measurements
of qualitative and quantitative aspects of cutaneous sensations
with electrophysiological measurements from single cutaneous nerve
fibers in order to examine the codes used by the central nervous
system in the processing of the information from the skin. In the
present report data on the correlation between psychophysical measurements of touch and thermal sensations and unit activity in the
human skin nerves will be described.

METHODS

Our electrophysiological recording technique is similar to
that used by the other groups with minor modifications (see Järvilehto, Hämäläinen, and Laurinen, 1976, for details). One of the
modifications is to use a micromanipulator to insert the electrode
into the nerve. The use of a micromanipulator allows very fine
electrodes to be used and, with small adjustments, an optimal recording position may be found for the electrode. It is also possible at times to recover a unit that has been lost.

The recording site in all our experiments is the superficial
branch of the radial nerve at the left wrist. In both psychophysical experiments and unit recording situations the skin of the
back of the hand is stimulated by mechanical or thermal stimuli.
Mechanical stimulation is carried out by plexiglass probes connected
to the moving coil of an electromechanical vibrator (the diameter
of the tip is usually 2 mm). Movements of the probe are sensed by
an accelerometer that is connected to integrating circuits for displacement measurements. The stimulus amplitude may be controlled
by the subject or by the experimenter. Thermal stimulation is applied by a Marstock stimulator (Fruhstorfer, Lindblom, and Schmidt,
1976) working according to the Peltier principle. The stimulator
has an area of 2 cm^2 and different rates of cooling and warming
may be applied by controlling the direction and amount of the current

flow through the stimulator. The amplified recording from the nerve is stored on magnetic tape along with stimulus information, trigger pulses, responses of the subject and comments of the experimenter.

To summarize our approach, we start with psychophysical measurements of the dependence of the sensations of the subject on some parameters of tactile or thermal stimuli. We also try to obtain data of the physiological properties of human cutaneous receptors to screen the best candidates for coding of the sensations. Then we combine the psychophysical measurements with the unit recording from the radial nerve. Our psychophysical research is not restricted only to quantitative aspects of the sensations, but we also try to determine qualitative changes in the sensations. This type of measurement is difficult, and it is important to further develop psychophysical methods for this purpose.

CHARACTERISTICS OF THE FIBER SAMPLE

Figure 1 shows the relative distribution of different types of fibers in a sample of 226 fibers so far identified in the radial nerve. The fibers were classified as SA or RA fibers according to the persistence of their discharge during a constant pressure stimulus (usually a von Frey hair of 2.0 g). Then possible subtypes of SA fibers (SA I or SA II) were determined on the basis of the receptive field characteristics and their responsiveness to skin stretching (Chambers, Andres, Düring, and Iggo, 1972). The column labeled as "Sp" indicates the proportion of fibers that had a resting discharge, but no receptive field on the skin, and the group "Oth" includes units supplying hair follicles, thermoreceptive fibers and proprioceptive fibers.

The lower histogram in Fig. 1 presents the distribution of the conduction velocities of 69 fibers. All fibers belong to the A-fiber group with a mean conduction velocity of 24.7 m/sec. There were no significant differences between the conduction velocities of SA and RA fibers or between the subgroups of SA fibers.

PERIPHERAL CODING OF TOUCH SENSATIONS

Psychophysical Observations

Hämäläinen (1978; unpublished master's thesis) in our laboratory has determined absolute and touch thresholds as well as estimation of the sensation magnitude for short touch pulses applied to the hairy or glabrous skin of the human hand. Both the velocity and the stimulation areas of the pulses were varied; here only the results in respect to different velocities are summarized.

The pulses were given by feeding one-cycle sinusoids (frequency 20, 60 or 250 Hz) from a function generator to the vibrator. The thresholds were measured by the method of production in which the subject was first required to set the stimulus amplitude so that

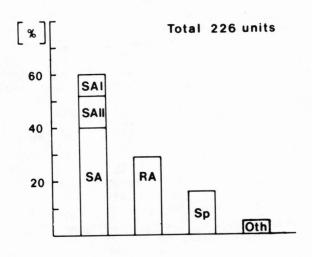

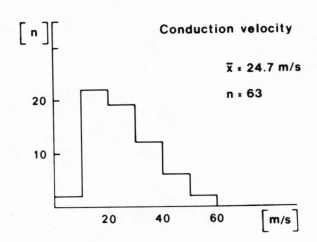

Fig. 1. Upper diagram: Relative distribution of different types of fibers in a sample of 226 units identified in the superficial branch of the radial nerve. SA = slowly adapting, RA = rapidly adapting, Sp = spontaneous, Oth = others. Lower diagram: Conduction velocity distribution of 69 SA and RA fibers, $\bar{x}$ = mean, n = number of fibers.

the stimulus was just noticeable (absolute threshold) and then to increase the amplitude until he had a distinct touch sensation (touch threshold). The latter threshold was determined, because the sensation at the absolute threshold had usually an obscure quality related to tickle rather than touch. The setting of the stimulus amplitude was started from both sub- and supraliminal amplitudes and the mean of the two settings was used as a threshold estimate. After threshold measurements, magnitude estimates of the sensations elecited by pulses at different frequencies and with amplitudes from 50 to 950 μm were carried out. Each frequency-amplitude combination was presented three times randomly during the stimulus series and the mean of the estimates was used. The

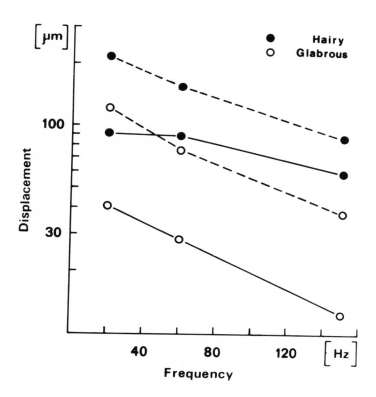

Fig. 2.   Absolute and touch thresholds as a function of the pulse frequency on the hairy (black dots) and glabrous (open dots) skin of the hand. Continuous line = absolute threshold, broken line = touch threshold. Each point is a mean of 32 measurements.

estimates were standardized by giving a value of 100 to the estimate for 150 Hz and 950 µm stimulus and by calculating the other
estimates in relation to this value.

Figure 2 presents absolute and touch thresholds as a function
of the pulse frequency for both hairy and glabrous skin. Both
thresholds were significantly higher for the hairy skin at each
frequency (p < .01, sign test), but on both skin areas the thresholds decreased as a function of the pulse frequency. The difference between the thresholds obtained by slowest and fastest
pulse frequencies was statistically significant.

The relation between magnitude estimates and pulse amplitude
at different pulse frequencies could be described by power functions
(Fig. 3), the exponents of which varied between 0.81 and 1.25.

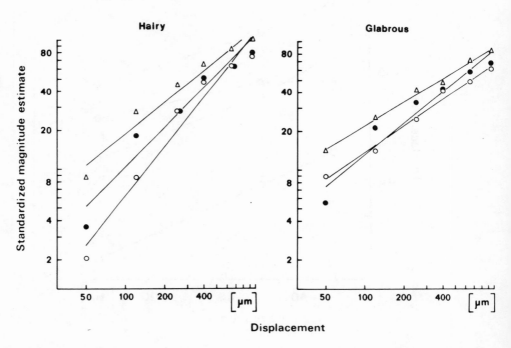

Fig. 3.   Estimates of sensation magnitude for touch pulses as a
           function of the displacement amplitude of the pulse on
           the hairy and glabrous skin of the hand. Each standard-
           ized function gives the relation for one pulse frequency;
           triangles = 150 Hz, black dots = 60 Hz, open dots = 20 Hz.

Pulse frequency had a significant effect on the magnitude estimate
on both skin areas, which is demonstrated in Fig. 4 showing equi-
sensation contours for pulse amplitude and frequency at standardized sensation levels of 20, 40 and 60. On both skin areas lower
pulse amplitudes were needed at higher pulse frequency to produce
sensations of equal magnitude. The sensitivity difference between
the skin areas disappeared at the highest sensation level, shown
in Fig. 4.

    The differences between the sensibility of the hairy and gla-
brous skin correspond to the results obtained by vibratory stimulation (Verrillo, 1968). The thresholds for the glabrous skin are
somewhat higher than those reported by Lindblom (1974) for comparable tactile pulses applied to the finger pulp. This difference

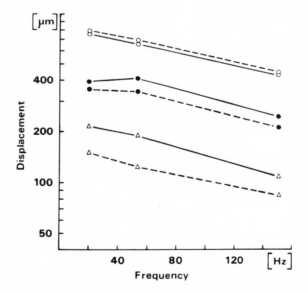

Fig. 4.   Equi-sensation contours relating pulse frequency and
          amplitude for three different standardized sensation
          levels (lowest = 20, middle = 40, uppermost = 60).
          Values interpolated from the functions in Fig. 3.   Con-
          tinuous line = hairy skin, broken line = glabrous skin.

may be partly due to the different stimulation site that here was
the thenar eminence. There is convincing evidence that the sensation threshold in the glabrous skin corresponds to the mechanical
threshold of sensitive RA receptors (Vallbo, this symposium), the
number of which decreases proximally in the glabrous skin of the
hand (Johansson, this symposium). Therefore, the probability of
hitting such a receptor may be smaller, proximally.

The available data on physiological properties of human cutaneous receptors are insufficient to unequivocally explain the psychophysical results on the basis of activity in certain receptors or
receptor groups. The results raise two primary questions that may
be answered by the simultaneous measurements of sensations and unit
activity. These are: (a) Which fibers code the threshold information in the hairy skin and what is the code? (b) What is the code
for the magnitude estimates and how can the effect of pulse frequency on the thresholds and magnitude estimates be explained?

Mechanoreceptive Unit Activity Correlated with Sensations

In recording unit activity from the radial nerve with simultaneous sensation measurements the same stimuli were used as in psychophysical experiments. Each stimulus was repeated five times with a
repetition rate of 1/sec. After each stimulus train the subject
gave an average estimate on the magnitude of the sensation. Since
the threshold measurements had to be carried out quickly, the production method was not used. Rather, the thresholds were simply
determined by slowly increasing the stimulus amplitude until the
subject reported a weak sensation. Mechanical thresholds of the
fibers were determined by adjusting the stimulus amplitude so that
a single impulse was elicited. Touch thresholds were usually not
measured.

Both threshold measurements and estimates of sensation magnitude were obtained together with the responses of the fiber for
12 SA and 8 RA fibers. In addition, either threshold measurements
or estimates of sensation magnitude were obtained for 17 SA and 5
RA fibers. In data processing the estimates of sensation magnitude
were standardized by setting the estimates given for the stimulus
with 150 Hz frequency and 650 μm amplitude as 100 and calculating
the other estimates in relation to this value. Responses of the
fibers during the stimuli were plotted, the number of impulses in
the responses was counted, and the intervals between the spikes were
measured with an accuracy of 0.5 msec.

Thresholds. Figure 5 presents the mechanical thresholds of 14
RA and 19 SA fibers with the means of simultaneously measured absolute sensation thresholds at each pulse frequency. The thresholds

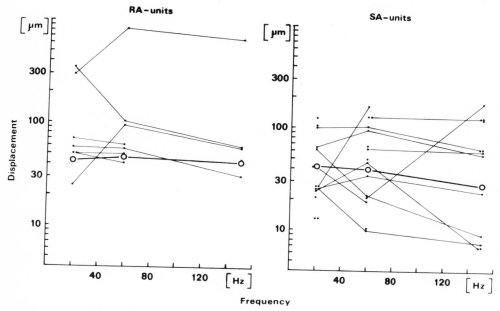

Fig. 5. Mechanical thresholds of RA and SA fibers (small dots)
as a function of the pulse frequency compared with the
means of simultaneously measured absolute sensation
thresholds (large open dots). Values measured for the
same fiber are connected by the thin line.

of several SA fibers coincided well with the subjective thresholds;
for all single measurements the same threshold values were obtained
in 50 per cent of the measurements at different frequencies, whereas
only 2 RA fibers had, at 20 Hz, mechanical thresholds that were
identical with the sensation thresholds. For 6 SA fibers the threshold decreased with increasing pulse frequency.

These measurements allow a tentative answer to some of the
questions posed by the psychophysical results. The threshold information in the hairy skin is coded mainly by SA fibers and the code
is a single impulse in the fiber. The decrease of the threshold
value with increasing pulse frequency is simply explained by the
decreasing mechanical thresholds of the fibers. RA fibers and several SA fibers seem not to be able to code threshold information.
They could, however, participate in the coding of the touch threshold which seems to presuppose activation of the fibers with higher
thresholds or larger number of impulses in fibers coding the threshold information. The data indicate that the sensitivity difference

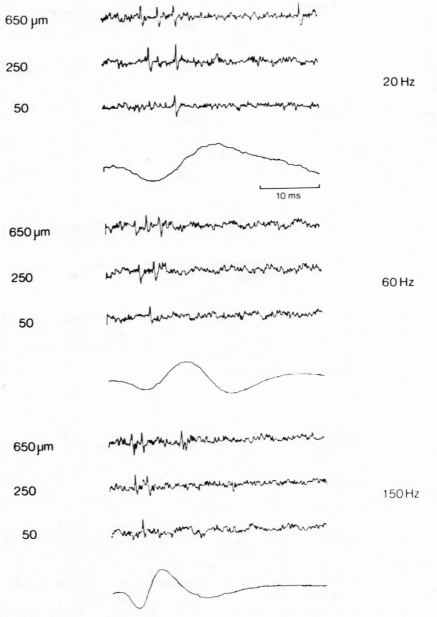

Fig. 6.   Response of an SA fiber to mechanical pulses of varying
          amplitude and frequency. Displacement amplitude on the
          right of each recording, pulse frequency on the left.
          The trace below each group of recordings shows the dis-
          placement of the stimulus probe (towards the skin upwards).

between the hairy and glabrous skin is probably not only due to higher density of receptors in the glabrous skin, but also to lower thresholds of individual receptors located in the glabrous skin.

Codes for estimation of sensation magnitude. Figure 6 shows the response of an SA fiber to pulses with varying frequency and amplitude. The fiber responded maximally with three impulses. The maximum number of impulses was seven for all fibers studied. The number of impulses clearly depends on the amplitude of the stimulus. Both displacement amplitude and pulse frequency affect the latency of the first impulse as well as the inter-spike-intervals. The response of the fibers to repeated identical stimuli were usually extremely constant especially at the higher pulse amplitudes; the maximum variation of the latency or of the first inter-spike-interval usually did not exceed 1 msec.

The estimation of the sensation magnitude during recording of

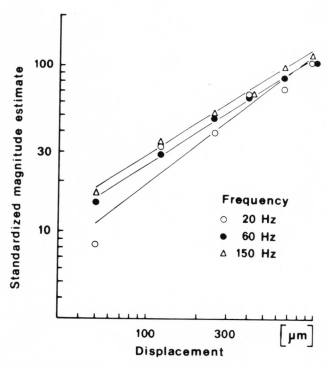

Fig. 7. Standardized magnitude estimation functions for the touch pulses obtained during simultaneous unit recording. Hairy skin.

the unit activity was similar to that in psychophysical experiments.
Figure 7 shows the pooled standardized magnitude estimation functions for each pulse frequency. The exponents of the functions
were 0.65 (150 Hz), 0.67 (60 Hz) and 0.80 (20 Hz). Larger estimates
were obtained with higher pulse frequencies.

The first possible code for the magnitude estimate could be
the number of impulses elicited in a single fiber as indicated by
the response of the fiber in Fig. 6. Figure 8 presents the relation
between the number of impulses and the magnitude estimate for one
RA and one SA I fiber at pulse frequencies of 20 and 150 Hz. The
relation is indeed monotonic and may be described by straight lines
which are different for different frequencies. A linear relation
between the number of impulses and the magnitude estimate was obtained for other 9 SA and 4 RA fibers at one or several of the
pulse frequencies. It was a typical feature of the fibers that
they usually had an optimal frequency at which a maximum number of
spikes were elicited. The number of spikes was also in linear

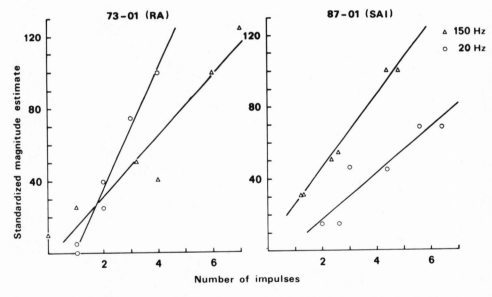

Fig. 8.   Relation between the number of impulses elicited by
          touch impulses of 150 and 20 Hz in a single RA (left)
          and SA I (right) fiber and the simultaneously obtained
          estimates of sensation magnitude. Number of impulses
          for each point is a mean of 5 repetitive responses.
          Symbols indicated in the right upper corner.

relation to the magnitude estimate at this frequency. The fibers could be divided in three groups on the basis of their response maxima and the monotonic relation between the number of impulses and the magnitude estimate: (a) Those responding best at lower frequencies (6 SA fibers). (b) Those responding best at 150 Hz (3 SA, 2 RA fibers). (c) Those for which no optimal frequency could be determined (1 SA and 2 RA fibers).

As the fibers usually responded with several impulses at higher stimulus amplitudes, another code for the intensity of the sensation could be the inter-spike-interval. Basically, the same results were obtained when the length of the first inter-spike-interval was used in place of the number of impulses. For several fibers a linear relation was seen between the magnitude estimate and the length of the first inter-spike-interval, but the interval did not unequivocally determine the magnitude estimate at different frequencies. Fibers had optimal responding frequencies that corresponded to those at which they also elicited the maximum number of spikes.

These findings indicate that a single fiber may be able to code the intensive aspect of short tactile stimulation at the frequency for which it is tuned on the basis of the number of impulses elicited in the fiber and/or on the basis of the first inter-spike-interval. As quite a few spikes are usually elicited, it is probable that in coding of the sensation magnitude, recruitment of additional fibers in the population with stronger stimuli is also involved (cf. Johnson, 1974). SA fibers seem to be tuned for a broad range of frequencies, whereas RA fibers code mainly high-frequency stimuli. Thus the larger magnitude estimates obtained by higher pulse frequencies could be due to activation of RA fibers in addition to SA fibers.

OBSERVATIONS IN THERMAL SENSATIONS

Cold Sensations

At the present we have obtained recordings from 3 receptors responding to warming of the skin and 4 receptors responding to cooling by an increase in their firing rate. For one cold fiber simultaneous sensation measurements were obtained. This fiber had a spot-like receptive field at the base of the index finger and it did not respond to mechanical stimulation.

Figure 9 represents responses of the fiber of different types of thermal stimulation. The upper part of the figure presents the response of the fiber to a sudden cold stimulus of 10.6°C that was

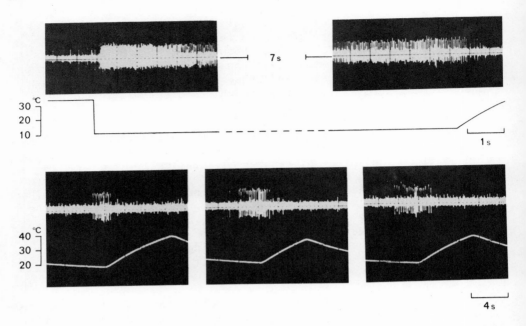

Fig. 9.   Responses of a single cold fiber to different types of
          thermal stimulation. The lines below the recording in-
          dicate the temperature changes of the stimulator rela-
          tive to the calibration on the left. For details see
          the text.

maintained for several seconds. In the beginning a vigorous burst
of impulses, exceeding 80 imp/sec, may be seen and the discharge
adapted during maintained stimulus temperature. During warming
the fiber stopped firing.

     The lower part of the figure demonstrates a testing sequence
during which the subject maintained the temperature of the stimulator at a neutral level by reversing the direction of the temperature change when he felt cool or warm. The response of the subject to cooling was invariably preceded by several impulses, usually
10, on the average. As the stimulator was touching the skin over
an area of about 1 cm^2 we estimate that about 10 cold spots were
activated by the cooling. If each of these spots were served by
a single cold fiber it is possible to state, on the basis of this
single experiment, that the number of impulses necessary for the
threshold sensation of cold is about 100. This figure agrees with
our earlier estimates that were based on recording activity from
single cold fibers in cat and on comparing activity changes to
threshold values of single cold spots in man (Järvilehto, 1973).

Paradoxical Heat

A second type of thermal sensation that we have examined is the paradoxical heat described initially by Eisenlohr (1879: cited in Long, 1977). This is a sensation of heat or warm that sometimes occurs when lowering the skin temperature. In the pilot experiments we found that this sensation was easily elicited if, before testing, the skin temperature was raised to heat pain threshold.

Vartiainen (unpublished master's thesis), in our laboratory, examined this phenomenon more closely. In his experiment, Vartiainen first determined that the indifferent temperature range for the subjects was between 29.1° and 35.7°C, on the average. The temperature of the stimulator (area 2 cm^2) was then lowered several times from the indifferent temperature to 14°C with a mean rate of change of 0.6°C/sec and the reports of the subjects were recorded. From 288 cooling trials in 18 subjects, paradoxical heat was reported 44 times, i.e., in 15 percent of the trials. The temperatures at which the sensations occurred ranged from 14° to 21°C. Before the next session, the heat pain threshold of the subject was determined and the temperature was again lowered several times from the indifferent temperature to 14°C. Now reports of paradoxical heat occurred in 32 percent of the trials and if the pain threshold was measured twice, positive reports occurred in 42 percent of the trials. The range of the temperatures at which the sensation occurred was also higher, being from 20° to 27°C, on the average.

These observations show that heating of the skin facilitates the appearance of paradoxical heat sensations during cooling the skin. One of the simplest explanations of the phenomenon was that heating increased the responsiveness of some peripheral nerve fibers to cooling, the activity of which would form the neural basis of heat sensation.

We have tested 11 SA fibers by heating and cooling and one of them seemed to respond to both types of stimulation. The signal-to-noise ratio of the recording was, however, too small for a detailed analysis. From the other fibers only one responded to cooling and the activity of the others was unaffected by the changes in the skin temperature. Thus it seems that the mechanoreceptive fibers are unlikely candidates for mediating the paradoxical heat sensation. Whether this sensation has an explanation based on the activity in the peripheral nerve fibers has to be solved by further recordings.

SUMMARY

Microelectrode measurements from human skin nerves may give quite conclusive evidence about the coding of cutaneous sensations

by the receptors in the skin if they are combined with psychophysical
analysis of the cutaneous sensations. In the present study attempts
to examine coding of touch and thermal sensations are described.
Psychophysical experiments with short pulses combined with unit recordings from the radial nerve indicated that the threshold information for touch on the hairy skin is coded mainly by SA fibers
and the code is a single impulse. No single code for the intensive aspect of the touch sensation could be shown, but the results
indicated that in a single fiber the number of impulses as well as
the inter-spike-interval may code the magnitude of the sensation.
The recruitment of fiber population probably also has significance.
Simultaneous measurements of cold sensation thresholds with activity in a single cold fiber indicated that at threshold the number
of impulses entering the central nervous system along specific cold
fibers is about 100. Finally, preliminary observations on paradoxical heat sensations are reported.

ACKNOWLEDGEMENT

This work was supported by the Finnish Academy.

REFERENCES

Chambers, M.R., Andres, K.H., Düring, M. & Iggo, A. The structure
    and function of the slowly adapting type II mechanoreceptor in
    hairy skin. Quarterly Journal of Experimental Physiology, 1972,
    57, 417-445.
Fruhstorfer, H., Lindblom, U. & Schmidt, W.G. Method for quanti-
    tative estimation of thermal thresholds in patients. Journal
    of Neurology, Neurosurgery and Psychiatry, 1976, 39, 1071-1075.
Hagbarth, K.E. & Vallbo, A.B. Mechanoreceptor activity recorded
    percutaneously with semimicroelectrodes in human peripheral
    nerves. Acta Physiologica Scandinavica, 1967, 69, 121-122.
Järvilehto, T. Neural coding in the temperature sense. Human
    reactions to temperature changes as compared with activity in
    single peripheral cold fibers in the cat. Annales Academie
    Scientiarum Fennicae; Series B, 1973, 184, 1-71.
Järvilehto, T. Neural basis of cutaneous sensations analyzed
    by microelectric measurements from human peripheral nerves -
    a review. Scandinavian Journal of Psychology, 1977, 18, 348-359.
Johnson, K.O. Reconstruction of population response to a vibratory
    stimulus in quickly adapting mechanoreceptive fiber population
    innervating glabrous skin of the monkey. Journal of Neurophy-
    siology, 1974, 37, 48-72.
Lindblom, U. Touch perception threshold in human glabrous skin in
    terms of displacement amplitude on stimulation with single me-
    chanical pulses. Brain Research, 1974, 82, 205-210.

Long, R.R.   Sensitivity of cutaneous cold fibers to noxious heat:
    Paradoxical cold discharge. Journal of Neurophysiology, 1977,
    40, 489-502.
Verrillo, R.T.   A duplex mechanism of mechanoreception.   In D.R.
    Kenshalo (Ed.) The skin senses. Thomas: Springfield, Ill.,
    1968.

DISCUSSION

DR. KONIETZNY: I am interested in your conduction velocity measurements. As you know, it is easy to measure conduction velocity when the single fiber preparation method is used. When the receptive field is stimulated electrically with a high current more than one action potential can be initiated. How can one be sure that the action potential is in the same nerve as that derived from mechanical stimulation. Drs. Torebjörk and Hallin (1974) have developed a very good method, that we also are now using. I think that this method solves this problem.

DR. JÄRVILEHTO: We did not use electrical stimulation for these measurements. Our measurements of conduction velocity seem somewhat low. We used either fast mechanical pulses of high amplitude or we measured, from the recordings, the latency of the spike. They are pretty low, generally.

DR. LINDBLOM: I was surprised that you could get so many action potentials from relatively short pulses. You had up to six action potentials produced by a 120 Hz stimulus. Was that right?

DR. JÄRVILEHTO: No, not six, but three.

DR. LINDBLOM: The duration of the rising phase of the most rapid stimulus you used would not be more than about 4 msec. From the time the first impulse is initiated there would not be enough time for so many more impulses to be recruited during the rising phase. Could it be an oscillation in the stimulus that makes the rapid discharge?

DR. JÄRVILEHTO: No, it does not oscillate.

DR. LINDBLOM: We used a 100 Hz stimulus and assumed that each stimulus would not give more than 1 or 2 impulses, and that touch magnitude was related to the recruitment of units. That is, touch magnitude was related to spatial summation rather than to the number of impulses per unit. But the data is somewhat different, and the conclusions are somewhat different on that point. Anyhow, I have one question about the type of sensation which was evoked by these stimuli. It seems as if you had two types of sensations, while we found a continuous type of sensation. It may be that we were not observant enough. You say that at threshold there was one type of sensation, and that suprathreshold stimulation aroused a tactile sensation. Was that right?

DR. JÄRVILEHTO: Yes, I would say that if you measure the absolute threshold for touch, then one is not measuring actually touch. If one measures the minimal amplitude needed, so that the subject just notices something, I would not call it touch. I would call it itch or something else.

DR. FRANZÉN: First, I have a short comment on the way you treat your data. If you look at your distribution of conduction velocities, it is extremely skewed and I think that was a contraindication for use of the mean. The median might have been better.
The second matter is that your functions agree very well with the data I showed. But if you use, say, a 20 Hz pulse of about 100 µm skin indentation, that will correspond to about 8 mm/sec, maybe we are dealing with different things. The function here is contaminated by recruitment of units and the pattern in the neural discharge. But you looked at it in terms of impulses/sec. I do not think it is appropriate to correlate the subjective function with the impulse frequency, with this kind of stimulus.

DR. JÄRVILEHTO: I am not correlating it with the impulse frequency, but with the number of impulses elicited. I did not say that there are not many others. These stimuli are recruiting more units, but I think it is important that the magnitude estimates are based just on this activity in a population of units. Single units seem to be able to carry the information that is necessary. That has been shown also for pressure stimuli by Mountcastle, (Werner, G. & Mountcastle, V. B. 1965) for example.

DR. HENSEL: Just a short question, did you also try to stimulate with a smaller area cold stimulus, or did you use only your thermode with 2 cm^2 area? This would be interesting, otherwise you assume a linear summation.

DR. JÄRVILEHTO: No.

REFERENCES

Torebjörk, H. E. & Hallin, R. G. Response in human A and C fibers to repeated electrical intradermal stimulation. Journal of Neurology, Neurosurgery and Psychiatry, 1974, 37, 653-664.
Werner, G. & Mountcastle, V. B. Neural activity in mechanoreceptive cutaneous afferents: Stimulus-response relations, Weber functions, and information transmission. Journal of Neurophysiology, 1965, 28, 359-397.

COINCIDENCE AND CAUSE: A DISCUSSION ON CORRELATIONS BETWEEN ACTIVITY

IN PRIMARY AFFERENTS AND PERCEPTIVE EXPERIENCE IN CUTANEOUS SENSIBILITY

Å. B. Vallbo and R. S. Johansson

Department of Physiology, University of Umeå

S-90187 Umeå Sweden

The method of recording naturally occurring activity from peripheral nerves in waking human subjects was first presented in 1966 (Vallbo and Hagbarth, 1967). This recording technique allows the afferent activity in the single units to be assessed with an extreme accuracy while, at the same time, the subject's experience of the stimuli may be explored with psychophysical methods. This approach opens the possibility (a) to define exactly the functional properties of primary afferent units in man and (b) to assess directly whether a correlation exists between a defined property of the afferent activity, and an element of the perceptive experience. It seems that these kinds of studies may narrow the gap, so far inconceivable, between biophysical events in the nervous system and perceptive phenomena within the mind, and thereby contribute to an understanding of the mechanisms by which the human brain brings into existence the product which we introspectively experience as consciousness.

The present report is a discussion of some problems and pitfalls in the study of psychoneural correlates in tactile sensibility, particularly as seen in relation to this recording technique. On the other hand, other experimental approaches which feasibly may be combined with this technique will not be considered , such as blocking of selected groups of nerve fibers with local anaesthetics or compression, nor artificial activation of nerve fibers by electrical stimulation.

The fundamental work on psychoneural correlates in tactile sensibility by Mountcastle's group and others was largely based on neurophysiological data extracted from subhuman primates and psychophysical data collected from human subjects (Werner and

Mountcastle, 1965; Mountcastle, Talbot, and Kornhuber, 1966; Mountcastle, 1967; Talbot, Darian-Smith, Kornhuber, and Mountcastle,
1968; Harrington and Merzenich, 1970). The assumption was adopted
that man and subhuman primates are equipped with mechanosensitive
units which have the same functional properties in relevant respects.

One very important achievement which has been reached by the
method of recording single units in man is a description of the
functional properties of the afferent units in man. Four different
types of mechanoreceptive units have been demonstrated in the
glabrous skin of the human hand: RA, PC, SA I and SA II (Knibestöl
and Vallbo, 1970; Johansson, 1978). Their nerve fibers very
likely belong to the Aα group implying that they have large diameters. Available evidence indicates that there are no low threshold mechanosensitive units with small myelinated or unmyelinated
fibers in the glabrous skin area (Burgess and Perl, 1973;
Georgopoulos, 1976; Kumazawa and Perl, 1977). This consideration
justifies the conclusion, at the present stage, that RA, PC, SA I
and SA II units are the ones which primarily account for the
tactile sensibility of the human hand.

The findings reported so far support the notion that the
mechanoreceptive units are functionally similar in man and monkey.
However, it is important to point out that the descriptions of the
unit types in man as well as in subhuman primates are by no means
comprehensive and the analyses have often been focused on different
functional properties of the units. For instance, one of the unit
types described in the human glabrous skin (SA II) has not yet been
clearly demonstrated in this area in the monkey. Moreover, the
properties of the receptive fields of the separate types of mechanoreceptive units have not been analyzed in the monkey, in such detail, as in man (Johansson, 1978). On the other hand, the adaptive
properties of the units and their responses to sinusoidal vibration
which have been carefully analyzed in other species have not been
much studied in man (Talbot et al., 1968; Iggo and Muir, 1969;
Chambers, Andres, Duering, and Iggo, 1972; Konietzny and Hensel,
1977). A lot of experimental work remains to be done before it can
be assessed to what extent the functional properties of tactile
sensory units are in fact identical in man and monkey. In experiments aiming at a comparison of neural and psychophysical data
it may be deleterious to extrapolate from subhuman primates to man
because small differences in functional properties of the afferent
units in the two species may account for a crucial difference in
afferent input even though the same stimulus is used.

A number of questions seem profitable to attack with the
method of recording naturally occurring activity in human peripheral nerves in combination with psychophysical tests. It is

reasonable to separate the questions into two groups.

One group is concerned with the causal relation between neural elements and perceptive elements. These questions have the following general structure: "Which neural element is required for the production of the perceptive element". By neural element in this context is implied any component or any property of the afferent impulse activity such as which units are activated, the pattern of impulse activity in the individual afferent units, or amount of afferent activity required as well as quantities describing relations between several inputs. The term perceptive element is used to denote the percept itself, i.e. whether it is there or not, or a component or a property of the percept, e.g., its intensity or location, as well as relations between components or properties of several percepts.

Another group of questions are concerned with the processing of the sensory signal within the central nervous system. These questions may have the following general structure: "In which respect is the sensory signal modified at the levels intervening between the primary afferents and the compartment where the perceptive experience is produced?" Examples are :"How much information is lost before the signal reaches the perceptive level" (cf. Vallbo and Johansson, 1976), and "Which kind of interference may occur in the central processing between two sensory messages?"

Before a question of this structure can be answered it has to be established that the neural and the perceptive element considered are causally related. This is the logic behind a separation of the problems in the two main groups.

It should be emphasized that a causal relationship in this context implies that the neural element is essential for the production of the perceptive element. On the other hand, it does not imply that the two are necessarily associated. The subject's attention and his decision criteria are of course factors which may profoundly affect the strength of association between the two phenomena in an actual experimental study.

Whenever problems concerning psychoneural correlates are considered the structure of the analysis is heavily dependent on the kind of neural activity recorded. Three kinds of situations may be considered. (a) Recordings of multiunit activity allow, to a certain extent, the assessment of alterations of activity from one instance to another whereas quantitization is largely impossible. Such recordings may still be useful for more general questions regarding which groups of nerve fibers are active when a particular perceptive experience is produced, particularly when combined with blocking of sets of fibers with local anaesthetics or compression (cf. Torebjörk and Hallin, 1973). When activity from a single

afferent unit is recorded it seems essential to differentiate between two kinds of situations. (b) One is when the activity of the
single fiber is assumed to represent or contain only a fraction of
the total neural element which is related to the perceptive element.
In such cases the recording monitors the activity in one out of a
number of simultaneously active units. (c) A clearly different
situation is when the experiment is based on the assumption that
the single unit whose impulses are recorded provides the total
neural element essential for a perceptive element and that no other
relevant unit is active.

When a coincidence between the presence of a neural element
and a perceptive element has been experimentally established it remains to be assessed whether a causal relation between the two
phenomena prevails or not, and on the other hand when a dissociation
has been found, it remains to be assessed in which respects a causal
relation can be excluded. This step in the analysis may entail considerable difficulties and pitfalls.

When a poor correlation is found in an experimental study between the activity of a single afferent and a perceptive element
the immediate conclusion one tends to draw is that the perceptive
element is not dependent on neural activity recorded. However,
this conclusion may not always be correct because the afferent impulses of the unit may not reach the central nervous system because

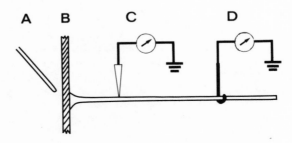

Fig. 1.   Schematic diagram of the experimental arrangements to test
          whether the impulses recorded with a tungsten needle
          electrode (C) propagate beyond the recording site or not.
          Mechanical stimuli were delivered with a glass rod or a
          drawing brush (A) to the skin (B). Nerve impulses in a
          single fiber of a skin mechanosensitive unit were re-
          corded with a tungsten needle electrode (C) inserted into
          the nerve and the activity of the whole nerve trunk was re-
          corded with a hook electrode further proximal on the same
          nerve (D). (Vallbo, 1976).

they are blocked by injury at the recording site. The recording electrode has a fairly large tip in relation to the nerve fibers and there are indications that a myelinated fiber is often damaged when single unit activity is recorded. The problem of propagation block was studied in experiments when the electrodes developed for percutaneous recording from human nerves were used to record afferent activity from nerves in cats and frogs (Vallbo, 1976).

The experimental situation is schematically shown in Fig. 1. The skin (B) was stimulated mechanically with a blunt instrument (A) and afferent impulses were set up in the nerve. Activity from a single unit was recorded with a needle electrode (C). Farther away from the skin the activity from the whole nerve trunk was recorded (D). When the triggering of the oscilloscope beams was suitably arranged a display, as shown in Fig. 2, was obtained. In this figure the upper trace shows the activity recorded with the

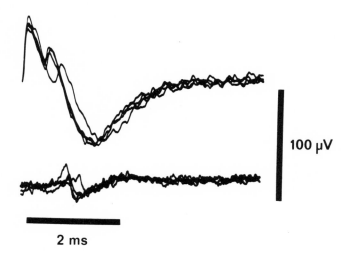

100 µV

2 ms

Fig. 2.   Four nerve impulses recorded from an afferent with a tungsten needle electrode (upper trace) and a hook electrode connected to the nerve trunk (lower trace). Arrangements are as in Fig. 1. The two oscilloscope beams were triggered by the rising phase of the impulses. It may be noticed that the impulses seen by the tungsten needle electrode have double peaks and that in one of the four impulses the second peak is delayed. This was associated with a delay also of the conducted impulse as seen in the lower trace. Upward deflections indicate positive signals at the tungsten needle electrode. (Modified from Vallbo, 1976).

needle electrode, and the lower trace the activity recorded farther
up along the nerve trunk. It may be seen that all four impulses
elicited by the stimulus in this case did propagate beyond the
recording site.

It was found that impulse block can be predicted in Aα fibers
with a high degree of probability from the shape of the impulse.
There are essentially three different shapes as shown in Fig. 3.
Negative impulses (A) are blocked in 10 percent whereas positive
and double peaked spikes (B) are never blocked. Positive and single
peaked spike (C) may be of two different natures, one is blocked
and the other is not. Sample records to demonstrate this are shown
in Fig. 4. During an experiment the spike shape usually alters
with time and from these alterations it is mostly possible to decide whether the single peaked spike is of the kind which is
blocked or not. A single peaked positive spike which later changes
into a double peaked spike is propagaged beyond the recording site,
whereas, a single peaked spike which has developed from a double
peaked spike does not propagate. In all, it was possible to predict

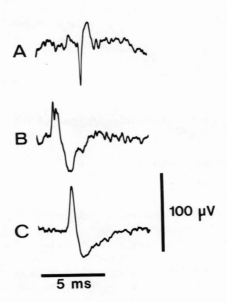

Fig. 3.   Three main types of impulse shapes as seen by the tungsten
           needle electrode inserted into a peripheral nerve. Up-
           ward deflections represent positive signals at the needle
           electrode. (Modified from Vallbo, 1976).

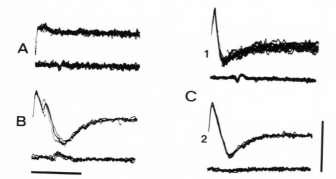

Fig. 4.   Unitary impulse propagation and block related to shape of
          impulse recorded with tungsten needle electrodes. The
          traces are arranged as in Fig. 2 and the electrode
          arrangements are as in Fig. 1. It may be seen that
          propagation is unimpaired in A and B. The impulses seen
          by the needle electrode were negative or positive with a
          double peak. When the impulse shape was positive with a
          single peak as in C, propagation was unimpaired in C1 and
          blocked in C2. Calibrations. Time: 2.5 msec for C2, 5
          msec for the other records. Amplitude: 100 μV except
          for upper trace in C1 where calibration bar represents
          50 μV. (Modified from Vallbo, 1976).

from the shape of the spike and its alteration, whether the impulse
is blocked or not, in 97 percent of the cases. In most recordings
(about 80 percent) of single impulses with tungsten needle electrodes the propagation was unimpaired during at least part of the
recording period.

     The two peaks of a doubled peaked positive spike were shown
to represent activities in two adjacent nodes of the fiber. Due
to injury by the electrode tip the activities are abnormally separated in time. Another point of interest is that the block develops
exactly when the second peak disappears, i.e. when the double
peaked spike turns into a single peaked spike. The fact that this
moment can be exactly defined provides an additional possibility
to assess the relevance of the impulses in this particular unit
for a perceptive phenomenon.

Providing the propagation of the impulse is unimpaired a negative finding concerning a psychoneural correlation often allows a clear conclusion. For instance, when it is demonstrated that a sinusoidal stimulation gives a clear modulation of the discharge of SA units but does not give a perceptive experience of a tactile stimulus which varies in intensity over time (Talbot, et al., 1968; Harrington and Merzenich, 1970; Konietzny and Hensel, 1977) then it is justified to conclude that the neural element consisting of a low frequency modulation of the discharge of SA units as found in the experiments is not relevant for any perceptive experience. However, the conclusion must be strictly limited to elements analyzed and any extrapolations may be fallacious. For instance when a unit is excited but no psychophysical response can be demonstrated this may be due to the input being subthreshold for a response. Still the kind of activity recorded in the peripheral nerve may be the critical one for the production of the type of sensation considered, but a summation of more activity may be required.

When a coincidence is found between a neural and a perceptive element it is tempting to conclude that the neural element is the essential input required for the perceptive element. However, this is of course not justified before other alternatives have been excluded. Often the analysis of activity in one set of single afferents must be supplemented with accurate information of the activity present in parallel channels. Consider the experiment when scaling of the amplitudes of rectangular skin indentations is studied (Werner and Mountcastle, 1965; Mountcastle, et al., 1966; Mountcastle, 1967; Harrington and Merzenich, 1970; Knibestöl and Vallbo, 1976). There are probably a number of neural variables which vary monotonically with the stimulus amplitude as well as with the subject's estimates, e.g. (a) the total number of impulses of single slowly adapting units (SA I or SA II), (b) the number of impulses during the dynamic, initial phase of indentation in these afferents, (c) the number of impulses during the static phase (Knibestöl, 1975), (d) the total number of slowly adapting units activated, (e) the total number of impulses from the whole population of these units during the initial or the static phase or during both these phases, (f) the impulse frequency or the number of impulses from single rapidly adapting units (RA or PC) etc.

A firm knowledge of the total population of afferents from the appropriate skin area and the functional properties of the units may be required to see which alternatives must be considered and to design crucial experiments to investigate these alternatives. Generally when more than one neural element is found to coincide with the presence of one and the same perceptive element there are several alternative interpretations. When, for instance, it is found that the threshold of detection of small skin indentations

matches the thresholds of two different kinds of units, RA and PC
(Vallbo and Johansson, 1976), there are four alternatives. (a)
The necessary input is provided by the PC units alone. (b) The
necessary input is provided by the RA units alone. (c) Activation
of both RA and PC units is required for the detection of the stimuli,
i.e. an input consisting of a combination of the two is essential.
(d) Finally there is the possibility that either RA units alone or
PC units alone may provide the crucial input. If this is the case
it would be of interest to analyse whether the perceptive experience
is identical in the two cases or whether the two kinds of units
give rise to different percepts. These considerations touch upon
a very basic problem with regard to the central processing of
neural input from the skin, namely whether all components of the
total neural input produced by a stimulus is required for the perceptive experience or to what extent there are redundant components
in the total neural input from the perceptive point of view.

     When the functional properties of more than one kind of
afferents are found to match a perceptive variable it may be essential to analyse the relative and absolute frequency of occurrence
of the different kinds of units as well as the sizes of their receptive field. From such analyses it may be possible to infer that
the likelihood is much larger for one of the unit types to account
for the perceptive phenomenon.

     In summary it may be concluded that an analysis of activity
in single cutaneous afferents in man is a very attractive approach
to many problems concerning psychoneural correlates from the point
of view that exact quantitative information is obtained. However,
it seems that in most studies the activity elicited by the stimulus
in other parallel units besides the one recorded must be considered.
A firm knowledge of the input in these fibers are required. Adequate information on this point is often possible to achieve only
by estimating the population properties. There is usually no short
cut to arrive at such estimates but to synthetize a model on the
basis of a single unit sample and morphological data concerning the
absolute number of nerve fibers distributed to the skin region considered.

     An analysis of the population properties of a set of units is
often a tedious procedure but it is probably worthwhile in studies
on human subjects considering the unique potentialities available
when neurophysiological recordings with extremely high resolution
capacity are combined with psychophysical methods in the same subjects.

SUMMARY

     The method of recording activity from human nerves with in-
traneural needle electrodes allows the input to the central nervous

system to be assessed with an extreme accuracy while, at the same
time, the subject's experience of the stimuli may be explored with
psychophysical methods. This approach opens the possibility (a) to
define exactly the functional properties of primary afferent units
in man and (b) to assess directly whether a correlation exists between a neuronal element, defined as a component or a property of
the afferent activity, and an element of the perceptive experience.

When a correlation has been established or refuted there remains to be assessed whether a causal relation between the two
phenomena prevails or whether a causal relation can be excluded.
This step may entail considerable difficulties and several pitfalls.
In most cases the assessment of a coincidence must be supplemented
with an accurate information of the activity present in parallel
channels. So far, there is no other way to obtain this information
than by an inference of the properties of the population of units.
The possibility of a conduction block at the site of recording from
a single fiber should be considered. When a coincidence between a
neuronal element is lacking the possibility of the input being subthreshold for a psychophysical response must be considered.

Once a causal relation has been established, the analysis may
be pursued to define in which respects the sensory signal is modified within the parts of the system intervening between the primary
afferents and the level of consciousness.

The studies performed so far emphasize the importance of an
accurate control of the stimulus parameters and a firm knowledge
of the relevant population properties in studies when activity of
a single unit is related to an element of the perceptive experience.

ACKNOWLEDGMENTS

This study was supported by the Swedish Medical Research
Council (project no. 04X-3548).

REFERENCES

Burgess, P. R., & Perl, E. R. Cutaneous mechanoreceptors and no-
        ciceptors. In A. Iggo (Ed.), Handbook of sensory physiology
        (Vol. II). Berlin: Springer, 1973.
Chambers, M. R., Andres, K. H., v. Duering, M., & Iggo, A. The
        structure and function of the slowly adapting type II mechano-
        receptor in hairy skin. Quarterly Journal of Experimental
        Physiology, 1972, 57, 417-445.
Georgopoulos, A. P. Functional properties of primary afferent units
        probably related to pain mechanisms in primate glabrous skin.
        Journal of Neurophysiology, 1976, 39, 71-83.

Harrington, T. & Merzenich, M. M. Neural coding in the sense of touch: Human sensation of skin indentation compared with the responses of slowly adapting mechanoreceptive afferents innervating the hairy skin of monkeys. Experimental Brain Research, 1970, 10, 251-264.

Iggo, A. & Muir, A. R. The structure and function of a slowly adapting touch corpuscle in hairy skin. Journal of Physiology (London), 1969, 200, 763-796.

Johansson, R. S. Tactile sensibility in the human hand: Receptive field characteristics of mechanoreceptor units in the glabrous skin. Journal of Physiology (London), 1978, 281, 101-123.

Knibestöl, M. Stimulus-response functions of slowly adapting mechanoreceptors in the human glabrous skin area. Journal of Physiology (London), 1975, 245, 63-80.

Knibestöl, M. & Vallbo, Å. B. Single unit analysis of mechanoreceptor activity from the human glabrous skin. Acta Physiologica Scandinavica, 1970, 80, 178-195.

Knibestöl, M. & Vallbo, Å. B. Stimulus-response functions of primary afferents and psychophysical intensity estimation on mechanical skin stimulation in the human hand. In Y. Zotterman (Ed.), Sensory functions of the skin in primates. Oxford: Pergamon Press, 1976.

Konietzny, F., & Hensel, H. Response of rapidly and slowly adapting mechanoreceptors and vibratory sensitivity in human hairy skin. Pflügers Archiv, 1977, 368, 39-44.

Kumazawa, T. & Perl, E. R. Primate cutaneous sensory units with unmyelinated (C) afferent fibres. Journal of Neurophysiology, 1977, 40, 1325-1338.

Mountcastle, V. B. The problem of sensing and the neural coding of sensory events. In G. C. Quarton, T. Melnechuk, & F. O. Schmitt (Eds.), The neurosciences. New York: Rockefeller University Press, 1967.

Mountcastle, V. B., Talbot, W. H., & Kornhuber, H. H. The neural transformation of mechanical stimuli delivered to the monkey's hand. In A. V. S. de Reuck, & J. Knight (Eds.), Touch, heat and pain. London: Ciba Foundation Symposium, Churchill, 1966.

Talbot, W. H., Darian-Smith, I., Kornhuber, H. H., & Mountcastle, V. B. The sense of flutter-vibration: Comparison of the human capacity with response patterns of mechano-receptive afferents from the monkey hand. Journal of Neurophysiology, 1968, 31, 301-334.

Torebjörk, H. E. & Hallin, R. G. Perceptual changes accompanying controlled preferential blocking of A and C fibre responses in intact human skin nerves. Experimental Brain Research, 1973, 16, 321-332.

Vallbo, Å. B. Prediction of propagation block on the basis of impulse shape in single unit recordings from human nerves. Acta Physiologica Scandinavica, 1976, 97, 66-74.

Vallbo, Å. B., & Hagbarth, K.E. Impulses recorded with micro-
     electrodes in human muscle nerves during stimulation of
     mechanoreceptors and voluntary contractions. Electroen-
     cephalography and Clinical Neurophysiology, 1967, 23, 392.
Vallbo, Å. B., & Johansson, R. S. Skin mechanoreceptors in the
     human hand: Neural and psychophysical thresholds. In Y.
     Zotterman (Ed.), Sensory functions of the skin of primates.
     Oxford: Pergamon Press, 1976.
Werner, G., & Mountcastle, V. B. Neural activity in mechano-
     receptive cutaneous afferents: stimulus-response relations,
     Weber functions and information transmission. Journal of
     Neurophysiology, 1965, 28, 359-397.

DISCUSSION

DR. ZOTTERMAN: What would happen if your electrode sticks into the node of Ranvier?

DR. VALLBO: I think this would be very traumatizing to the fiber. The probability of blocking would be higher if you penetrate the nodal membrane with such a course electrode.

DR. FRANZEN: As I pointed out this finding (evidence of neural activity without an accompanying sensation [see p. 39]) was not only true for the tactile system, but also for the visual system. This has also been confirmed in studies that Libet, et al. (1975) carried out. He found that you could see a response on the exposed cortex although the patient did not report any sensation. I think there is a lot of evidence that my conclusions are correct. The second point deals with the problem of changes in threshold. For instance, in the patients that we have studied, one can see that the threshold goes up tremendously. It seems very unlikely then that only the low threshold fibers are gone and only high threshold fibers are left. In one patient it was raised more than 10 fold (Franzén and Lindblom, 1976). How would you explain that?

DR. VALLBO: My main point was that we are probably dealing with two different systems (Verrillo, 1963). Your stimulus is a very sharp rising indentation which I suspect would excite a large number of PC units. If the PC-system requires summation from a number of units to reach consciousness, it seems feasable that activity from one or several units might reach cortex, but does not give a positive psychophysical response. Whereas, in the other system (RA-system) the evidence indicated that a subject can detect psychophysically, activity from a single unit.

REFERENCES

Franzén, O. & Lindblom, U. Tactile intensity functions in patients with sutured peripheral nerve. In Y. Zotterman (Ed.), Sensory functions of the skin in primates, with special reference to man. Oxford, New York: Pergamon Press, 1976.

Libet, B., Alberts, W. W., Wright, E. W., Jr., Lewis, M., & Feinstein, B. Cortical representation of evoked potentials relative to conscious sensory responses, and of somatosensory qualities in man. In H. H. Kornhuber (Ed.), The somatosensory system. Stuttgart: Georg Thieme, 1975.

Verrillo, R. T. Effect of contractor area on the vibrotactile threshold. Journal of Acoustical Society of America, 1963, 35, 1962-1966.

ACTIVITY IN C NOCICEPTORS AND SENSATION

H. Erik Torebjörk

Department of Clinical Neurophysiology, University

Hospital, 75014 Uppsala, Sweden

Afferent unmyelinated (C) fibers are numerous in our peripheral cutaneous nerves, and they convey important messages about noxious skin stimuli and temperature changes in the skin. It is now possible to study in detail the discharge pattern of individual C units in human cutaneous nerves in situ (Torebjörk and Hallin, 1970) and to correlate directly the afferent discharge in different types of C units with sensation (e.g. Hallin and Torebjörk, 1970; van Hees and Gybels, 1972; Torebjörk, 1974; Konietzny and Hensel, 1975). This report will summarize briefly the physiological properties of C nociceptors in normal and injured skin in man, with reference to sensations evoked by various impulse patterns in these nociceptors.

IDENTIFICATION OF SINGLE C UNITS

C-unit potentials have been recorded with lacquer insulated tungsten semimicroelectrodes inserted percutaneously into the radial, peroneal or saphenous nerves in alert, healthy subjects. The C-fiber spikes appeared as all-or-none phenomena in responses to electrical or natural skin stimuli (Fig. 1), and several afferent C-units in a particular recording site could be identified as independent elements with separate receptive fields and individual conduction velocities (Torebjörk and Hallin, 1970, 1974a). These findings suggest that the C-fiber spikes derived from activity in single axons, and no signs of electrical interaction between adjacent axons have been observed. Some anatomical observations support this interpretation. Gasser (1955) followed the course of unmyelinated fibers in the saphenous nerve of the cat and found a continous interchange of axons between Schwann cell bundles. He came to the conclusion that unmyelinated axons ran in close association for only small distances, that were probably too short to allow for any cross excitation. In cutaneous nerves in man, the unmyelinated axons are enwrapped individually in small Schwann cell processes, each enclosing one or two axons which run separately, to reunite only near the nuclear region of the next Schwann cell in the chain (Ochoa, 1976). This arrangement might serve to prevent suprathreshold interaction between unmyelinated axons under normal conditions.

CLASSIFICATION OF C-UNITS

The uninsulated tip of the recording electrode usually picks up impulses from numerous fibers within a nerve fascicle, and the identification of a particular unit may be difficult if several units with similar potential waveforms interfere with each other. To overcome this problem, a special technique was developed (Hallin and Torebjörk, 1974; Torebjörk and Hallin, 1976a) which considerably facilitates the classification of various types of C-units. The method is based on the observation that repetitive firing caused a slowing of impulse conduction in unmyelinated fibers when the firing frequency was increased, and a slow recovery occurred when the frequency was lowered (Torebjork and Hallin, 1974b), (see also Fig. 1 D).

The technique works as follows: a number of C units are activated at a low (0.3 Hz) constant frequency by electrical stimulation through needle electrodes which are inserted intradermally 2 to 5 mm apart from each other. At this low frequency the latencies of C-fiber deflections are relatively constant. If a C unit is then also activated by physiological stimuli, a transient slowing of conduction will serve as a sensitive index of increased firing in that particular unit.

In this way it was possible to differentiate orthodromic impulses in afferent C-units, which were only activated from defined receptive fields in the skin, from antidromic impulses in sympathetic afferent C-units, which were activated by various psychological tests that increased the sympathetic outflow. Furthermore, a qualitative classification and an estimate of the relative occurrence of different types of afferent C-units could be made by observing their responsiveness to various types of skin stimuli (Torebjörk and Hallin, 1976b). Finally, the extents of the unitary receptive fields could be mapped with a high degree of reliability, since it was possible to determine if one and the same unit was activated by stimuli in different skin spots.

MULTISENSITIVE OR "POLYMODAL" NOCICEPTORS WITH C FIBERS

About two hundred afferent C-units have been studied in non-glabrous skin on the dorsum of the hand and forearm, as well as on

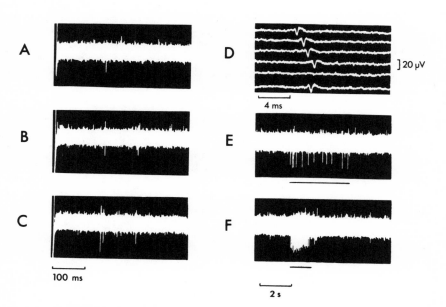

Fig. 1. Identification of single C-units in the intact radial
nerve in conscious man. Recording is at wrist level.

A-C: Recruitment of 3 individual C-units at increasing
strength of electrical stimulation (1 Hz) in the skin on
the dorsum of the hand. Conduction velocities were 0.84,
0.79 and 0.48 m/sex, respectively.

D: All-or-none responses in a single unit to electrical
stimulation (3 Hz). Note the progressive increase in
latency during repetitive activation, and the decrease in
excitability leading to a drop-out of the response. Also
note the recovery of latency after the block. These phenomena have been used for identification of single C units
in multi-unit recordings (see text).

E-F: C-nociceptor response to firm pressure (E) and painful heat (F) applied to the receptive skin field on the
dorsum of the hand. (Modified from Torebjörk and Hallin,
1970, with permission).

the dorsum of the foot and the lateral calf. The majority of these
were multisensitive nociceptors, which had the unique capacity to
give graded responses to mechanical, thermal and chemical stimuli
in the painful intensity range (van Hees and Gybels, 1972;
Torebjörk and Hallin, 1974a; Torebjörk, 1974; Torebjörk and Hallin,
1976b). In many respects, these nociceptors in man resemble the
so called "polymodal" nociceptors with C-fibers identified in
hairy skin of the cat (Bessou and Perl, 1969) and monkey (Beitel
and Dubner, 1976; Kumazawa and Perl, 1977).

The receptive skin areas of human C-nociceptors could extend from
less than 1 mm^2 up to 1 cm^2 and often were complex with several (2
to 7) point-like receptive maxima surrounded by areas of relative
insensitivity. The mosaic of sensitive spots of different C-units
did often overlap, so that even a pointed noxious stimulus could
activate several nociceptors. The complexity of the receptive
fields probably reflects peripheral branching of the parent axons.

The most sensitive C-nociceptors on the dorsum of the foot had
mechanical thresholds of about 0.7 g to stimulation with von Frey's
hairs. This, according to Strughold (1924), is the mean threshold
for the most sensitive "pain spots" in the skin of the foot. The
C-nociceptors were not spontaneously active at normal temperature
in undamaged skin. Many of them started to respond at skin temperatures of 43 to 45°C, and they were typically activated by painful heat. Rapid cooling (by ether or chlorethyl evaporation) below 20°C induced sparse activity in some of the units. Chemical
irritants, such as histamine or acetic acid elicited prolonged,
irregular activity, that correlated with sensations of pain or
itch.

The C-nociceptors showed a slow or intermediate adaptation to
constant mechanical stimuli as compared with rapidly and slowly
adapting mechanoreceptors with A-fibers in human skin. Some of the
units could continue to discharge at a low frequency for several
seconds after the stimulus had been withdrawn (Fig. 2B). Such
afterdischarges correlated with poorly described aftersensations,
following, for instance, a firm scratch on the skin. In general,
the discharge frequency of the C-nociceptors increased with increasing stimulus intensities, until receptor inactivation occurred due to discharge damage. Noxious stimuli, threatening to
damage the skin, could elicit short bursts of impulses with minimal
spike intervals equivalent to rates of 40 to 115 imp/sec (Torebjörk,
1974). However, during maintained stimulation the impulse frequency decreased; the mean frequency over 10 to 15 sec of noxious
heat stimulation being only a few impulses/sec (van Hees, 1976).
On repeated stimulation at short intervals, the receptor responses
as well as the after-discharges decreased as an indication of
"fatigue" (Fig. 2C). Apparently, the C-nociceptors have a limited
capacity to maintain high frequency activity for long periods of
time.

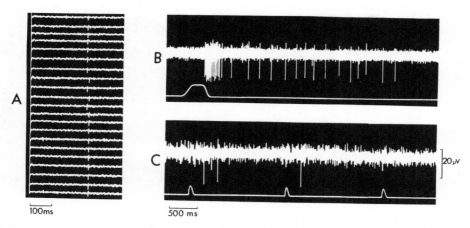

Fig. 2.   Some characteristics of an afferent C-unit, responding to
          mechanical and painful heat stimuli, recorded from the
          saphenous nerve. Receptive field (about 1 cm^2) in hairy
          skin near the ankle. Conduction velocity about 0.9 m/sec.

          A: Bimodal latency distribution of C-unit responses to
          intradermal electrical stimulation (0.5 Hz) of constant
          intensity indicates peripheral branching of the parent
          axon.

          B: The discharge pattern was characterized by a burst of
          impulses at application of blunt pressure (strain gauge
          signal indicated in lower trace), evident adaption on
          continous stimulation, and low frequency after-discharges
          after removal of the stimulus.

SENSITIZATION OF NOCICEPTORS IN HUMAN SKIN

     A superficial burn in the skin usually produces local hyper-
algesia, i.e. a painful oversensitivity to mechanical and thermal
stimuli. Preliminary attempts have been made to study the neurophysiological basis of this hyperalgesia in man (Torebjörk and
Hallin, 1977; Torebjörk and Hallin, 1978).

     Superficial burns were produced in the receptive fields of
C-nociceptor units by heat stimuli of 50°C applied to an area of
about 6 mm^2 on the dorsum of the hand or foot for 1.5 min. During
the first 5 to 8 min after heating, the C-unit responses were
typically reduced both to thermal and mechanical stimuli as compared with the responses before heating. This period of

desensitization corresponded with a period of hypoalgesia. During
the succeeding hour, some (but not all) of the C-nociceptors exhibited lower thresholds and enhanced responses to thermal and
mechanical stimuli as compared with controls before heating. During this period of sensitization the subjects reported hyperalgesia.

The desensitization immediately following the burn lesion might
be due to receptor fatigue after intense activation and/or partial
damage of the receptors. Prolonged heating for more than 3 min at
50°C could completely depress the responsiveness of some C-nociceptors for at least 1 hr probably as an indication of receptor
damage. The observed increase in the C-receptor responses was
possibly due to a release of algogenic substances, which could act
on reactive nerve endings.

It is of interest to note, the sensitization of C-nociceptors,
previously described in the skin of the rat (Witt and Griffin,
1962), in the cat (Bessou and Perl, 1969; Beck, Handwerker, and
Zimmermann,1974) and in monkey (Beitel and Dubner, 1976; Croze,
Duclaux and Kenshalo, 1976; Kumazawa and Perl, 1977), occurs also
in man. The parallel time courses between the desensitization of
C-nociceptors and the subjects' reports of hypo- and hyperalgesia,
respectively, suggest a contribution from C-nociceptors in the
production of hyperalgesia. However, a sensitization occurred not
only in some of the C-nociceptors but also in other nociceptors
supplied by fibers with higher conduction velocities (A-fibers).
This conclusion was based on the observation that the subjects reported pain in response to previously non-painful stimuli applied
to the sensitized skin on the foot even before the afferent C-fiber
signals reached the recording electrode in the peroneal nerve at
knee level. Obviously, the hyperalgesia following a burn can not
be explained only by sensitization of C-nociceptors, and we have to
look for more direct evidence of sensitization of human nociceptors
supplied by myelinated fibers, as described for the cat by
Fitzgerald and Lynn (1977) and for the monkey by Meyer, Campbell,
and LaMotte (1977) and LaMotte (this Symposium).

ACTIVITY IN C RECEPTORS AND SENSATION

Previous experiments with controlled selective nerve blocks in
alert man have shown that C-fibers mediate signals perceived as
warmth, heat, and delayed pain (Torebjörk and Hallin, 1973;
Mackenzie, Burke, Skuse, and Lethlean, 1975; Hallin and Torebjörk,
1976). Specific C "warm" receptors have been identified as reasonable candidates to signal warmth (Konietzny and Hensel, 1975;
Torebjörk and Hallin, 1976b). The C-nociceptors, which are activated by various kinds of stimuli that threaten to damage the skin
are obviously capable of signalling delayed pain. However, single
impulses from individual C receptors need not necessarily reach

consciousness (Torebjörk and Hallin, 1974a). Van Hees (1976) has tried to quantify the number of impulses that are necessary to evoke a pain sensation by heat stimuli. He calculated the mean impulse frequency in single C-polymodal nociceptors during periods of skin heating for up to 15 sec. Mean impulse frequencies below 0.3/sec were reported as nonpainful, whereas discharge frequencies exceeding 0.4/sec were mostly accompanied by pain. Discharges exceeding 1.5/sec were invariably associated with strong pain.

Many stimuli, that activate the C-nociceptors, also evoke impulses in other types of receptors and fibers, and the nociceptive message may very well be blocked or modified in the sensory processing of the afferent signals at central levels. Thus, repeated impulses from C-nociceptors need not be painful if they are elicited by, for instance, mechanical stimuli that cause simultaneous activation of mechanoreceptors with large myelinated fibers. After blocking of impulse transmission in myelinated fibers by nerve compression, identical mechanical stimuli, inducing approximately the same afferent inflow in unmyelinated fibers, are perceived as more painful than before the block. C-nociceptors are excited at low frequency by stimuli perceived as itch or heat. It is suggested the afferent signals from the C-nociceptors may contribute to a more or less painful component of such composite sensations, that probably results from activation of more than one receptor type.

SUMMARY

The relevance, to man, of the extensive work on C-nociceptors in animals is enhanced by the finding that there are C-receptors in human skin that, in several respects, resemble those found in the cat and the monkey. The relevance of this finding to the laboratory animals may also be important, from ethical points of view, inasmuch as human experimenters realize that their victims have, at least in part, a peripheral neural apparatus for pain that has similarities with their own.

The multisensitive C-nociceptors in human skin can be activated by various modes of stimulation, such as mechanical, thermal or chemical, that threaten to damage the skin, and signals from these nociceptors can give rise to a sensory modality of (delayed) pain. However, not only are the nociceptive signals modulated by interfering activity in the central nervous system, the activity of the nociceptors can be modulated in the periphery by previous activity (fatigue) or moderate tissue damage (sensitization). It is anticipated that further insight into the mechanisms for modulation of the nociceptive input from the periphery could be used for the relief of pain.

ACKNOWLEDGEMENTS

   This work was supported by the Swedish Medical Research Council, Grant No B 80-14X-05206-03A.

REFERENCES

Beck, P. W., Handwerker, H. O., & Zimmermann,M.   Nervous outflow
     from the cat's foot during noxious heat stimulation. Brain
     Research, 1974, 67, 373-386.
Beitel, R. E. & Dubner, R.   Response of unmyelinated (C) polymodal
     nociceptors to thermal stimuli applied to monkey's face.
     Journal of Neurophysiology, 1976, 39, 1160-1175.
Bessou, P. & Perl, E. R.   Response of cutaneous sensory units with
     unmyelinated fibers to noxious stimuli. Journal of Neuro-
     physiology, 1969, 32, 1025-1043.
Croze, S., Duclaux, R., & Kenshalo, D. R.   The thermal sensitivity
     of the polymodal nociceptors in the monkey. Journal of Phy-
     siology (London), 1976, 263, 539-562.
Fitzgerald, M. & Lynn, B.   The sensitization of high threshold
     mechanoreceptors with myelinated axons by repeated heating.
     Journal of Physiology (London), 1977, 365, 549-563.
Gasser, H. S.   Properties of dorsal root unmedullated fibers on the
     two sides of the ganglion. Journal of General Physiology,
     1955, 38, 709-728.
Hallin, R. G. & Torebjörk, H. E.   Afferent and efferent C units re-
     corded from human skin nerves in situ. Acta Societatis Medi-
     corum Upsaliensis, 1970, 75, 277-281.
Hallin, R. G. & Torebjörk, H. E.   Methods to differentiate elec-
     trically induced afferent and sympathetic C unit responses in
     human cutaneous nerves. Acta Physiologica Scandinavica, 1974,
     92, 318-331.
Hallin, R. G. & Torebjörk, H. E.   Studies on cutaneous A and C
     fiber afferents, skin nerve blocks and perception. In Y.
     Zotterman (Ed.), Sensory functions of the skin in primates.
     Oxford: Pergamon Press, 1976.
Hees, van, J.   Human C fiber input during painful and nonpainful
     skin stimulation with radiant heat. In J. J. Bonica & D.
     Albé-Fessard (Eds.), Advances in pain research and therapy.
     (Vol. 1), New York: Raven Press, 1976.
Hees, van, J. & Gybels, J. M.   Pain related to single afferent C
     fibers from human skin. Brain Research, 1972, 48, 397-400.
Konietzny, F. & Hensel, H.   Warm fiber activity in human skin
     nerves. Pflügers Archiv, 1975, 359, 265-267.
Kumazawa, T. & Perl, E. R.   Primate cutaneous sensory units with
     unmyelinated (C) afferent fibers. Journal of Neurophysiology,
     1977, 40, 1325-1338.

Mackenzie, R. A., Burke, D., Skuse, N. F., & Lethlean, A. K. Fiber function and perception during cutaneous nerve block. Journal of Neurology, Neurosurgery, and Psychiatry, 1975, 38, 865-873.

Meyer, R. A., Campbell, J. N., & LaMotte, R. H. Sensitization of A-delta nociceptive afferents to noxious radiant heat delivered to the monkey hand. Neuroscience Abstracts 7th Annual Meeting, 1973, 3, 487.

Ochoa, J. The unmyelinated nerve fiber. In D. N. Landon (Ed.), The peripheral nerve. London: Chapman and Hall, 1976.

Strughold, H. Uber die Dichte and Schwellen der Schmertzpunkte der Epidermis in den verschiedenen Körperregionen. Zeitschrift für Biologie, 1924, 80, 367-380.

Torebjörk, H. E. Afferent C units responding to mechanical, thermal and chemical stimuli in human non-glabrous skin. Acta Physiologica Scandinavica, 1974, 92, 374-390.

Torebjörk, H. E. & Hallin, R. G. C-fiber units recorded from human sensory nerve fascicles in situ. Acta Societatis Medicorum Upsaliensis, 1970, 75, 81-84.

Torebjörk, H. E. and Hallin, R. G. Perceptual changes accompanying controlled preferential blocking of A and C fiber responses in intact human skin nerves. Experimental Brain Research, 1973, 16, 321-332.

Torebjörk, H. E. & Hallin, R. G. Identification of afferent C units in intact human skin nerves. Brain Research, 1974a, 67, 387-403.

Torebjörk, H. E. & Hallin, R. G. Responses in human A and C fibers to repeated electrical intradermal stimulation. Journal of Neurology, Neurosurgery, and Psychiatry, 1974b, 37, 653-664.

Torebjörk, H. E. and Hallin, R. G. A new method for classification of C-unit activity in intact human skin nerves. In J. J. Bonica & D. Albé-Fessard (Eds.), Advances in pain research and therapy (Vol. 1), New York: Raven Press, 1976a.

Torebjörk, H. E. & Hallin, R. G. Skin receptors supplied by unmyelinated (C) fibers in man. In Y. Zotterman (Ed.), Sensory functions of the skin in primates. Oxford: Pergamon Press, 1976b.

Torebjörk, H. E. & Hallin, R. G. Sensitization of polymodal nociceptors with C fibers in man. Proceedings of the International Union of Physiological Sciences, 1977, 13, 758.

Torebjörk, H. E. & Hallin, R. G. Recordings of impulses in unmyelinated nerve fibers in man; afferent C fiber activity. Acta Anaesthesiologica Scandinavica, 1978, 70, 124-129.

Witt, J. & Griffin, J. P. Afferent cutaneous C-fiber reactivity to repeated thermal stimuli. Nature, 1962, 194, 776-777.

DISCUSSION

DR. JOHANSSON: I would like to ask a technical question. You say that these C-fibers did not show any spontaneous activity, and were not sensitive to weak mechanical stimulation nor to mild cooling or warming. How do you search for these units; what do you do?

DR. TOREBJORK: The first thing is that the recording electrode should be in good enough condition that it can record signals from C-fibers. To test this, I use synchronized signals in the sympathetic outflow to check the recording electrode. If the recordings are performed in a skin nerve, I will induce sympathetic reflex activity in efferent unmyelinated fibers by snapping my fingers or shouting at the subject or having him solve a mathematical problem. That is enough to induce considerable synchronized multi-fiber activity in C-fibers in the sympathetic system. As for the muscle nerves, one must look for another type of sympathetic activity in which the impulses are synchronized and which is easily identified by bursts of impulses waxing and waning with the respiration and mostly associated with the heart beats. When the electrode capacity has been checked I start to look for C-fiber units. I screen the receptive field as tested by touch stimuli when I know that I have signals from afferent A-fibers. I start with very light touch stimuli and mild cooling and mild warming. Then sometimes a warm receptor will appear. But, using this method, I have never seen any low threshold C-mechanoreceptor of the type I was referring to before. I start these testing maneuvers very lightly in order not to fatigue the receptors. When, in this way, I do not find any low threshold receptors I go on with stronger stimuli, for instance, scratching the skin with a piece of bristle or something like that. What I am particularly looking for then are the after-discharges at the end of the scratching. The C-fibers often show these after-discharges, in contrast to large A-fibers. Finally when I have found an area from which I have elicited these after-discharges, I use electrical stimulation in this area of the receptive field to check that I have C-fibers in my recording, as measured by the latency of the responses to the cutaneous test shocks. The electrical stimulation can continue in combination with physiological stimuli to check the specific type of receptor. That method has been described.

DR. IGGO: The results you've presented go a long way to resolving what did seem to be a very paradoxical situation. When single C-fibers became available in the cat it was immediately apparent that they were responding to a variety of different kinds of natural stimulation, light mechanical stimulation or mild heating or mild cooling or severe damaging intensities of stimulation and so on. In the work done in the late 1950's and early 60's the results coming from the cat seemed very difficult indeed to fit with the expectations from work done in man on peripheral nerve block and so on. It is really very interesting to find that your results have in fact shown that all the work on the cat might as well not have been done, except, perhaps, to give you some idea of what to look for. Because, you have, more or less, unless somebody comes along and upsets your results, established that the nonmyelinated afferents in man have the characteristics that had been predicted for nociceptors of a generalized sensitivity to a wide variety of noxious stimuli, and not, as I had expected would be found, quite a variety of different sorts of nociceptors. Could I now ask you a question? The warm fibers can be readily distinguished from the nociceptors?

DR. TOREBJÖRK: Yes.

DR. IGGO: In the monkey, one difference between the presumed warm fibers, and the nociceptors with the C-fiber axons is the size of the receptor field. In general in the monkey, in my experience, the warm fibers have quite tiny receptor fields whereas the nociceptors have a rather large receptor field. Do you find a similar kind of organization in man?

DR. TOREBJÖRK: The number of receptor fields innervated by specific warm fibers that I have investigated is limited but so far they are small, whereas the considerable number of the C-fiber nociceptor receptive fields are large and may be rather complex, as I showed.

DR. HENSEL: I think that this corresponds with our finding that the specific warm fibers have small almost "point-like" receptive fields. I have another question concerning the blocking of C-fibers by local anaesthetics. I have some doubts that a local anaesthetic will block first the C-fiber and then the others. There is some experimental evidence that the situation might be different. I was very surprised when applying a local anaesthetic to a multi-fiber preparation of the infraorbital nerve in the cat that contained unmyelinated warm fibers and small myelinated cold fibers. The local anaesthetic blocked first the whole group of cold fibers, warm fibers continued to fire after several minutes they too were blocked. The warm fiber discharge reappeared first and later the discharge of the cold fibers. I do not know how to explain that.

DR. TOREBJÖRK: In a more or less didactic lecture of this type, I have to generalize. I am very well aware that there are exceptions to the general rule that I described here. That has been pointed out in a paper by Hallin and myself, where we pointed out the difficulty in using local anaesthetics to estimate the relative importance of different fiber groups in sensation. Because the order of blocking is not always as constant as I had described and that might be, in part, due to heterogeneous infiltration of the anaesthetic in and among the fasiculi in the nerve, and also among the nerve fibers in the nerve. There appears to be quite a lot of exceptions to this general rule of blocking.

DR. ZOTTERMAN: We have now a rather great opportunity to discuss a problem that has been around for 50 years. What is the problem of the neural background tickle. We have here people who can record from single nerve fibers in humans and Perl, who together with Burgess recorded a lot of low threshold C fibers in the dorsal ganglion of the cat. That, of course, strengthens my old belief that tickle is modulated by specific C-fibers. I had the opportunity to examine a patient who had been operated on for trigeminal neuralgia. He could feel the touch of cotton wool on both sides of his face but no pain on the operated side. Also he could feel no tickle on the operated side. So superficial tickle was lost and I want you to see what correlate you can give for this. What happened in this man when you tickle?

DR. TOREBJÖRK: We have not found the tickle unit yet, but maybe Professor Perl has in the monkey.

DR. PERL: This is a question that could have been anticipated. I think there are several problems as well as some possible suggestions. The kind of sensory unit that Professor Zotterman was referring to is the C-mechanoreceptor that I believe was probably first seen by him in some multi-unit records back in 1939, and then subsequently described in Iggo's paper of 1960, in which he found a number of C units that had very low thresholds of mechanical stimuli and large receptive fields that change with the intensity of the stimulation. Our observations of these units suggested that they did have some interesting characteristics. They showed a considerable discharge for very slowly moving stimuli, the type of stimulus that is well known from common experience to provoke tickle in man. The trouble is that Dr. Torebjörk cannot find these in man, and we do not see these units in monkeys. At least they are so rare that we were suspicious of their occurrence. The most distally distributed nerves had far fewer than the more proximal nerves. There is one possibility that such C-units do exist in man, but they are only present in more proximal nerves. That does not explain, however, why we have tickle from the palm of our hand. That is clearly an area where tickle is readily illicited and, yet, an is clearly an area where tickle is readily elicited and, yet, an devoid to these C-mechanoreceptors. The only explanation that we might offer at this moment is something from some experiments that Dan Trevino and Ellen Lite, and that I have been doing on second order units in the spinal cord. That is that there are a significant number of units in the substantia gelatinosa that receive an excitation from slowly conducting myelinated fibers and that have most peculiar responses. They habituate very easily to repeated stimuli, they have a definite predilection to very slowly moving mechanical disturbances across the surface of the skin, and they have no input from the more rapidly conducting myelinated fibers. We have no idea where they project. We know that they are substantia gelatinosa neurons, without question, because we have filled them and have nice Golgi type pictures of them. They are very distinctive and are different from the units that have other kinds of afferent input. So there is a possible explanation to suggest that perhaps there is a substantial central processing as well as some special receptor characteristics in the periphery. The slowly conducting myelinated fibers that project upon these units are responsive to very gentle mechanical stimuli. They were called D or delta hair follicle receptors by Iggo. They may or may not be hair follicle receptors. There is some question about that, but whatever they are, they are units that seem also to exist in the glabrous skin. At least something very similar to them exists in the transitional skin, in particular and it is possible that those people who are recording from slowly conducting myelinated fibers in man, if that ever becomes a regular possibility, we will see whether they occur in sufficient numbers to perhaps offer an explanation.

DR. LAMOTTE: Equal in mystery is the sensation of itch, and I wonder if during your recordings of these substantia gelatinosa neurons, Dr. Perl, if you happened to notice any response to a stimulus that might provoke itch. The reason I ask this is that after-discharges usually do not last very long in primary afferent fibers, at least not as long as a tickle can last. There is a specific phenomenon that you might look at. It is very easy to evoke itch in human transitional skin around the wrist. If you poke a 25 micron wire into the skin you get a pricking pain, then 1 or 2 sec later you get an explosion of itch sensation that lasts several seconds and it is best evoked in the hairy skin of the wrist. It can be gotten in the glabrous skin but the itch sensation only lasts a few seconds. So it is possible to study itch without histamine or other drugs and so forth. The itch is totally eliminated by rubbing and you can rub before you do it and you will only get the pricking sensation and not the itch .

DR. TOREBJÖRK: I was very interested by your finding. Actually the itch sensation can also be easily induced by a von Frey hair, especially if you waddle it a bit in the skin. That induces C-fiber activity regularly, as I've shown here.

INTENSIVE AND TEMPORAL DETERMINANTS OF THERMAL PAIN

Robert H. LaMotte, Department of Anesthesiology

Yale University School of Medicine, 333 Cedar Street

New Haven, Connecticut 06510

The search for peripheral neural determinants of pain is aided by the attempt to correlate measurements of pain sensation with neural activity in peripheral afferent nerve fibers. Those fibers that respond only to noxious stimulation of their receptive fields are called "nociceptive afferents" and their distal endings, "nociceptors". The word "nociceptive" is derived from the Latin word for "injury"; yet a biologically useful function of neural activity in nociceptive afferents may be to evoke pain in order to signal the threat of injury before it actually occurs (Burgess and Perl, 1973). Evidence for this comes from the close correlation between neural activity in nociceptive afferents in the peripheral nerve of conscious humans and simultaneous reports of pain during noxious stimulation of the skin (Torebjörk and Hallin, 1974; van Hees and Gybels, 1972). Heating the skin is an effective method of quantifying noxious stimulation. It is well known that the magnitude of pain, evoked by heating the skin, is determined to a large extent by the stimulus temperature. Much less is known about the temporal determinants of pain and the way is which the duration and frequency of heating interact with intensity to influence the magnitude of pain. I will describe our analyses of these variables in psychophysical studies in humans, and in studies of heat-sensitive nociceptors in the monkey.

THERMAL INJURY AND THE ACUTE INFLAMMATORY REACTION

The relation between intensive and temporal parameters of stimulation has been examined in studies of cutaneous thermal injury. A mild local injury results, within seconds, in the release of chemical mediators which act primarily on the microcirculation and trigger one or more signs of an acute inflammatory

327

reaction (Ryan and Majno, 1977). These signs include heat and
erythema (produced by vasodilation), swelling (caused by an increase in vascular permeability), and pain. Which of these signs
occur, and how many, will depend in part upon the type of injury,
its severity, and the characteristics of the skin, such as the type
of vascularization. The latter differs for different loci on the
body and from one species to the next (Sevitt, 1957; Wilhelm and
Mason, 1960). Table 1 illustrates some of the time-dependent consequences of thermal stimuli of different temperatures applied to
the skin of humans and certain animals. This information was taken
from studies in which the skin was heated rapidly to achieve a
desired temperature and this temperature then held constant for the
stated duration. The table shows that the presence or absence of
certain signs of inflammation, and the occurrence of irreversible
cellular damage (transepidermal necrosis), depend not only upon
the intensity of the stimulus, but also upon its duration and the
number and rate of stimulations. For example, a continuous stimulation of 49°C, to the pig (whose skin is similar to man's), must
last about 9 min for transepidermal necrosis to occur. Stimulation of 49°C for 3 min produces only erythema, a reversible condition (although histological analysis will reveal some epidermal
cells that are irreversibly affected) (Moritz and Henriques, 1947)
yet, if this stimulus is followed by two more stimuli, each of 3
min duration, at 24 and 48 min, transepidermal necrosis occurs.

The data presented in Table 1 encourage speculation about the
relation between pain, injury, and the responses of nociceptors.
The most successful attempt to link pain with injury was Hardy's
thermochemical model which related the magnitude of pain to the
rate of tissue damage (Hardy, 1953). However, it is necessary to
modify his original model in order to account for the transient
pain (and responses in a few nociceptors) evoked by temperatures
below 49°C where the possibility of injury is essentially nonexist-
ent (Hardy, Stolwijk, Hammel, and Murgatroyd, 1965; Hardy, Stolwijk,
and Hoffman, 1968). Indeed, a conclusion of practical importance
from Table 1 is that if short durations of thermal stimuli are
used, it is possible to evoke intense pain without injury, Hardy
predicted that very intense pain, between 9 and 10 on the "dol"
scale of pain, could be evoked without tissue damage for relatively
short durations of 5 sec or less at constant temperatures (Hardy,
1953).

RESPONSE SPECIFICITY OF NOCICEPTORS

The existence of nociceptors as a class separate from other
classes of cutaneous receptors and the existence of nociceptors
with myelinated and unmyelinated axons were predicted in the early
work of Zotterman (Zotterman, 1933; Zotterman, 1936). There is
now considerable evidence that nociceptors with either type of
axon can be classified further into subgroups based upon differences
in the specificity of their responses to certain forms of stimulus

Table 1   Selected effects of heating the skin.

STIMULUS TEMPERATURE* AT SKIN SURFACE (C°)	DURATION OF STIMULIS*	RESULTS
≥ 55	≥ 30 SEC.	Inactivation of Many Nociceptive Afferents (Monkey, Cat) (Burgess & Perl, 1973; Fitzgerald & Lynn, 1977)
53	40 SEC.	Minimal Increase in Permeability of Dermal Vessels (Guinea Pig) (Sevitt, 1964)
	20-30 SEC.	Erthema Only (Guinea Pig, Human) (Sevitt, 1964) Sensitization of AMH Nociceptors*** (Monkey) (Campbell et al., in press; Meyer et al., 1977)
50	8 MIN.	Minimal Increases in Permeability of Dermal Vessels (Guinea Pig) (Sevitt, 1964)
49	3 SEC; Fast Rise Time From Base of 38° to 49°C in 300 MSEC.	Some C-Polymodal Nociceptors Respond in 300 Msec (Monkey) (LaMotte & Campbell, 1978)
	9 MIN**	Transepidermal Necrosis (Pig) (Moritz & Henriques, 1947)
	3 MIN: THEN Again 24 and 48 MIN Later.	With Single Application: Erythema, But No Macroscopic Epidermal Injury; After Repeating, Transepidermal Necrosis (Pig) (Moritz & Henriques, 1947)
47	5 MIN.	Pain Increases; May Reach Plateau; Erythema (Man (Fig. 11)
45	5 MIN.	Pain May Decrease or Disappear; Then Increases (Man) (Fig. 11)
44	6 HOURS.***	Transepidermal Necrosis (Man) (Moritz & Henriques, 1947)
43-44	3 SEC.	Mean Threshold in C-Polymodal Nociceptors (Monkey and Pain Threshold (Man) When Base Temp = 38°C (Glab. Skin) (LaMotte & Campbell, 1978)
43	5 MIN.	Initial Pain Disappears (Fig. 11)
36-41	5 MIN.	Thresholds for a Few C-Polymodal Nociceptors (Monkey) (Beitel & Dubner, 1976a; LaMotte & Campbell, 1978) and Pain Threshold (Man) When Base Temp. = 31-35°C (Hairy Skin) (Hardy, et al., 1965; Lele, Weddell & Williams, 1954).

*   Values subject to errors inherent in the various methods of temperature
     measurement and control.
**   Minimal durations.
*** Mechanosensitive nociceptors with A-fibers that sensitize to heat (see
     text)

energy (Burgess and Perl, 1973; Georgopoulos, 1976). The diversity
of nociceptor response to different types of stimuli is summarized
in Table 2 by a list of studies that were carried out in cat, monkey and man. There are nociceptors that respond only to thermal
and not to mechanical stimulation, or to the converse, while others
respond to various combination of thermal and mechanical stimulation such as to cold and mechanical stimuli but not to heat, and
so on. Some of these nociceptors have myelinated axons (A fibers)
while others have unmyelinated axons (C fibers). The results of
the studies referenced in Table 2 support several generalizations:
(a) there are no overall differences between myelinated and unmyelinated nociceptive afferents as to the type of stimuli to which
they will respond (Georgopoulos, 1976); (b) afferents innervating
the hairy, and glabrous, skin are responsive to the same types of
stimuli; (c) few differences have been found between properties of
the same type of nociceptor in cat, monkey and man. The latter
statement is important for establishing the validity of correlations between studies of monkey and man; and (d) nociceptors can
be classified most conveniently on the basis of their response
specificities for different forms of energy impinging upon the
skin; it seems reasonable to predict that nociceptors will be
found for all categories in Table 2.

Additional classifications of nociceptors based upon differences in their chemoreceptive properties have been omitted from
Table 2 for simplification. It is well known, however, that nociceptors may be sensitive to certain chemicals, externally applied
(Keele and Armstrong, 1964; Szolcsanyi, 1976; Szolcsanyi, 1977) or,
to one or more chemical mediators (e.g., histamine and proteases)
or their by-products (e.g. kinins) that are released following
tissue injury (Beck and Handwerker, 1974; Handwerker, 1976; Keele
and Armstrong, 1964; Szolcsanyi, 1976; Szolcsanyi, 1977; Torebjörk
and Hallin, 1974; van Hees and Gybels, 1972). Thus, nociceptors
may be activated in at least two ways, one of which is direct, in
response to a specific type (or types) of energy, externally
applied; the other way, indirect in response to substances released internally as a result of tissue damage. Both types of
activation would provide input to a receptor that encodes the
intensity of painful stimulation of the skin.

EXPERIMENTAL STUDIES OF PAIN

Described here are the results of some studies in which recordings of neural activity in single nociceptive afferents in
monkeys are related to psychophysical measurements of pain in humans. The C-polymodal nociceptors and one class of A-fiber nociceptors were studied in detail. In one series of experiments, when
the skin of human subjects was heated repetitively, there was a
suppression of pain (a reduction in magnitude during intermittent

Table 2   Nociceptive afferents studied in primate and cat.

STIMULUS SPECIFICITY	TYPE OF SKIN			
	GLABROUS		HAIRY	
	C-FIBERS	A-FIBERS	C-Fibers	A-FIBERS

Mechanical (Mech.,)	Monkey:
	  Georgopoulos, 1976
	  LaMotte & Campbell, 1978
	Cat:
	  [c]Beck et al., 1974
		Campbell et al, Sub.
		Georgopoulous, 1976
		Perl, 1968
		
		[c]Beck et al., 1974
			Kumazawa & Perl, 1977
			LaMotte & Campbell, 1978
			
			[c]Beck et al., 1974
			Bessou & Perl, 1969
				[c]Dubner & Hu, 1977a
				Perl, 1968
				
				[c]Beck et al., 1974
				Burgess & Perl, 1967
				Burgess et al., 1968
				Hunt & McIntyre, 1960

Mechanothermal: Mech + Heat (polymodal)	Monkey:
	  Georgopoulos, 1976
	  LaMotte & Campbell, 1978
	Human:
	
	Cat:
	  [c]Beck et al., 1974
		Campbell et al., Sub.
		Georgopoulos, 1976
			Beitel & Dubner, 1976a
			Croze et al., 1976
			Kumazawa & Perl, 1977
			LaMotte & Campbell, 1978
			Torebjörk & Hallin, 1974
			Torebjörk & Hallin, 1976
			Van Hees & Gybels, 1972
			
			[c]Beck et al., 1974
			Bessou & Perl, 1965
			Iggo, 1959
				[c]Campbell et al., Sub.
				Dubner & Hu, 1977a
				
				[*]Fitzgerald & Lynn, 1977

Mech + Cold	Monkey:
	  Georgopoulos, 1976
	  LaMotte & Campbell, 1978
	Cat:
		Georgopoulos, 1976	Iggo, 1959
			Iriuchijima & Zotterman, 1960	

Mech + Heat	Monkey:
	  Georgopoulos, 1976
	  LaMotte & Campbell, 1978
	Human:
	Cat:
		Georgopoulos, 1976	LaMotte & Campbell, 1978
			
			Torebjörk & Hallin, 1976
			Bessou & Perl, 1969
			Iggo, 1959
			Iriuchijima & Zotterman, 1960
				Iggo & Ogawa, 1971
				Kumazawa & Perl, 1977

Thermal: Heat	Monkey:
	  Georgopoulos, 1976
	Cat:
	  [c]Beck et al., 1974
		Georgopoulos, 1976	[c]Beck et al., 1974	

Cold	Monkey:	[d]LaMotte & Thalhammer Unpublished		[d]LaMotte & Thalhammer, Unpublished
Heat + Cold	Monkey: Georgopoulos, 1976 Cat:	Georgopoulos, 1976		

[c]Sensitivity to cold was not tested.
[*]These fibers, most of which were intially unresponsive to heat, became "sensitized" following repeated presentations of noxious heat.
[d]These fibers had no spontaneous activity, and responded only to cold, with increasing rates of discharge, as stimulus temperature was decreased over the range of 20 to 0°C or lower. Conduction velocity ranged from 3 to 10 m/sec (n=4).

stimulation). This was compared with the well-known <u>fatigue</u> that
can occur in the responses of nociceptors in monkeys <u>during</u> repetitive stimulation. In other experiments certain conditions
were determined under which, instead of suppression, <u>hyperalgesia</u>
(an increase in pain sensibility) occurred in humans and <u>sensitiza-</u>
<u>tion</u> of nociceptors to heat developed in monkeys. In another
series of experiments the skin was heated for 5 min to a constant
temperature; the <u>adaptation</u> of pain (a reduction in sensory magnitude during a sustained stimulation) at lower temperatures, was
compared with the development of hyperalgesia at higher temperatures. Drs. Campbell and Meyer collaborated with me on certain
phases of this work (Campbell, Meyer, and LaMotte, in press; LaMotte
and Campbell, 1978; Meyer, Campbell, and LaMotte, 1977).

     Stimulus temperature was controlled at the surface of the
skin in either of two ways: (a) with a radiant heat source provided by a CO_2 infrared laser; the power to the laser was controlled to maintain the desired surface skin temperature via feedback from a radiometer that remotely sensed skin temperature
(LaMotte and Campbell, 1978; Meyer, Walker, and Mountcastle, 1976)
or (b) with a contact stimulator that maintained the temperature
of a silver plate pressed against the skin; the other side of the
plate was warmed by heating cool circulating fluid; the temperature,
recorded by a thermocouple at the interface between the skin, and
the thermode plate, was held constant by feedback control (Darian-
Smith, Johnson, LaMotte, Shigenaga, Kenins, and Champness, in
press; Hilder, Ramey, Darian-Smith, Johnson, and Dally, 1974). All
results except those illustrated in Fig. 1, 5A and 10, were obtained with the contact thermal stimulator.

A SCALE OF SUBJECTIVE THERMAL INTENSITY

     In the first series of psychophysical experiments, a scale
of subjective thermal intensity was derived using the radiant heat
stimulator. Stimuli of 40-50°C, each 3 sec in duration and 7.5
mm in diameter, were randomly delivered to the glabrous skin of
the hand superimposed on a base-temperature ("adapting temperature")
of 38°C. Four human subjects categorized the sensation evoked by
each stimulus as warmth, heat, or pain, that was either faint, moderate, strong, or very strong. These categorizations were given
numerical values and then transformed so that the values represented responses to the stimuli on an equal-interval scale, according to the method of successive intervals (Torgerson, 1958).

     The scale in Fig. 1 is the first of its kind in which the
magnitude of thermal sensation is related to stimulus temperature,
held constant at the surface of the skin during radiant heating.
The perceived magnitude of radiant heat is a slightly positively
accelerating function of stimulus temperature. The low end of the
scale is "anchored" to the detection threshold for warming. We

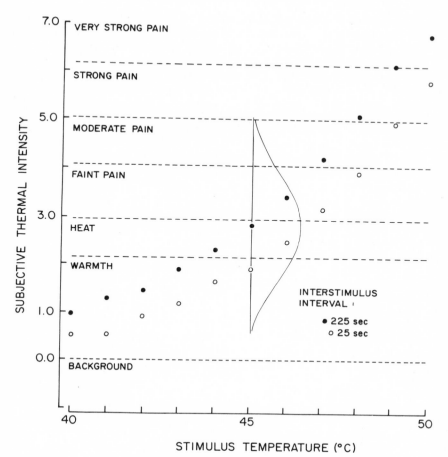

Fig. 1. A scale of the subjective intensity of radiant heat. Four
         subjects categorized the magnitude of thermal sensations
         evoked by radiant heat delivered to the glabrous skin of
         the hand.   The category ratings were used to construct an
         equal-interval scale using the method of successive in-
         terval Torebjörk & Hallin, 1977).   Closed circles repre-
         sent scale values obtained when the mean interstimulus
         interval (ISI) was 225 sec. Open circles designate scale
         values with a mean ISI of 25 sec. The dashed lines are
         the obtained boundaries between each category. Each stimu-
         lus scale value represents the mean of the normal distri-
         bution of category responses obtained for a given stimulus
         temperature and ISI. Distance along the ordinate is pro-
         vided in standard-deviation units.

         The distribution of responses to the 45°C stimulus de-
         livered under the long ISI condition is illustrated and

is representative of the other distributions. The boundary for heat intersects this distribution at a point that
is 0.13 standard deviation units above the distribution mean
thereby indicating that 55% of the response of the 45°C stimulus under the long ISI condition were choices of "heat" or
less while 45% were judgments of "faint pain" or greater.

The scale shows that the magnitude of warm and painful
sensation depends not only upon stimulus temperature but
also upon the rate of stimulus delivery. A more rapid
delivery suppresses subjective thermal intensity (from
LaMotte and Campbell, 1978).

also obtained a slightly positively accelerating function when subjects used numbers of their own choosing and made ratio judgments
of subjective magnitude (unpublished observations). The advantages of this category scale are the following: (a) we can state
precisely the frequency with which a subject assigns each of these
labels to each stimulus temperature (see legend of Fig. 1). It is
noteworthy that stimulus temperatures as high as 47°C may occasionally evoke sensations of warmth without pain, in agreement with
the results of another psychophysical study (Hardy et al., 1968)
and with evidence from neurophysiological studies that warm fiber
afferents may still be active at temperatures of 47 to 49°C (Darian-
Smith et al., in press; LaMotte and Campbell, 1978; Sumino, Dubner,
and Starkman, 1973); (b) we can estimate how well subjects can
discriminate one stimulus from another, on the basis of the number
of standard deviations on the ordinate that separates two stimuli
on the abscissa; (c) we can state how the magnitude of warmth and
pain, evoked by stimulations of the same spot on the skin vary as
a function of two interstimulus intervals; the scale of Fig. 1
shows that the more rapid delivery suppresses subjective thermal
intensity.

   In a parallel series of experiments in the anesthetized monkey, we delivered the same radiant heat stimuli to the receptive
fields of mechanothermal nociceptors: most of these were C-fiber
polymodal nociceptors (CPNs). The cumulative number of impulses
evoked in each CPN during each stimulus was plotted against the
temperature of the stimulus. Typically, the resulting intensity-
response function was slightly positively accelerating in agreement
with the results of previous studies of these fibers in the monkey
(e.g., Beitel and Dubner, 1976b). Furthermore, these functions increased monotonically over the range of temperatures described by
humans as increasingly painful (45 to 50°C). Thus, neural activity
in the population of CPNs increases in a parallel fashion with
judgments of increasing magnitude of pain, and thus may encode the
intensity of pain (LaMotte and Campbell, 1978). These results are
consistent with those obtained by comparing judgments of pain in
humans with simultaneous recordings from CPNs in the same subjects

(Torebjörk and Hallin, 1974; van Hees and Gybels, 1972). To this
we have added another observation: the magnitude of pain and the
magnitude of response of CPNs depend not only upon stimulus intensity but also upon stimulus history. Specifically, we find the
magnitude of pain sensations in humans and the cumulative number
of impulses evoked in CPNs by each stimulus varies inversely with
the number, delivery rate and intensity of preceding stimulations
(LaMotte and Campbell, 1978). Some of these and additional findings are documented in the following paragraphs.

THE EFFECTS OF SUPPRESSION AND FATIGUE UPON TEMPERATURE THRESHOLDS

The suppressive effects of preceding stimuli have a number
of consequences that provide additional support for the hypothesis
that activity in CPNs encode the intensity of painful stimulation
of the skin. Firstly, the threshold response to heat of CPNs is
lowest in unstimulated skin, but then is elevated, with repeated
thermal stimulations, by an amount related to the intensities of
stimulation and the interstimulus intervals. In glabrous skin
adapted to 38°C and not previously stimulated with higher temperatures, the threshold for 34 CPNs innervating the glabrous skin of
the monkey averaged 43.6°C, while the threshold for pain (one
stimulus per day) in humans varied between 42 and 44°C (LaMotte
and Campbell, 1978). In hairy skin, and with a lower temperature
of adaptation, thresholds can be as low as 36°C (Hardy et al.,
1965; LaMotte and Campbell, 1978; Lele, Weddell and Williams,
1954). When stimuli of different intensities are applied twice
every minute to the same locus on the glabrous skin, the threshold
for pain in humans (see Fig. 1) and the fiber threshold in monkeys
may be elevated as high as 47°C.

It is apparent from the data in Table 1 and Fig. 1, that the
threshold for pain can vary over at least a range of 11°C from
36 to 47°C depending upon such differences as locus on the body
(Hardy, Wolff, and Goodell, 1952), stimulus duration, base temperature (i.e., prior adaptation) and the effects of preceding stimuli
delivered to the same spot on the skin. Thus, it is risky to compare results obtained by one investigator with those of another unless, in each case, the above conditions are precisely specified.

THE TEMPORAL COURSE OF DEVELOPMENT OF SUPPRESSION AND FATIGUE

The suppressive effects of preceding stimulations has been
observed in experiments wherein stimuli of the same temperature
are delivered repeatedly to the same spot on the skin (LaMotte and
Campbell, 1978; Price and Dubner, 1977; Price, Hu, Dubner, and
Gracely, 1977). In one series of experiments, a stimulus of 49°C
and 3 sec duration was delivered every 28 sec to the human hand and
to the cutaneous receptive fields of CPNs in the monkey. The

magnitude of pain evoked in humans decreased with each stimulation
in parallel with a decrease in the number of impulses evoked in
monkey CPNs. The magnitude of pain and the impulse-count in CPNs
decreased the greatest amount during the first two stimulations,
after which a plateau in response magnitude was reached (LaMotte
and Campbell, 1978). These findings confirm those of other
studies in which either the fatigue of nociceptors in monkeys or
the suppression of pain in humans was observed during repetitive
stimulation of the skin (e.g., Price et al., 1977).

        At relatively high temperatures of stimulation, the phenomenon
of fatigue prevents those CPNs directly under the thermal stimulus
from signaling the increasing "threat of injury". An example is
provided by the responses of a CPN to a 50°C, 10 sec duration
stimulus repeated every 30 sec (Fig. 1). Fatigue is not merely
the result of injury to the receptor as might be hypothesized
following delivery of higher temperatures (Beitel and Dubner, 1976a).
A result such as that in Fig. 2 is usually reproducible following
a 10 to 20 min interval without stimulation. Further, the same
temporal course of fatigue in CPN response is found using stimuli
of lower temperatures, including those that are non-injurious to
the skin, such as 45°C, 3 sec in duration, presented every 28 sec.

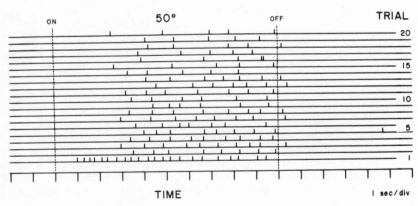

Fig. 2. Responses of a C-polymodal nociceptive afferent, inner-
         vating the monkey palm, to a series of 50°C stimuli. Heat
         pulses of 10 sec duration were delivered every 30 sec with
         the contact thermal stimulator. Base temperature, between
         successive stimuli, was 38°C. Each horizontal line re-
         presents one trial. Each small vertical mark represents
         a single nerve impulse. The dashed vertical lines mark
         the time between onset of the stimulus and the onset of
         cooling. (LaMotte and Thalhammer, unpublished observation).

RECOVERY CYCLES FOR FATIGUE AND SUPPRESSION

In earlier neurophysiological experiments the recovery cycle of fatigue was determined for a few CPNs (LaMotte and Campbell, 1978). Most fibers recovered to nearly 100 percent during a 10 min stimulus-free interval following a 49°C stimulus. Recently, I have studied the recovery cycle of the suppression of subjective intensity in humans following repeated stimulations of 47°C. I used a procedure that measured the change in the magnitude of thermal sensations as a function of time. A similar procedure has been used in studies of tingling (Gernandt and Zotterman, 1946) and chemogenic pain (Keele and Armstrong, 1964). Three subjects made category judgments of the magnitude of warmth and pain using a scale of 0 to 30 with 6 verbal labels: 1 to 4 = "warmth", 5 to 9 = "heat", 10 to 14 = "faint pain", 15 to 19 = "moderate pain", 20 to 24 = "strong pain" 25 to 29 = "very strong pain" and 30 to 35 = an additional category, if needed. Before, during, and following each stimulus, the subjects indicated perceived intensity continuously by moving a lever-potentiometer along side the numerical scale. Voltage analogs of the subjects' response and the stimulus temperature were collected via PDP 11/40 computer and presented in real-time on a high resolution graphic display (VT-11) (Digital Equipment Corp.); stimulus control, and data analyses were carried out by the same computer. The computer programs were written by Dr. David Stagg. The subject could not see the screen and received no feedback during the experiment.

In the first experiment, a 5 sec stimulus of 47°C was delivered repeatedly to the same spot on the volar forearm every 30 sec for 6 trials. Typical results obtained during the first 6 presentations are illustrated in Fig. 3. The magnitude of sensation during a stimulus reached a maximum near the end of the stimulus (heating) but occasionally continued after the onset of cooling. The greatest category rating occurred during the first presentation of the stimulus (top, Fig. 3). The pain evoked during the first two trials was no longer present by the fourth trial. After 6 trials, a 5 min waiting period ensued without further stimulation after which the sequence was repeated; this was followed a 10 min interval and then a third sequence of 6 stimulations. The recovery from suppression was nearly complete following the 10 min interval as indicated by the results of the same subject (bottom, Fig. 3) and by the maximum category ratings of each stimulus, averaged for the 3 subjects and shown in Fig. 4. The averaged rating on the first trial after the 10 min interval was 90 percent of that obtained on the first trial at the beginning of the experiment. These results emphasize the importance of allowing very long intervals between successive stimulations of the same locus on the skin in experiments where temporal interactions are to be entirely avoided.

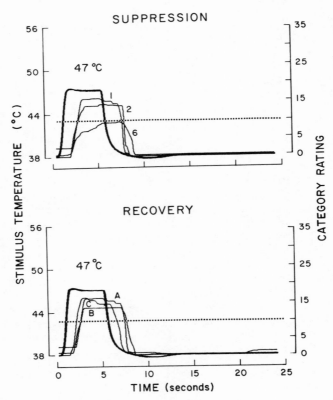

Fig. 3. Continuous category ratings of the magnitude of thermal sensations, during and immediately following a stimulus of 47°C delivered every 30 sec to the thenar eminence of the hand. The voltage analogs of stimulus temperature for 3 different presentations are superimposed (dark lines). The subject rated the intensity by moving a lever-potentiometer along a numerical scale (position indicated by the thin lines) (see text). The dashed line marks the threshold for pain. A: Intentsity-time ratings of the first, second and sixth presentation of the stimulus. Note that the subjective intensity was suppressed on the 6th trial to the extent that pain was no longer evoked. B: Intensity-time ratings of the first presentation of the stimulus in a series of 6 where the first series was presented without prior stimulation (A); the series was repeated after a 5 min pause (B) and then repeated again after a 10 min pause (C). Note that there was more recovery from suppression following the 10 min interval.

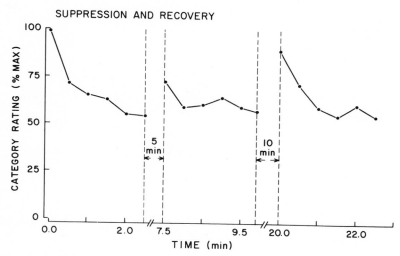

Fig. 4. Suppression and recovery of subjective intensity during
         repetitions of a 47°C stimulus. The maximum intensity-
         rating of each presentation of a 47°C stimulus was ob-
         tained from data of the type shown in Fig. 3 and averaged
         for 3 subjects. These averages are expressed as a per-
         cent of the maximum response obtained. Note that the
         ratings of intensity decreased with successive presen-
         tations within each series of 6 trials (suppression).
         Recovery from suppression was nearly complete after the
         10 min stimulus-free interval.

CONSEQUENCES OF CHANGES IN THE RANGE OF STIMULUS TEMPERATURES

        A characteristic of fatigue in CPNs is that it is graded in
direct proportion to the intensity of preceding stimuli. A parallel
phenomenon occurs in the psychophysical setting. The magnitude of
thermal sensation evoked in humans and the number of impulses evoked
in monkeys CPNs by a heating stimulus varies inversely with the
temperature of the preceding stimulus delivered earlier (LaMotte
and Campbell, 1978). The number of impulses evoked in CPNs by a
stimulus also depends upon the context in which the stimulus is
presented; specifically it depends on the range of stimulus temperatures used. In one experiment, stimuli of 41 to 49°C (in 2°
steps) were randomly presented in the receptive fields of CPNs in
the monkey followed, after a 10 min pause, by a second set of
stimuli randomly delivered and ranging from 45 to 53°C in 2° steps.
The intensity-response functions of CPNs shifted along the

temperature axis without a change in slope, following a change from
one range of intensities to the other (see Fig. 5A). A shift in
the function from left to right along the temperature axis, when
the range of stimulus temperatures shifted from low (41 to 49°C)
to high (45 to 53°C), is due presumably to the suppressive effects
of 51 and 53°C. A stimulus within the upper range had to be about
3°C higher than a stimulus within the lower range in order to evoke
the same response.

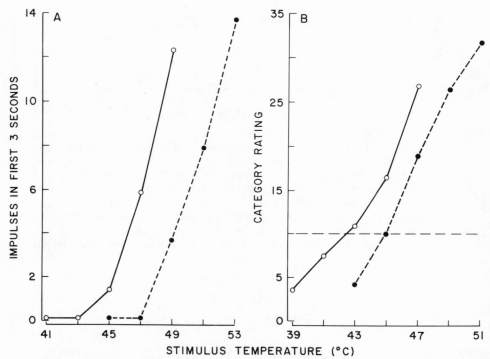

Fig. 5.   Shifts in the intensity-response functions with changes
           in the range of stimulus temperatures. A: Intensity-
           response functions averaged for 3 C-polymodal nociceptive
           afferents innervating the monkey palm. Stimuli of 3 sec
           duration, were randomly presented and ranged in 2°C steps
           either from 41°C to 49°C (solid line) or from 45°C to 53°C
           (dashed line) (From LaMotte and Campbell, 1978). B: Mag-
           nitude of warmth and pain in one subject as a function of
           stimulus temperature and temperature range. Stimuli of 5
           sec duration were randomly presented to the thenar eminence
           of the hand and ranged in 2°C steps either from 39 to 47°C
           (solid line) or from 43 to 51°C (dashed line). The hori-
           zontal dashed lines designate the threshold for pain.

I obtained an analogous result in a phychophysical experiment wherein human subjects made continuous category ratings of stimuli with the lever-potentiometer. The stimuli ranged in 2° steps of intensity either from 39 to 47°C, on certain days of testing, or from 43 to 51°C on the other days. Subjects were not informed as to the nature of any variations in the stimuli. They were instructed to judge each sensation on an "absolute" and not a "relative" scale of sensory magnitude. The maximum category ratings obtained in response to each stimulus, for one subject, are shown in the ordinate of Fig. 5B. The psychophysical function is shifted without a change in slope, in correspondence with the shift in temperature range. Stimuli of 43 to 47°C were judged as lesser in magnitude when presented in context with 49 and 51°C. The implication from the data in Fig. 5 is that the fatigue of CPNs may serve to maintain the slope of the intensity-response functions of nociceptors afferents despite upward shifts in the range of stimulus intensities. This, in turn, may contribute to a constancy in discriminative judgements of pain, from one "working range" of temperatures to the next, thereby increasing the range of intensities over which discriminative capacity is maintained. In the visual system an analagous shift, by an entirely different neural mechanism (viz. synaptic), of the intensity-response curves of bipolar cells along the intensity axis occurs as the intensity of the surround illumination is increased (Thibos and Werlin, 1978). This mechanism is thought to be important for maintaining contrast sensitivity to local differences in intensity despite wide variations in ambient intensity.

TEMPORAL PROFILES OF THERMAL SENSATIONS THAT DIFFER IN MAGNITUDE

Stimuli of different temperatures evoke sensations that differ not only in magnitude but also in duration. Each category rating in Fig. 5B was the maximum height of a curve that was an average of several curves each depicting a continuous rating of sensory magnitude as a function of time. These intensity-time profiles, obtained for the two temperature ranges, are shown in Fig. 6. Stimuli from each range that evoked similar maximum category ratings also elicited similar intensity-time profiles. Within a given range of temperatures, not only does the peak category rating increase as a function of stimulus temperature but there is also a corresponding decrease in the latency of pain and an increase in the duration of sensation. These events correspond with an increase in area under the intensity-time curve with increasing stimulus temperature. Thus, even though the temperature is cooled back to base temperature within 2 to 3 sec after each stimulus (as illustrated for a typical stimulus in Fig. 3), there is still a considerable after-sensation. This after-sensation may be a function of central summation, as suggested by the recordings of long after-discharges in the responses of dorsal horn neurons in the monkey or cat, and the typical absence of such after-discharges in nociceptive afferents (Price and Dubner, 1977; Zimmermann and Handwerker, 1974), e.g., Fig. 2.

Intensity-time judgments, not common in most scaling studies, are useful for measurements of the magnitude of sensations that change with the passage of time. Otherwise, the experimenter cannot be certain from a single numerical estimate whether the subject reported only the peak magnitude, or whether he integrated magnitude over time; the choice of one over the other may influence the slope of the psychophysical function for perceived magnitude.

Some of the variables that influence the magnitude of thermal sensation may be summarized in the following. When a single spot on the skin is heated repetitively with non-injurious stimuli, the magnitude of thermal sensations evoked will depend partly upon stimulus temperature and partly upon the degree of temporal interaction, the latter manifested as a suppression of sensory magnitude. The magnitude of sensation evoked by a given stimulus temperature is greatest in unstimulated skin and is suppressed during repetitive

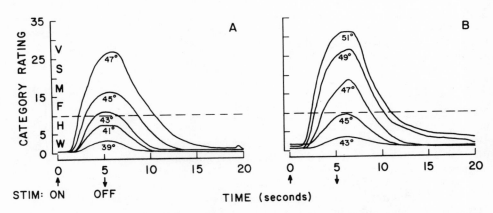

Fig. 6.   Subjective intensity-time ratings of stimuli that varied over two ranges of temperature: 39 to 47°C (A) and 43 to 51°C (B). Along the ordinate are the first letters of each response category: W = warmth, H = heat and F,M,S, and V designate, respectively, pain that is faint, moderate, strong or very strong. The dashed line designates the threshold for pain. Arrows mark the time between onset of the stimulus and the onset of cooling back to the base temperature of 38°C. Each curve is the average of individual curves obtained for one subject from 25 stimulus presentations (standard errors of the mean varied from 0.4 to 1.0).

stimulation by an amount directly related to the number, delivery
rate and intensities of prior stimulations. The psychophysical
function relating sensory magnitude to stimulus temperature will
shift upward along the temperature axis with an increase in delivery rate (Fig. 1) or with an upward shift in the range of temperatures used as stimuli (Fig. 5B). Analogous effects of repetitive
stimulation have been observed in the responses of CPNs in the
monkey but more studies are needed of other classes of heat-sensitive nociceptors. Most of the psychophysical experiments upon
which the statements about suppression are based employed stimuli
of short duration (5 sec) of less than 51°C delivered no more than
twice per minute. The experiments to be described next were directed toward understanding the conditions under which a stimulus of
longer duration or higher intensity will lead to the opposite of
suppression, namely an <u>increase</u> in the sensory magnitude of thermal
sensations.

HYPERALGESIA DURING INTERMITTANT STIMULATION

It is well known that heat, of sufficient duration and/or intensity applied to the skin, can evoke a state of hyperalgesia under
which pain threshold is lowered and the magnitude of pain evoked
by suprathreshold stimuli is increased. In the following experiments, I studied the temporal course of changes in the perceived
magnitude of heat applied to the skin of human subjects following
exposure to different durations of a conditioning stimulus (CS).
The CS was presented for either 5, 30, or 60 sec. Four subjects
made continuous ratings of the magnitude of thermal sensations
throughout a 35 min period during which a sequence of 3 test stimuli
(39, 41, and 43°C) was presented once before the CS, and than again
at 10 sec, and 5, 10, 20, and 30 min after the CS. Within each sequence the stimuli, each of 5 sec duration, were delivered every
30 sec with the contact thermal stimulator. The base temperature
between stimuli was maintained at 38°C. The subjects were not informed as to when any stimulus would be delivered or what intensities and durations of stimulation would be employed. The responses
of one subject, during a stimulus sequence delivered to the thenar
eminence of the hand, are shown in Fig. 7 (see legend for further
details). The maximum category rating obtained in response to each
stimulation was averaged for three runs from each subject. The results from each subject were very similar. The mean maximum ratings from the volar forearm are plotted in Fig. 8 as a function of
time before and after a CS of 50°C lasting 60 sec. The "background"
sensation was taken as the category rating just prior to the onset
of a stimulus. The ratings of pain and warmth were typically suppressed immediately following the CS. However, after 5 min had
elapsed, the ratings were significantly higher than they were prior
to the CS, and remained elevated until the end of testing. Following the initial suppression, the threshold decreased by approximately

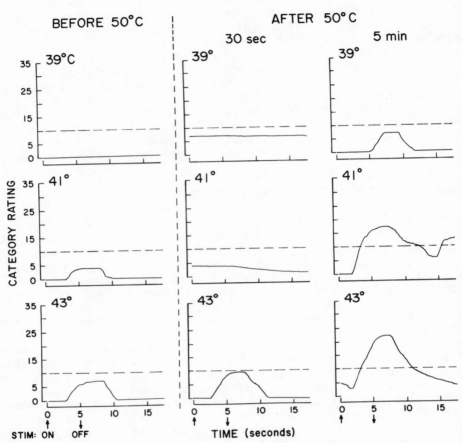

Fig. 7.   Development of hyperalgesia following a conditioning
          stimulus. Subjective intensity-time ratings by one sub-
          ject are shown from a run in which a sequence of 3 test
          stimuli (39, 41 and 43°C) was presented before, and 30
          sec and 5 min after, a conditioning stimulus (CS) of 50°C
          (60 sec duration). Dashed lines designate the threshold
          for pain and the arrows mark the duration of each stimulus.
          Hyperalgesia is indicated by the increase in subjective
          ratings of each stimulus after an elapsed time of 3 min.

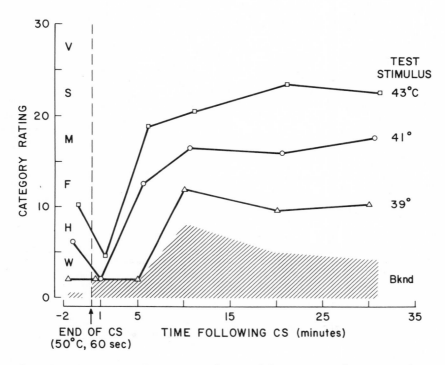

Fig. 8.   Development of suppression and hyperalgesia following a
conditioning stimulus (CS). Category ratings are the
maxima of intensity-time curves of the kind shown in Fig.
7, averaged for 4 subjects. Stimuli of 39, 41, and 43°C
were delivered before and at successive intervals of time
after a CS of 50°C (for 60 sec). Along the ordinate are
the first letters of the category labels (see legend, Fig.
6). The shaded area designates the magnitude of "background" sensation (Bknd)-which was the mean category
rating prior to each stimulus.

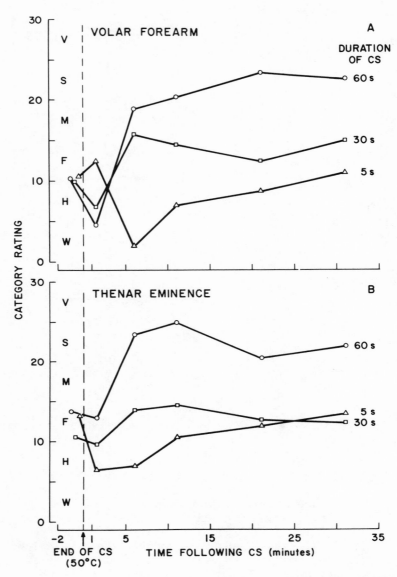

Fig. 9.   Development of suppression and hyperalgesia following con-
           ditioning stimuli (CS) of different durations. Category
           ratings are the maxima of intensity-time curves, averaged
           for 4 subjects, obtained in response to a stimulus of 43°C
           presented before and after a CS of 50°C. Data for three
           different durations of the CS are shown for stimuli de-
           livered to the volar forearm (A) or the thenar eminence
           of the hand (B).

4°C, indicating the development of hyperalgesia. Here we are speaking of <u>primary</u> hyperalgesia (Hardy, et al., 1952) in the erythralgic skin (Lewis, 1942) directly beneath the probe, as opposed to secondary hyperalgesia (Hardy, et al., 1952), Lewis' region of "nocifensor tenderness" (Lewis, 1936), that may develop over a much wider area surrounding the probe. The decrease in pain threshold was accompanied by an increase in "background" sensations that were commonly labeled as "heat" or occasionally "faint pain." The stimulus of 43°C, usually only faintly painful to normal skin, evoked ratings of "strong pain" 10 min after the CS. The 39°C stimulus which, prior to the CS, elicited barely perceptible sensations of "warmth," was subsequently reported as painful. Whenever the 39°C stimulus failed to evoke any sensation prior to the CS, it subsequently elicited a sensation of pain or, less often, warmth 5 min and 10 min after the CS (see Fig. 7, first row).

The above experiments were repeated for shorter durations of the CS on the thenar eminence of the hand and on the volar forearm. The maximum category ratings in response to the 43°C stimulus were averaged for the 4 subjects and are displayed in Fig. 9. The 5 sec CS commonly resulted only in suppression and the elimination of pain, followed by a slow recovery over the next 30 min. The suppression following a CS of 30 or 60 sec was usually reversed by the development of hyperalgesia 2 to 5 min after the CS. The results obtained for hairy and glabrous skin were similar. Thus, the duration of the CS determined whether only suppression would occur or whether suppression would be replaced by hyperalgesia.

SENSITIZATION OF NOCICEPTORS DURING INTERMITTANT STIMULATION

There is considerable evidence from neurophysiological studies that CPNs innervating the hairy skin in cats, monkeys and humans can be sensitized to heat following exposure to relatively high intensities and long durations of heating (Beitel and Dubner, 1976b; Bessou and Perl, 1969; Kumazawa and Perl, 1977; Perl, Kumazawa, Lynn, and Kenins, 1976; Torebjörk and Hallin, 1973). Sensitization is usually characterized by one or more of the following: the development of a low rate of spontaneous activity; decreased threshold temperature; and, for suprathreshold stimuli, a decrease in the latency of response and an increase in the number of impulses evoked. Some investigators have found that a staircase of increasing stimulus temperatures will sensitize most CPNs in cat and monkey (Bessou and Perl, 1969; Kumazawa and Perl, 1977; Perl et al., 1976). Other investigators have employed a variety of procedures to sensitize CPNs to heat. In one study, the threshold temperatures for some but evidently not all CPNs decreased by 2 to 4°C over a period of several minutes following a sensitizing stimulus such as 48°C for 30 sec (Beitel and Dubner, 1976b). This result is in agreement with that obtained in our human psychophysical experiments. A closer confirmation is provided by percut-

aneous recordings from CPNs from the peripheral nerve of alert
human subjects. Torebjörk and Hallin (1976) found that a CS of
50°C lasting 1 to 2 min, was followed by a fatigue of the responses
of CPNs to heat and a corresponding suppression of evoked pain that
lasted from 5 to 10 min; this was then followed by a sensitization
of the CPN response and by corresponding verbal reports of hyperalgesia that continued over the next hour. These results correlate
very well with those illustrated in Figs. 8 and 9.

Recently we applied the stimulus conditions used in these
psychophysical experiments to our neurophysiological studies of
CPNs innervating the monkey hand (LaMotte and Thalhammer, unpub.
observation). Although the results are preliminary, we found CPNs
that demonstrated a change in sensitivity to heat, following a CS
of 50°C for 60 sec, that paralleled the change in thermal sensiti-
ity observed in our human psychophysical studies. That is, responsiveness was suppressed immediately after termination of the
CS followed after 5 to 10 min by a lowering of threshold by 2 to
6°C. We have also observed CPNs that were only fatigued by heating and did not show signs of sensitization.

Repeated presentations of stimuli with temperatures as high
as 53°C typically evoke fatigue in CPNs (see Fig. 2) at least during the course of stimulation. Conversely, such stimuli may evoke
exactly the opposite response in another group of nociceptive
afferents (Campbell, et al., in press; Meyer, et al., 1977). The
number of impulses evoked in the latter by successive presentations
of 53°C increased and, following a pause of 5 or 10 min, their
threshold temperature was greatly decreased. These fibers were
myelinated, mechanosensitive nociceptive afferents that commonly
did not respond to heating stimuli of less than 50°C (3 sec). As
shown by Fitzgerald and Lynn (1977) for the cat and by Campbell
et al., (in press), and Meyer, et al., (1977) for the monkey,
these fibers become more sensitive to heat following repeated heat-
ings of relatively high intensity. For brevity, these fibers may
be called AMHs (A-fibers, primarily mechanosensitive but can be
sensitized to heat) to distinguish them from other mechanosensitive
nociceptive afferents than do not respond to heating, even with
temperatures that blister the skin (Meyer, et al., 1977). The
AMHs are more appropriately classified as "A-fibers" than "A-delta
fibers" because their mean conduction velocity in the monkey is
31 ± 1.5 m/sec (range: 5-53 m/sec, N=37). The AMHs may develop
a remarkable degree of sensitization, as illustrated for one fiber
in Fig. 10. Note the development of a considerable after-discharge
lasting, in some cases, many seconds after the stimulus returned
to base temperature. There was often a development of spontaneous
activity which was suppressed by cooling as are spontaneous sensations of pain in humans following a cutaneous burn (Lewis and
Hess, 1933). Before sensitization, 86 percent of the AMHs had
thresholds greater than 50°C; after sensitization, threshold tem-

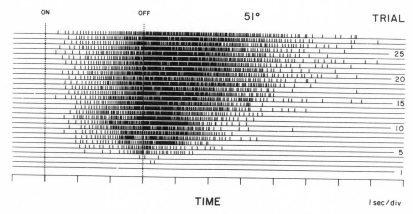

Fig. 10.   Responses of a myelinated mechanosensitive nociceptive
           afferent, innervating the monkey palm, to radiant heat
           pulses of 51°C. Stimuli of 3 sec duration were delivered
           every 28 sec from a base temperature of 38°C (format is
           the same as that for Fig. 2). This fiber initially re-
           sponded to noxious mechanical stimulation but not to
           noxious heat of less than 51°C. Following repeated
           stimulation of its receptive field with 51°C, it became
           sensitized to heat and its threshold temperature dropped
           subsequently to 39°C (Campbell, Meyer and LaMotte, un-
           published observations).

perature decreased for all fibers and 66 percent of these were
less than 44°C. We have yet to determine the temporal course of
changes in sensitivity of AMHs to heat following a conditioning
stimulus of the kind used in the psychophysical experiments described above.

     The AMHs are probably of a different class of A-fibers from
those described as initially sensitive to heat (thresholds similar
to those of CPNs) in normal skin in monkeys, for example the "A-
delta heat nociceptive afferents of Dubner, Price, Beitel, and Hu
(1977) and possibly those A-delta fibers of Iggo and Ogawa (1971)
and some of those described by Georgopoulos (1976). In a psychophysical study, very short latencies of response to a pricking
sensation, evoked in humans by radiant heat stimuli with very fast
rise-times, indicated the existence of heat nociceptors with myelinated axons and very short latencies of response in normal skin
(Campbell and LaMotte, 1977). In contrast, the response latencies
of AMHs are relatively long, even after sensitization, e.g., 1 to
3 sec in sensitized skin (Campbell, et al., in press).

Thus, neural activity in subpopulations of AMHs and CPNs probably contributes to the development of hyperalgesia following a
sensitizing stimulus such as that used in the present psychophysical
studies. There may also be other nociceptive afferents that contribute to hyperalgesia (see Table 2) including those that are
sensitive only to noxious heat (Beck, Handwerker and Zimmermann,
1974; Georgopoulos, 1976).

ADAPTATION AND HYPERALGESIA DURING SUSTAINED STIMULATION

Most of the stimuli in the above experiments were of short
duration and intermittently delivered to the skin. In the next
series of experiments, only one stimulus is delivered in order to
determine the temporal course of the adaptation of pain. Three
subjects continuously rated the magnitude of thermal sensation
throughout a 5 min stimulation of either 43, 45 or 47°C. All
stimuli were presented with the contact thermal stimulator from a
base temperature maintained at 38°C for 2 min prior to testing.
Figure 11 presents the results during one run and the averages from
several runs for stimuli delivered to the volar forearm. Similar
results were obtained for stimuli delivered to the glabrous skin
of the hand. We conclude from these results, and those obtained
in experiments with other temperatures, the following: (a) stimulus temperatures of 42 to 44°C, delivered from a base temperature
of 38°C, typically evoke a transient sensation of pain that disappears (adaptation); (b) pain evoked by 45°C decreases or disappears, in most instances after 30 to 60 sec, only to return later
and increase slightly near the end of stimulation; and (c) the
pain evoked by higher temperatures increases gradually and usually
continues to do so until the termination of the stimulus. Thus,
adaptation is followed or replaced by hyperalgesia during sustained stimulations of 45°C or greater. None of these stimuli resulted in edema. The erythema lasted several hours follwoing the
5 min, 45°C stimulus but as long as several days after the 5 min,
47°C stimulus.

The results illustrated in Fig. 11 confirm and extend those
obtained in an earlier study from subjects who rated the intensity
of pain during 30 sec immersions of the whole hand in a water bath
of controlled temperature (Hardy, et al., 1968).

RESPONSE OF NOCICEPTORS DURING SUSTAINED STIMULATION

A number of neurophysiological studies of the monkey and cat
have characterized the temporal profile of the response of CPNs
during continuous stimulation of heat with durations as short as
3 sec or as long as 4 min (Beitel and Dubner, 1976b; Bessou and
Perl, 1969; Croze, Duclaux, and Kenshalo, 1976; LaMotte and Campbell, 1978). The pattern of discharge evoked by stimulation of a

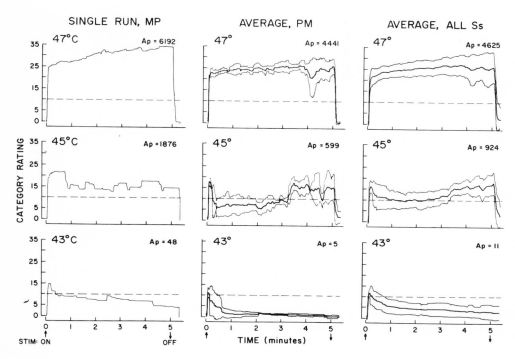

Fig. 11.   Continuous ratings of the magnitude of thermal sensations
during stimulations of constant temperature, each lasting
5 min. The category scale is identical to that described
for earlier figures; the dashed line marks the threshold
for pain. The temperature of each stimulus, delivered
to the volar forearm, is given in the left corner of
each graph and the area of pain (between the rating
curve and the dotted line) (A_p) is given in the right
corner in arbitrary units of rating x time. Stimulus
duration is designated by the arrows. Left column: results of a single run at each temperature for subject
MP. Middle column: average of 3 runs (dark, middle line)
with one standard deviation of the mean (S.D.) indicated
above and below by the thinner lines, for subject PM.
Right column: grand mean (±1 S.D.) of 9 runs, 3 con-
tributed from each of 3 subjects.

CPN that is not already fatigued is an initially high frequency of discharge at the beginning of the stimulus, followed by a decrease to a low rate that usually continues until the end of stimulation; the fiber may even cease to respond before the end of a long-duration stimulation if the stimulus temperature is greater than 50°C (e.g., Bietel and Dubner, 1976c). This pattern of discharge correlates with the occurrence of pain and its subsequent disappearance during stimuli of less than 45°C (e.g., Fig. 11). Here one must assume that the residual, low rate of activity is not sufficient to evoke pain. This same pattern of increase and subsequent decrease in frequency cannot account for the increase in pain that occurs at higher temperatures unless an additional mechanism is postulated. However, there have been occasional observations of gradual increases in the rate of discharge of CPNs (Croze, et al., 1976) and "C-heat nociceptors" (Beck, Handwerker, and Zimmermann,1974) during sustained stimulations of several minutes.

Activity in the AMHs may also contribute to an increase in pain since the frequency of response in this type of fiber typically increases to a plateau during a stimulation that lasts at least 20 sec (Campbell, et al., in press). We have yet to test these fibers with stimuli of longer durations; however, if they continue to respond at the same frequency of discharge for longer periods of time, they would provide one peripheral neural determinant of hyperalgesia during continuous stimulation.

THERMAL INJURY AND NOCICEPTOR SENSITIZATION

The long response latencies of AMHs to heat and the gradual increase in their discharge rates during sustained heating with 53°C suggest that their endings may be sensitized to heat by the action of chemical mediators released by injured cells or by substances that appear following an increase in vascular permeability. In the case of CPNs, it is unlikely that sensitization is dependent solely upon the release of substance from the blood, for CPNs can be sensitized to heat in the artifically perfused rabbit ear (Perl, et al., 1976). Also, sensitization of CPNs and AMHs is not solely dependent upon a change in vascular permeability since neither type of nociceptor is effectively sensitized by noxious mechanical stimulation (Bessou and Perl, 1969; Campbell, et al., in press; Fitzgerald and Lynn, 1977) even though such stimulation increases vascular permeability (Handwerker, 1976). Chemical mediators released from damaged cells might sensitize nociceptors. If this is the case, then the diffusion from injured cells to nociceptor endings must be localized to the site of injury, at least for CPNs. Thus, when a ring is burned around the receptive field of a CPN neither an enhanced responsiveness to heat nor the development of spontaneous activity occurs (Croze, et al., 1976). Similarly, heating one part of the receptive field of a CPN in human subjects resulted in suppression and sensitization in that area while sensitivity to heat in remaining parts of the receptive field of the same fiber remained unaltered (Torebjörk and Hallin, 1977). These experiments have yet to be carried out for AMHs and other types of nociceptors.

Just as nociceptors are selective in their immediate responses to different forms of stimulation from the external world (see Table 2) so are they differentially responsive to local conditions, with the skin, associated with injury and the inflammatory reaction. The degree of sensitization following local injury differs even for fibers within the same class. For example, sustained noxious heating of the skin will sensitize some CPNs and some A-fiber mechanosensitive nociceptors to heat but others in each class are not affected (Beck, et al., 1974; Campbell, et al., in press; Croze, et al., 1976; Dubner, et al., 1977). Once nociceptors in each class become sensitized to heat, some of them will also become more sensitive to mechanical stimulation while others will not (Bessou and Perl, 1969; Campbell, et al., in press). Other differences are class-dependent. For example, heat-sensitized CPNs develop a sensitivity to noxious cold (Bessou and Perl, 1969), a sensitivity they do not have in normal skin, whereas activity in sensitized AMHs is suppressed by cold (Campbell, et al., in press). Nociceptors also differ in their responsiveness to certain chemical stimuli that are present in injured tissue. Histamine excites CPNs but apparently not AMHs (Fjällbrant and Iggo, 1961; Lynn, 1977). Thus, it is probable that injury and inflammation do not have the same generalized effect on the sensitivities of all nociceptors. Rather, the consequences of thermal injury may be highly specific for each nociceptor.

CONCLUSION

Nociceptors differ in their selectivity of response to different forms of energy impinging upon the skin. They also differ in their susceptibility to changes in sensitivity during the development of the inflammatory reaction to local injury. When non-injurious heating stimuli of short duration are repetitively delivered to the same spot on the skin, both the magnitude of pain evoked in humans and the amount of activity in at least one class of nociceptors, the CPNs, depend not only upon the temperatures of the stimuli but also upon temporal interactions between stimuli. At lower stimulus temperatures, of short durations, these interactions are largely characterized as a suppression of pain and a fatigue of nociceptor response. The amount by which pain and nociceptor response are suppressed by prior stimulations is directly related to the intensities of these stimuli and to their rate of delivery.

During a sustained stimulation, lasting 5 min, the temporal
course of the onset and adaptation of pain at temperatures of 45°C
or less is paralleled by a similar temporal profile in the discharge pattern of CPNs. At higher temperatures, pain does not
adapt, and the development of hyperalgesia that can occur may be
accompanied by the enhanced responsiveness of nociceptors, most
notably the AMHs. The possible relations between sensitization of
nociceptors and certain phases of the inflammatory reaction to injury have yet to be determined. Further comparisons are also
needed between the temporal course of changes in the sensitivity
to pain and changes in the responsiveness of all classes of nociceptors.

REFERENCES

Beck, P. W., Handwerker, H. O., & Zimmermann, M. Nervous outflow
     from the cat's foot during noxious radiant heat stimulation.
     Brain Research, 1974, 67, 373-386.
Beck, P. W., & Handwerker, H. O. Bradykinin and serotonin effects
     on various types of cutaneous nerve fibres. Pflügers Archiv,
     1974, 347, 209-222.
Beitel, R. E., & Dubner, R. Fatigue and adaptation in unmyelinated
     (C) polymodal nociceptors to mechanical and thermal stimuli
     applied to the monkey's face. Brain Research, 1976a, 112,
     402-406.
Beitel, R. E., & Dubner, R. Response of unmyelinated (C) poly-
     modal nociceptors to thermal stimuli applied to monkey's face.
     Journal of Neurophysiology, 1976, 39, 1160-1175.
Beitel, R. E., & Dubner, R. Sensitization and depression of C-
     polymodal nociceptors by noxious heat applied to the monkey's
     face. In J. J. Bonica & D. Able-Fessard (Eds.), Advances in
     pain research and therapy (Vol. 1). New York: Raven Press,
     1976c.
Bessou, P., & Perl, E. R. Response of cutaneous sensory units with
     unmyelinated fibers to noxious stimuli. Journal of Neuro-
     physiology, 1969, 32, 1025-1043.
Burgess, P. R., & Perl, E. R. Cutaneous mechanoreceptors and no-
     ciceptors. In A. Iggo (Ed.), The somatosensory system.
     Berlin: Springer-Verlag, 1976.
Burgess, P. R., & Perl, E. R. Myelinated afferent fibers respond-
     ing specifically to noxious stimulation of the skin. Journal
     of Physiology (London), 1967, 190, 541-562.
Burgess, P. R., Petit, D., & Warren, R. M. Receptor types in cat
     hairy skin supplied by myelinated fibers. Journal of Neuro-
     physiology, 1968, 31, 833-848.
Campbell, J. N., & LaMotte, R. H. Reaction time to first pain in
     human subjects. Neuroscience Abstract 7th Annual Meeting,
     1977, 13, 478.

Campbell, J. N., Meyer, R. A., & LaMotte, R. H. Sensitization of myelinated nociceptive afferents that innervate the monkey hand. Journal of Neurophysiology (in press).

Croze, S., Duclaux, R., & Kenshalo, D. R. The thermal sensitivity of the polymodal nociceptors in the monkey. Journal of Physiology (London), 1976, 263, 539-562.

Darian-Smith, I., Johnson, K. O., LaMotte, C., Shigenaga, Y., Kenins, R., & Champness, P. Warm fibers innervating palmar and distal skin of the monkey: Responses to thermal stimuli. (in press).

Dubner, R., & Hu, J. W. Myelinated (Aδ) nociceptive afferents innervating the monkey's face. Journal of Dental Research, 1977, 56, A167.

Dubner, R., Price, D. D., Beitel, R. E., & Hu, J. W. Peripheral neural correlates of behavior in monkey and human related to sensory discriminative aspects of pain. In D. J. Anderson & B. Mathews (Eds.), Pain in the trigeminal region. Amsterdam: Elsevier, 1977.

Fitzgerald, M., & Lynn, B. The sensitization of high threshold mechanoreceptors with myelinated axons by repeated heating. Journal of Physiology (London), 1977, 365, 549-563.

Fjällbrant, N., & Iggo, A. The effect of histamine, 5-hydroxytryptamine and acetylcholine and cutaneous afferent fibres. Journal of Physiology (London), 1961, 156, 578-590.

Georgopoulos, A. P. Functional properties of primary afferent units probably related to pain mechanisms in primate glabrous skin. Journal of Neurophysiology, 1976, 39, 71-83.

Gernandt, B., & Zotterman, Y. The effect of respiratory changes upon the spontaneous injury discharge of afferent mammalian and human nerve fibers. Acta Physiologica Scandinavica, 1946, 11, 248-259.

Handwerker, H. O. Pharmacological modulation of the discharge of nociceptive C fibers. In Y. Zotterman (Ed.), Sensory functions of the skin in primates. Oxford: Pergamon Press, 1976.

Hardy, J. D. Thresholds of pain and reflex contraction as related to noxious stimulation. Journal of Applied Physiology, 1953, 5, 725-739.

Hardy, J. D., Stolwijk, J.A.J., Hammel, H. T., & Murgatroyd, D. Skin temperature and cutaneous pain during warm water immersion. Journal of Applied Physiology, 1965, 20, 1014-1021.

Hardy, J. D., Stolwijk, J.A.J., & Hoffman, D. Pain following step increase in skin temperature. In D. R. Kenshalo (Ed.), The skin senses. Springfield: Thomas, 1968.

Hardy, J. D., Wolff, H. G., & Goodell, H. Pain sensations and reactions. Baltimore: Williams and Wilkins, 1952.

Hees, J., van, & Gybels, J. M. Pain related to single afferent C fibers from human skin. Brain Research, 1972, 48, 397-400.

Hilder, R., Ramey, E., Darian-Smith, I., Johnson, K.O., & Dally, L.J. A contact stimulator for the study of cutaneous thermal sensibility. Journal of Applied Physiology, 1974, 37, 252-255.

Hunt, C. C., & McIntyre, A. K. An analysis of fiber diameter and
    receptor characterization of myelinated cutaneous afferents in
    cat. Journal of Physiology (London), 1960, 153, 99-112.
Iggo, A. Cutaneous heat and cold receptors with slowly conducting
    (C) afferent fibres. Quarterly Journal of Experimental
    Physiology, 1959, 44, 362-370.
Iggo, A. Cutaneous mechanoreceptors with afferent C fibres.
    Journal of Physiology (London), 1960, 152, 337-353.
Iggo, A., & Ogawa, H. Primate cutaneous thermal nociceptors.
    Journal of Physiology (London), 1971, 216, 77-78.
Iriuchijima, J., & Zotterman, Y. The specificity of afferent
    cutaneous C fibres in mammals. Acta Physiologica Scandinavica,
    1960, 49, 267-278.
Keele, C. A., & Armstrong, D. Substances producing pain and itch.
    Baltimore: Williams and Wilkins, 1965.
Kumazawa, T., & Perl, E. R. Primate cutaneous sensory units with
    unmyelinated (C) afferent fibers. Journal of Neurophysiology,
    1977, 40, 1325-1338.
LaMotte, R. H., & Campbell, J. N. Comparison of the responses of
    warm and nociceptive C fiber afferents in monkey with human
    judgements of thermal pain. Journal of Neurophysiology, 1978,
    41, 509-528.
Lele, P. P., Weddell, G., and Williams, C. M. The relationship
    between heat transfer, skin temperature and cutaneous sensi-
    bility. Journal of Physiology (London), 1954, 126, 206-234.
Lewis, T. Experiments relating to cutaneous hyperalgesia and its
    spread through somatic nerves. Clinical Science, 1936, 2,
    373-423.
Lewis, T. Pain. New York: MacMillan, 1942.
Lewis, T., & Hess, W. Pain derived from the skin and the mechanisms
    of its production. Clinical Science, 1933, 1, 39-61.
Lynn, B. Cutaneous hyperalgesia. British Medical Bulletin, 1977,
    33, 103-108.
Meyer, R. A., Walker, R. E., & Mountcastle, V. B. A laser stimula-
    tor for the study of cutaneous thermal and pain sensations.
    IEEE Transactions on Biomedical Engineering, 1976, 23, 54-60.
Meyer, R. A., Campbell, J. N., & LaMotte, R. H. Sensitization of
    A-delta nociceptive afferents to noxious radiant heat delivered
    to the monkey hand. Neuroscience Abstract 7th Annual Meeting,
    1977, 13, 487.
Moritz, A. R., & Henriques, F. C., Jr. Studies of thermal injury.
    II. The relative importance of time and surface temperature in
    the causation of cutaneous burns. American Journal of Pathology
    1947, 23, 695-720.
Perl, E. R. Myelinated afferent fibres innervating the primate
    skin and their response to noxious stimuli. Journal of Physio-
    logy (London), 1968, 197, 593-615.

Perl, E. R., Kumazawa, T., Lynn, B., & Kenins, P. Sensitization of high threshold receptors with unmyelinated (C) afferent fibers. In A. Iggo & O. B. Ilyinsky (Eds.), Somatosensory and visceral receptor mechanisms, Progress of Brain Research (Vol.43), Amsterdam: Elsevier, 1976.

Price, D. D., & Dubner, R. Mechanisms of first and second pain in the peripheral and central nervous systems. Journal of Investigative Dermatology, 1977, 69, 167-171.

Price, D. D., Hu, J. W., Dubner, R., & Gracely, R. H. Peripheral suppression of first pain and central summation of second pain evoked by noxious heat pulses. Pain, 1977, 3, 57-68.

Ryan, G. B., & Majno, G. Acute inflammation. American Journal of Pathology, 1977, 86, 185-274.

Sevitt, S. Burns, pathology and therapeutic applications. London: Butterworth, 1957.

Sevitt, S. Inflammatory changes in burned skin: Reversible and irreversible effects and their pathogenesis. In L. Thomas, J. W. Uhr & L. Grant (Eds.), Injury, inflammation and immunity. Baltimore: William and Wilkins, 1965.

Sumino, R., Dubner, R., & Starkman, S. Responses of small myelinated "warm" fibers to noxious heat stimuli applied to the monkey's face. Brain Research, 1973, 62, 260-263.

Szolcsanyi, J. On the specificity of pain-producing and sensory neuron blocking effects of capsaicin. In J. Knoll & E.S. Vizi (Eds.), Symposium on Analgesics. Budapest: Academiai Kiado, 1976.

Szolcsanyi, J. The local efferent function of capsaicin-sensitive C-nociceptors. Proceedings of International Union of Physiological Sciences, 1977, 13, 736.

Thibos, L. N., & Werblin, F. S. The response properties of the steady antagonistic surround in the mudpuppy retina. Journal of Physiology (London), 1978, 278, 79-99.

Torebjörk, H. E., & Hallin, R. G. Perceptual changes accompanying controlled preferential blocking of A and C fiber responses in intact human skin nerves. Experimental Brain Research, 1973, 16, 321-332.

Torebjörk, H. E., & Hallin, R. G. Identification of afferent C units in intact human skin nerves. Brain Research, 1974, 67, 387-403.

Torebjörk, H. E., & Hallin, R. G. Skin receptors supplied by unmyelinated (C) fibres in man. In Y. Zotterman (Ed.), Sensory functions of the skin in primates. Oxford: Pergamon Press,1976.

Torebjörk, E., & Hallin, R. G. Sensitization of polymodal nociceptors with C fibres in man. Proceedings of International Union of Physiological Sciences, 1977, 13, 758.

Torgerson, W.S. Theory and methods of scaling. New York: Wiley, 1958.

Wilhelm, D.L., & Mason, B. Vascular permeability changes in inflammation: the role of endogenous permeability factors in mild thermal injury. British Journal of Experimental Pathology, 1960, 41, 487-506.

Zimmermann, M., & Handwerker, H. O. Total afferent inflow and
    dorsal horn activity upon radiant heat stimulation to the cat's
    footpad. Advances in Neurology (Vol. 4), New York: Raven
    Press, 1974.
Zotterman, Y. Studies in the peripheral nervous mechanisms of pain.
    Acta Medica Scandinavica, 1933, 80, 185-242.
Zotterman, Y. Specific action potentials in the lingual nerve of
    the cat. Scandinavica Archiv Physiologica, 1936, 75, 105-119.

DISCUSSION

DR. STEVENS: About 10 years ago when I did a scaling experiment
with R. Adair and L. E. Marks, using a Hardy dolorimeter (Adair,
E. R., Stevens, J. C. and Marks, L. E., 1968); we got some order
out of that study, but we were dismayed at the tremendous variability of the magnitude estimates. We dreamed, at that time, of
having the marvelous stimulus control that you have. We thought
we would eliminate a lot of that variability if we could have a
constant background temperature and bring the temperature up to a
precise value and keep it there. But then I noticed from your
first figure that the dispersion of judgments around 45°C is very
wide. It includes some judgments of slightly warm, of moderately
warm, all the way up to rather painful. I have a couple of
questions about that. First, do you have any speculation on the
source of this variability? Second, does that dispersion include
judgments across subjects and is a good deal of the variability
possibly attributable to individual differences? And third, is the
dispersion significantly greater for the condition where the
stimuli came at the rate of one every 25 sec as opposed to one
every 225 sec? In other words, does the time factor significantly
influence the variation?

DR. LaMOTTE: No, to the third question. As for the first
question, we have shown that the scaling model is valid for individual subjects but here we have pooled the results of individual
subjects because the results were similar. A bit of the variability is due to pooling results obtained from different subjects,
but it is also due to (a) regional differences in the thermal
sensitivity of adjacent spots on the skin, and (b) temporal
interactions between the effects of repetitively stimulating the
same loci on the skin: for example, the category rating of any
stimulus is lowered ("supressed") in direct proportion to the
intensities of prior stimulations recently delivered to the same
spot (LaMotte & Campbell, 1978). If you were able to obtain the
scale from a single presentation to the same spot of the skin
each day over perhaps many days, you might be able to determine
how much of the variability is due to the effects of repeatedly
stimulating an area and how much due to forgetting from one day to
the next what category judgment to make.
   I do not have any idea of what causes the huge variability.
I think, probably, the most obvious reason is a cognitive variable - the capacity to make the same judgment from memory over
a time - would account for a lot of variability. If you presented
the same two stimuli over and over again on one day of testing you
would get a considerable reduction in variability.

DR. STEVENS: Possibly, but that strains my credulity a bit, because
the responses go all the way from mild warmth to very painful.

DR. LaMOTTE: I do not have a simple explanation. I think that is the best one I can come up with.

DR. PERL: As long as we are talking about the scale, I was sur- prized to see the nice, even divisions of the categories, parti- cularly that upper category. Intuitively, I cannot accept that the upper category was as narrow as you suggest.

DR. LaMOTTE: You are absolutely right. The boundary of the highest category cannot be determined by this method and neither can the lowest boundary. It remains open, you have to have more categories and more stimuli to do that.

DR. LINDBLOM: This investigation you have made of the responses over time is very important. I would like to ask you one question about the method and interpretation coming from the experiments. We use a contact thermode for tracking the heat pain threshold. The first stimulus then is often seen to be painful at a fairly low temperature, say $42^{\circ}C$, the next painful stimulus is at about $44^{\circ}C$ and then it levels off at about $45^{\circ}C$. We have thought that adapt- ation is partly responsible. Also, perhaps a shifting criterion is involved, so that the first pain is signalled at a lower in- tensity. But, as I understand you, this would rather reflect the neural event being decreased by successive stimuli. Nevertheless, I wonder if the suppression you found with the $45^{\circ}C$ stimuli might partly be due to a shift in the criterion so that the subjects jump from one category to another.

DR. LaMOTTE: We have studied this effect with a variety of pro- cedures. My own impression is that the effect is very little. For example, the intensities of preceding stimuli can influence category judgments. When stimuli are presented to nine different spots on the skin, and there is no way that the subject could remember the intensities of the preceding stimuli given four minutes earlier to each of nine spots, you get this suppressive effect. That kind of effect, is a little bit less than what I have shown for the first six trials (Fig. 3). These category ratings are modulated by the intensity of the preceding stimulus and I do not think that supression can be explained by any shift in response bias.

DR. FRANZEN: My first comment is with respect to variability in the data. There is an analogous situation in the study of vibratory and auditory pitch. There is a shift in the discrimination function and as we went from frequencies where it had nothing to do with pitch, to some point where you have a change in the quality of the sensation, then for both audition and vibration, the subjects reported some uncertainty as to the choice of appropriate criterion for their frequency matchings. You have a change in quality from warmth, to heat, and pain and I think that can very easily account for the variability in the data.

DR. HENSEL: How did you define your categories and how did you present the categories to your subjects? Did you present the scale and say that they should behave according to the scale or did they just report some spontaneous experience?

DR. LaMOTTE: Initially, we tried introspective experiments to determine those qualities of sensation that might be appropriate. But we found that on the glabrous skin of the hand we always evoked about the same quality of burning pain sensation and so we decided to choose purely intensive descriptors like faint, moderate, strong. Then we had to have something for non-painful so we chose heat and warmth and required the subjects to push buttons to indicate the category of response.

REFERENCES

Adair, E. R., Stevens, J. C., & Marks, L. E. Thermally induced pain, the doe scale, and the psychophysical power law. American Journal of Psychology, 1968, 81, 147-164.

LaMotte, R. H., & Campbell, J. N. Comparison of the responses of warm and nociceptive C fiber afferents in monkey with human judgements of thermal pain. Journal of Neurophysiology, 1978, 509-528.

AVERAGED EVOKED POTENTIALS AND SENSORY EXPERIENCE

Stephen W. Harkins, Medical Center, University of
Washington and Seattle Veterans Administration Hospital

Willie K. Dong, Department of Anesthesiology Medical
Center, University of Washington

Drawing relationships between stimulus parameters, physiological response of peripheral nerves and subsequent report of sensation is possible for the skin senses in man because of the accessibility of the peripheral somatosensory system (Gybels and van Hees, 1972). Such relationships, however, are more difficult to obtain when the physiological responses of the central nervous system are considered. One approach to this problem has been to determine the stimulus-response relation of central neural activity in animals and to correlate this relation to human psychophysical responses (Mountcastle and Darian-Smith, 1968; Mountcastle, Talbot, Sakata, and Hyvärinen, 1969). A second approach has been to directly relate central neural activity to psychophysical responses in human subjects. Franzén and Offenloch (1969), for example, have demonstrated a relation between magnitude of cortical evoked potentials and perceived stimulus intensity in man. Both cortical potentials and psychophysical responses were power functions of stimulus intensity.

Recently, brainstem evoked potentials to auditory (Jewett, 1970; Buchwald and Huang, 1975) and to somatosensory (Cracco and Cracco, 1976; Wiederholt and Iragui-Madoz, 1977) stimuli have been demonstrated. These "far-field" brain responses are reflections of sequential activation of relay nuclei in the afferent pathway. The distinction between far-field and near-field evoked potentials has been made to differentiate between the volume conduction of electrical activity over a relatively large distance versus potentials whose source is close to the active recording electrode (Jewett, 1970). From electrodes on the surface of scalp in man far-field potentials can be generally considered to reflect subcortical activity. These potentials are widely distributed, not

recorded from bipolar electrodes short distances apart and are
more sensitive to stimulus variables than subject variables
(Jewett, 1970; Sutton, 1969). Near-field potentials from scalp
electrodes can be generally considered to reflect cortical activity.
They are characterized by large differences in amplitude, polarity
or both at electrode positions a short distance apart. Usually
they are maximal over a limited area, reflecting their dependence
on proximity to their site of origin and these potentials are often
more sensitive to subject variables than stimulus variables
(Jewett, 1970; Jewett and Williston, 1971; Sutton, 1969). In this
chapter we deal exclusively with two recently described evoked
potentials to discrete afferent stimulation and focus on the relevance of these brain electrical events to sensation and perception
in man. The evoked potentials are far-field or brainstem somatosensory responses to radial nerve stimulation and pain related,
near-field or cortical responses to noxious electrical stimulation
of teeth.

Somatosensory Evoked Potentials

     When brief suprathreshold electrical shocks are delivered to
skin electrodes placed over peripheral nerves a complex evoked
potential can be observed in the averaged electroencephalogram
(EEG) recorded from scalp electrodes in man. These somatosensory
evoked potentials (SEPs) are time-locked to onset of the electrical
shock but due to the poor signal-to-noise ratio with respect to
spontaneous EEG activity they are unobservable on a trial-to-trial
basis. By use of laboratory computers it is now readily possible
to obtain summed or averaged evoked potentials.

     Until recently the earliest identified components of somato-
sensory evoked potentials were a triphasic negative-positive-
negative complex with peak latencies occurring at approximately
18, 20, and 30 msec respectively (Halliday, 1975). These potentials, illustrated in Fig. 1, are consistently observed following electrical stimulation of the radial or median nerve at the
wrist. With improvements in signal averaging techniques, certain
changes in electrode placement, and amplification (see Cracco,
1972; Cracco and Cracco, 1976) a series of early positive components
have been identified. These are thought to be far-field reflections of the subcortical neural activity evoked by the afferent
stimulus. They include a relatively large positive wave with a
latency of approximately 13 msec (P_1 in Fig. 1) (Cracco, 1972)
and several quite small potentials which have been demonstrated in
rat (Wiederholt and Iragui-Madoz, 1977), cat (Iragui-Madoz and
Wiederholt, 1977) and man (Cracco and Cracco, 1976; Chizppa, Choi,
and Young, 1978). The very early, nanovolt range potentials require averaging a large number of trials for reliable resolution.
The most reliable of these include the potentials labeled III and
IV in Fig. 1.

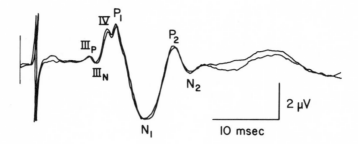

Fig. 1. Example of far and early near-field components of the
evoked potential to percutaneous electrical stimulation
of the radial nerve at the wrist. Two repeated measures
from the same subject are superimposed to illustrate reproducibility of the response. Two msec of baseline pre-
cedes onset of the shock artifact. Shock intensity of 1
mA below motor threshold and duration was 0.2 msec. The
electroencephalogram (EEG) was measured from a parasigital
lead placed over the hand representation of somatosensory
cortex referred to a lead at C5 - C6. Positively at the
cephalic lead is upward. The EEG was amplified using a
Grass P511 preamplifier at a gain of 5×10^4 (half amp.
filter settings of 30 Hz and 3k Hz). A Nicolet 1024
signal averager system was used to collect evoked potentials. Each trace is composed of 1024 responses. A grass
S88 stimulator with a stimulus isolation and constant
current unit were employed to deliver shocks. The components of the triphasic negative-positive-negative complex with peak latencies at approximately 18, 20, and 30
msec are labeled N_1, P_2, N_2 respectively. (See text).

     Evidence from lesion and microelectrode experiments indicate
that the components labeled III and IV reflect sequential activation
of subcoritcal nuclei that is volume conducted to surface electrodes
(Wiederholt and Iragui-Madoz, 1977; Dong and Harkins, 1978). Topographic studies in man (Cracco and Cracco, 1976) and lesion studies
in cat (Dong and Harkins, 1978) suggests that the positive wave at
approximately 13 msec (P_1) is also subcortical in origin. While
the specific sites of origin of these waves are not yet clearly
defined evidence to date indicates that Wave III arises from
either volume conducted peripheral nerve activity, dorsal column
activity and/or neural activity at the level of the dorsal column
nuclei (Cracco and Cracco, 1976; Dong and Harkins, 1978).

Component IV is thought to be generated at the level of the dorsal
column nuclei and/or medial lemniscus (Cracco and Cracco, 1976).
The P_1 response, in cat, is eliminated by thalamotomy but not removal of cortical areas SI or SII (Dong and Harkins, 1978).   It
is not clear if the diphasic $N_1 \rightarrow P_2$ component is subcortical or
cortical in origin but it does reach maximum amplitudes at central-
parietal scalp locations overlying the somesthetic cortical representation of the hand, suggesting at least a partial near-field
origin.

A relationship between several components of sensory evoked
potentials and sensory behavior in humans has recently been demonstrated (Ivanitsky and Strelets, 1977; Harkins and Chapman, 1978).
The study by Ivanitsky and Strelets (1977) involved evaluation of
somatosensory evoked potentials elicited by shocks to the anterior
forearm and accuracy of intensity discrimination of such shocks.
They found a significant correlation between discrimination
ability or d' derived from sensory decision theory (Green and
Swets, 1966; Swets, 1971) and amplitude of $N_1 \rightarrow P_2$ component.   They
suggest that amplitude of this component represents some form of
neural coding for stimulus intensity and subsequent sensory experience.

A pilot study was undertaken to evaluate if amplitude of the
early components studied by Ivanitsky and Strelets (1977) are related to stimulus intensity.   Figure 2 presents the results for
two subjects.   In this figure averaged evoked potentials to radial
nerve stimulation as a function of stimulus intensity are presented
on the left and peak-to-peak amplitudes of several components are
plotted against stimulus intensity on the right.   Between the
ranges of stimulus and pain thresholds, amplitude versus stimulus
intensity was acceptably fitted by a power function of the form
$Y = qx^k$ where x and y are intensity and amplitude respectively and
q and x are parameters free to vary between individuals and stimuli
(Stevens, 1975; Staddon, 1978).   Figure 3 illustrates these functions on log-log coordinates for amplitude of the $P_1 \rightarrow N_1$ component.
Slope of these functions is approximately 1.50 and two functions
are plotted for subject VL to illustrate within individual stability.
Similar functions (not graphed) were obtained for amplitude of the
$N_1 \rightarrow P_2$ component but not the $P_2 \rightarrow N_2$ component.

The levels of stimulations used by Ivanitsky and Strelets
(1977) averaged about 6 MA and thus were in the middle of the dynamic range of the amplitude intensity function for $P_1 \rightarrow N_1$ in
Fig. 3.   This suggests that these curves could be used to predict
subsequent discrimination performance.   On the basis of data such
as these, it can be hypothesized that discrimination performance
between shocks will be best at intensities where there is maximum
change in amplitude of the far-field and early near-field components

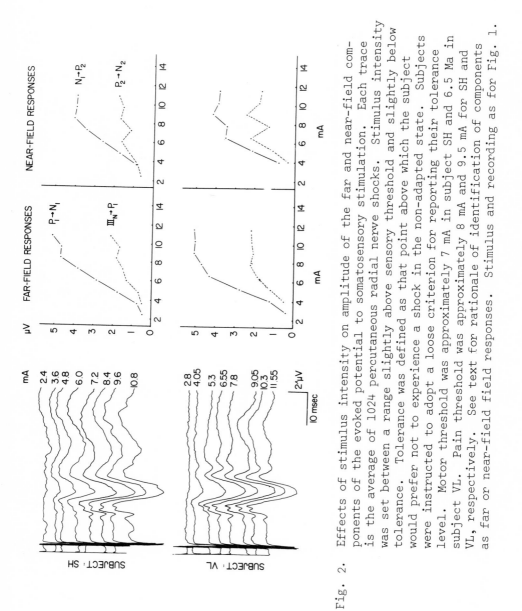

Fig. 2.   Effects of stimulus intensity on amplitude of the far and near-field components of the evoked potential to somatosensory stimulation. Each trace
is the average of 1024 percutaneous radial nerve shocks. Stimulus intensity
was set between a range slightly above sensory threshold and slightly below
tolerance. Tolerance was defined as that point above which the subject
would prefer not to experience a shock in the non-adapted state. Subjects
were instructed to adopt a loose criterion for reporting their tolerance
level. Motor threshold was approximately 7 mA in subject SH and 6.5 Ma in
subject VL. Pain threshold was approximately 8 mA and 9.5 mA for SH and
VL, respectively. See text for rationale of identification of components
as far or near-field field responses. Stimulus and recording as for Fig. 1.

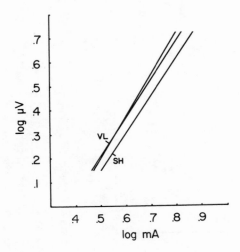

Fig. 3. Log-log coordinate plot of amplitude of the $P_1 \rightarrow N_1$ com-
         ponent versus stimulus intensity. Between ranges of
         sensory and pain thresholds these functions are accept-
         ably fitted by a power function. Two repeated runs on
         Subject VL illustrate stability of the intensity evoked
         potential amplitude relationship. Slopes of these func-
         tion for both subjects approximated 1.50. At pain thres-
         hold these functions become non-linear (not plotted, see
         Fig. 2). A power function relationship between intensity
         and amplitude was observed for the $N_1 \rightarrow P_2$ component but
         not the $P_2 \rightarrow N_2$ component. Amplitudes are peak-to-peak
         measures and therefore obscure the specific relationship
         of each individual component to stimulus intensity. The
         possible relationship of these components to psychophy-
         sical judgments of stimulus intensity are discussed in
         the text.

shown in Fig. 2 and 3. At higher levels of stimulation the response saturates and poor discrimination would be expected (Fig.
1). It was approximately at maximum amplitude of $P_1 \rightarrow N_1$ that
subjects began to report a noxious stinging or burning quality
which was due perhaps to recruitment of $A\delta$ fibers (Collins,
Nulsen, and Randt, 1960). Prior to onset of the noxious qualities
of the stimulus, subjects typically described the stimulus as a
thumping or tapping sensation. Such a change in sensory qualities
could increase discrimination even though the amplitude of these
components has reached a limit. It would appear that these early
brain responses originating from subcortical and primary cortical

receiving areas of the somatosensory afferent system reflect mainly Aβ activity. While the early components of somatosensory evoked potentials may not reflect Aδ fiber activity and, certainly not C-fiber activity, recent reports have focused on later evoked potential components in relation to pain report.

Pain Evoked Potentials

Attempts to relate middle and later components of event related evoked potentials to sensation and perception are fraught with technical (Vaughan, 1975a; 1975b; Sutton, 1969) and conceptual difficulties (Schwartz, 1976; Uttal, 1967). Nevertheless, reliable correlations between psychophysical measures and near-field components of somatosensory evoked potentials have been obtained (Rosner and Goff, 1967; Beck and Rosner, 1968; Ivanitsky and Strelets, 1977). While it is difficult at best to associate specific properties of averaged, scalp recorded evoked potentials to specific experiences it has been suggested that a late positive near-field component of the evoked response to noxious electrical stimulation of finger, toe and lip (Stowell, 1977), to noxious electrical stimulation of teeth (Chatrian, Farrell, Canfield, and Lettich, 1975; Chatrian, Canfield, Knauss, and Lettich, 1975), and to noxious laser stimulation of forearm (Carmon, Mor, and Goldberg, 1976a; 1976b) may be an objective, physiological correlate of subjective pain in man.

Recently, relationships among stimulus intensity, subjective report of pain and amplitude of late components of dental evoked potentials elicited by electrical stimulation of teeth has been reported (Harkins and Chapman, 1978). The tooth is a particularly interesting model to use in the study of acute, laboratory induced pain since it is innervated mainly by high threshold Aδ- and C-fibers which are thought to mediate nociceptive input (Mumford and Bowsher, 1976). Electrical tooth stimulation has been used successively in a number of laboratory studies of pain including evaluation of the effects of age (Harkins and Chapman, 1976; 1977), drugs (Chapman, Gehrig, and Wilson, 1975; Harkins, Benedetti, Chapman, and Colpitts, 1978), and acupuncture (Chapman, Chen, and Bonica, 1977) on pain perception.

While cutaneous somatosensory stimuli, such as electrical shock, can be painful this form of stimulation also produces substantial activation of low-threshold sensory afferents. Somatosensory evoked potentials to painful skin shock represent the combined influence of sensory receptors as well as activity from nociceptors. The early evoked potential components of such stimulation illustrated in Fig. 1 and 2 were, in fact, related to stimulus intensity in the non-painful range. The amplitude of these responses was near Δ maximum by the time the stimulus was reported to

be painful. The dental evoked potential (DEP), in turn, has a
much longer latency of onset than early SEP responses and is likely
a near-field reflection of cortical activity (Chatrian, Canfield,
et al., 1975; Harkins and Chapman, 1978).

Figure 4 illustrates the major components of the DEP and the
effects of stimulus intensity on component amplitude for one subject. Figures 5 and 6 illustrates the effect of stimulus intensity
on latency and amplitude of major components of the DEP. Amplitude
covaried with perceived pain intensity (and stimulus intensity)
suggesting that amplitude of the DEP may be a physiological correlate of acute pain in man. Latency did not vary with stimulus
intensity as illustrated in Fig. 5.

The fact that perceived pain intensity and amplitude of the
DEP covary suggests that differences in amplitude of the DEP may be
related to ability to discriminate noxious shocks of various intensities. Recently it has been demonstrated that pain threshold
for electrical stimulation of tooth pulp is invariant with age but
that elderly individuals have a deficit for discrimination (d') of
suprathreshold tooth shocks (Harkins and Chapman, 1976; 1977).
Figure 7 presents the DEP of a young person (age 24) on the left
and that of an elderly individual on the right (age 72). Note that
the DEP in response to a shock reported to be faintly painful is
quite similar in both the young and elderly subject. In the elderly
person note, however, that the amplitude to faintly painful shocks
tended to be near the maximum level of response evoked by strongly
painful shocks. The evoked potentials results suggests a decreased
differentiation of neural events to painful shocks in elderly persons and are consistent with the lack of an age effect on pain
threshold but a deficit in pain discrimination in elderly people
(Harkins and Chapman, 1976; 1977).

An attempt to evaluate more directly if amplitude of the DEP
is related to sensory/perceptual experience was recently undertaken
(Harkins, Benedetti, Chapman, and Colpitts, 1978). Volunteers were
asked to determine the shock level considered to be "Strong Pain."
Evoked potentials were measured at this level stimulation before
and after administration of 33 per cent nitrous oxide. The results (see Fig. 8) indicated a significant reduction in amplitude
of major DEP components and a decrease in report of pain from
strong to mild. Evaluation was also made of the affects of N_2O on
auditory EPs and while a reduction in the auditory potential was
observed it was not as large as that for the painful DEPs indicating a differential responsivity of the DEP to the effects of N_2O.
There was no change in subjective report of tone intensity during
N_2O intoxication.

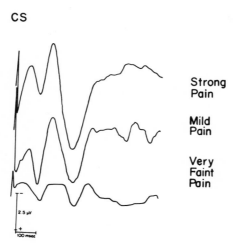

Fig. 4. Effects of stimulus intensity on amplitude of the dental evoked potential for one subject. Five msec shocks were delivered via a conductive rubber probe tip that the subject held against of a healthy, unfilled central incisor. EEG was measured from vertex (negative at vertex upward) referred to inion. Psychophysical determination of shock level necessary to elicit a verbal report of "very faint", "mild", or "strong" pain was determined by ascending trials. These levels were subsequently employed to obtain evoked potentials. Each trace is composed of 192 trials. Consistency of the subjective report of pain was assessed throughout each session. The earliest identifiable component that is consistent across subjects is a positive wave at approximately 100 msec which is followed by a negative-positive-negative complex with peak latencies at approximately 175, 200, and 350 msec, respectively. These components are labeled P100, N175, P260, and N350, respectively, in Figs. 5 and 6. Note that these components are considerably longer in latency and larger in amplitude than the far-field somatosensory evoked potentials to radial nerve stimulation. These potentials are likely near-field reflections of cortical activity. (Harkins and Chapman, 1978)

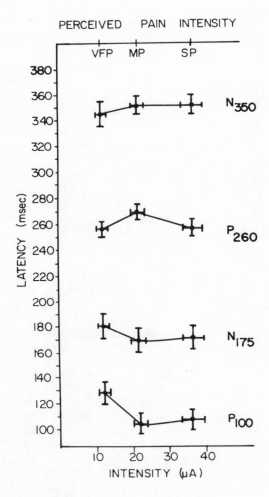

Fig. 5. Effects of stimulus intensity on latency of the four major
         components of the dental pain evoked potential in 11 young
         young subjects. With one exception (P100 from VFP to MP)
         there was no significant change in latency of these com-
         ponents with changes in stimulus intensity. Bars repre-
         sent standard error of the mean. Very faint pain = VFP;
         Mild pain = MP; Strong pain = SP; (Harkins and Chapman,
         1978).

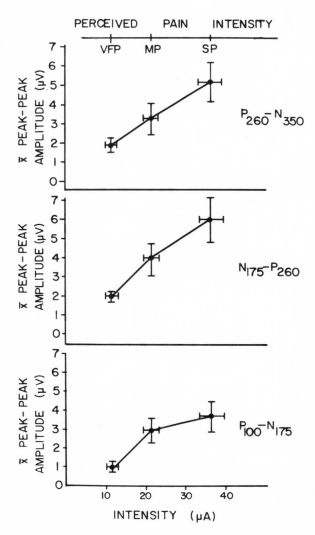

Fig. 6. Effects of stimulus intensity on latency of the peak-to-peak amplitudes of the four major components of the dental pain evoked potential in 11 young subjects. Amplitude was found to increase with stimulus intensity. Bars represent standard error of the mean. (Harkins and Chapman, 1978).

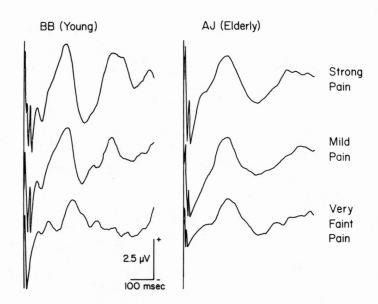

Fig. 7.   Effects of age on amplitude of the dental pain evoked
          potential. Note the change in amplitude across levels of
          pain report in the young subject and the lack of such a
          change in the elderly subject.

         Vaughn (1975b) has pointed out that there are at least four
criteria to be met in future studies attempting to relate sensory
experience and psychophysiological events such as evoked potentials.
These are: (a) precise control over the stimulus within a sufficient
intensity range to provide a meaningful interpretation of stimulus-
response relationships (see for example Fig. 2); (b) ideally, psychophysical and physiological measures should be obtained con-
currently; (c) within subject variability of both psychophysical
and psychophysiological measures should be assessed; and (d) topographic evaluation and multiple component analyses should be performed. These criteria hold particularly for studies attempting
to related specific perceptual experiences (such as pain) and
evoked potentials. No single study or sequence of studies to date
has met these precedural criteria. Nevertheless, the communality
across studies of late components to noxious stimulation (Chapman
and Harkins, 1978), the within subject stability of pain evoked
responses, the complete absence of such potentials in a patient with
congenital insensitivity to pain (Chatrian, Farrell, et al., 1975),

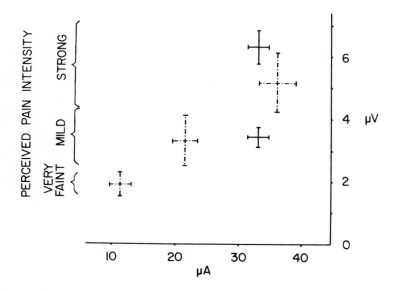

Fig. 8.   This figure represents a summary of the effects of stimulus
          intensity and an anesthetic (nitrous oxide) on peak-to-
          peak amplitude of the N175 → P260 response. Broken lines
          (redrawn from Fig. 6) show the relationship of stimulus
          intensity, perceived pain intensity and amplitude of the
          N175 → P260 component. Solid lines represent the ampli-
          tude of this component for a stimulus judged to be a
          strong pain before (top solid cross) administration of
          nitrous oxide. Following a twenty minute induction period
          of 33 percent nitrous oxide there was a significant re-
          duction in peak-to-peak amplitude that was accompanied by
          a change in pain report from strong to mild pain. These
          results indicate that amplitude of the dental pain evoked
          potential is more strongly related to subjective report
          than to the physical parameters of the stimulus. Broken
          limbs (redrawn from Harkins and Chapman, 1978) and solid
          lines (redrawn from Harkins, Benedetti, et al., 1978) re-
          present standard errors of the mean.

and the differential responsiveness of these evoked potentials to
low dosages of anesthetics (Harkins, Benedetti, et al., 1978) lend
strong circumstantial support to the contention that near-field
components of evoked potentials to noxious stimulation are related
to sensory experience and are an objective, non-verbal index of
acute pain in man.

SUMMARY

In this chapter we have dealt exclusively with two recently described evoked potentials. These are the far-field and early near-field responses to somatosensory stimulation and near-field responses to painful electrical stimulation of teeth. Circumstantial evidence was presented indicating that certain components of the very early responses may be related to sensory discrimination. It is clear that amplitude of several components is best described as a power function of stimulus intensity. Circumstantial evidence was presented indicating that certain components of later, near-field responses are related to the degree of pain experienced. The basic issue of whether averaged evoked potentials measured from scalp in man are directly related to certain perceptual experiences such as pain or rather are reflections of global, non-specific operations (Schwartz, 1976; Uttal, 1967) awaits further empirical evaluation.

ACKNOWLEDGEMENTS

This research was supported, in part, by USPHS Grants No. AG-00573 and GM 15991. The authors wish to thank Dr. M. Colpitts, Ms. B. Ashleman, and Ms. M. Warner for their assistance in recording and analysis of evoked potentials and Ms. J. Byce for her assistance in typing and editing.

REFERENCES

Beck, C., & Rosner, B. S. Magnitude scales and somatic evoked potentials to percutaneous electrical stimulation. Physiology and Behavior, 1968, 3, 947-953.

Buchwald, J. & Huang, C. Far-field acoustic response: Origins in the cat. Science, 1975, 189, 382-384.

Carmon, A., Mor, J., & Goldberg, J. Application of laser to psychophysiological study of pain in man. In J. J. Bonica & D. Albe-Fessard (Eds.), Advances in pain research and therapy (Vol. 1). New York: Raven Press, 1976a.

Carmon, A., Mor, J., & Goldberg, J. Evoked cerebral responses to noxious thermal stimuli in humans. Experimental Brain Research, 1966, 25, 103-107.

Chapman, C. R., Chen, A., & Bonica, J. Effects of intrasegmental electrical acupuncture on dental pain: Evaluation by threshold estimation and sensory decision theory. Pain, 1977, 3, 213-227.

Chapman, C. R., Gehrig, J., & Wilson, M. Acupuncture compared with 33 percent nitrous oxide for dental analgesia. Anesthesiology, 1975, 42, 532-537.

Chapman, C. R. & Harkins, S. W. Cerebral evoked responses as correlates of laboratory pain. In J. J. Bonica & J. C. Liebaskind (Eds.), Advances in pain research and therapy(Vol. III). New York: Raven Press, (In Press).

Chatrian, G. E., Canfield, R. C., Knauss, T. A., & Lettich, E. Cerebral responses to electrical tooth pulp stimulation in man. Neurology, 1975, 25, 745-757.

Chatrian, G. E., Farrell, D. F., Canfield, R. C., & Lettich, E. Congenital insensitivity to noxious stimuli. Archives of Neurology, 1975, 32, 141-145.

Chizppa, K. H., Choi, S. K., & Young, R. R. Short latency somato-sensory evoked potentials following median nerve stimulation in patients with neurological lesions. In J. E. Desmedt (Ed.) Progress in Clinical Neurophysiology. Basel: Karger, 1978.

Collins, W. F., Nulsen, F. E., & Randt, C. T. Relation of peri-pheral nerve fiber size and sensation in man. Archives of Neurology, 1960, 3, 381-385.

Cracco, R. Q. The initial positive potential of the human scalp-recorded somatosensory evoked response. Electroencephalo-graphy and Clinical Neurophysiology, 1972, 32, 623-629.

Cracco, R. Q. & Cracco, J. B. Somatosensory evoked potential in man: Far field potentials. Electroencephalography and Clinical Neurophysiology, 1976, 41, 460-466.

Dong, W. & Harkins, S. W. Origins of somatosensory near and far-field evoked potentials. (In preparation).

Frazén, O & Offenloch, K. Evoked response correlates of psycho-physical magnitude estimates for tactile stimulation in man. Experimental Brain Research, 1969, 8, 1-18.

Green, D. M. & Swets, J. A. Signal detection theory and psycho-physics. New York: Krieger, 1974 (Reprint of 1966 Edition).

Gybels, J. & Van Hees, J. Unit activity from mechanoreceptors in human peripheral nerve during intensity discrimination of touch. In G. G. Somjen (Ed.), Neurophysiology studied in man. Amsterdam: Excerpta Medica, 1972.

Halliday, A. M. Somatosensory evoked responses. In A. Redmond (Ed.), Handbook of electroencephalography and clinical neuro-physiology. Amsterdam: Elsevier, 1975.

Harkins, S. W., Benedetti, N., Chapman, C. R., & Colpitts, Y. Cerebral evoked potentials to noxious and non-noxious stimu-lation: Effects of nitrous oxide. (In Preparation).

Harkins, S. W. & Chapman, C. R. Detection and decision factors in pain perception in young and elderly men. Pain, 1976, 2, 253-264.

Harkins, S. W. & Chapman, C. R. The perception of induced dental pain in young and elderly women. Journal of Gerontology, 1977, 32, 428-435.

Harkins, S. W. & Chapman, C. R.   Cerebral evoked potentials to
    noxious dental stimulation: Relationship to subjective pain
    report. Psychophysiology, 1978, 15, 248-252.
Iraqui-Madoz, V. J. & Wiederholt, W. C.   Far-field somatosensory
    evoked potentials in the cat: Correlation with depth record-
    ing. Annals of Neurology, 1977, 1, 569-574.
Ivanitsky, A. J. & Strelets, V. B.   Brain evoked potentials and
    some mechanisms of perception. Electroencephalography and
    Clinical Neurophysiology, 1977, 43, 397-403.
Jewett, D. L.   Volume-conducted potentials in response to auditory
    stimuli as detected by averaging in the cat. Electroen-
    cephalography and Clinical Neurophysiology, 1970, 28, 609-
    618.
Jewett, D. L. & Williston, J. S.   Auditory-evoked far fields
    averaged from the scalp of humans. Brain, 1971, 94, 681-696.
Mountcastle, V. B. & Darian-Smith, I.   Neural mechanisms in somes-
    thesis.   In V. B. Mountcastle (Ed.), Medical physiology.   St.
    Louis: Mosby, 1968.
Mountcastle, V. B., Talbot, W. H., Sakata, H., & Hyvärinen. J.
    Cortical neuronal mechanisms in flutter-vibration studied in
    unanesthetized monkeys.   Neuronal periodicity and frequency
    discrimination. Journal of Neurophysiology, 1969, 32, 452-
    484.
Mumford, J. M., & Bowsher, D.   Pain and protopathic sensibility.
    A review with particular reference to the teeth. Pain, 1976,
    2, 223-244.
Rosner, B. S. & Goff, W. R.   Electrical responses of the nervous
    system and subjective scales of intensity.   In W. D. Neff
    (Ed.), Contributions to sensory physiology, (Vol. 2).   New
    York: Academic Press, 1967.
Schwartz, M.   Averaged evoked responses and the encoding of per-
    ception. Psychophysiology, 1976, 13, 546-553.
Staddon, J. E. R.   Theory of behavioral power functions. Psycho-
    logical Review, 1978, 85, 305-320.
Stevens, S. S.   Psychophysics. New York: Wiley, 1975.
Stowell, H.   Cerebral slow waves related to the perception of pain
    in man. Brain Research Bulletin, 1977, 2, 23-30.
Sutton, S.   The specification of psychological variables in an
    averaged evoked potential experiment.   In E. Donchin & D. B.
    Lindsley (Eds.), Average evoked potentials: Methods, results
    and evaluations.   Washington, D. C.:   NASA, 1969.
Swets, J. A.   The relative operating characteristic in psychology.
    Science, 1973, 183, 990-1000.
Uttal, W. R.   Evoked brain potentials: Signs of codes? Perspec-
    tives in Biology and Medicine, 1967, 10, 627-639.
Vaughan, H. G.   Psychological correlates of the association cortex
    potentials.   In A. Redmond, (Ed.), Handbook of electroen-
    cephalography and clinical neurophysiology, (Part A).   Amster-
    dam: Elsevier Scientific Publishing Co., 1975a.

Vaughan, H. G. Psychophysical relations of evoked responses. In
    A. Remond, (Ed.), Handbook of electroencephalography and
    clinical neurophysiology. (Part A) Amsterdam: Elsevier
    Scientific Publishing Co., 1975b.
Wiederholt, W. G., & Iragui-Madoz, V. J. Far-field somatosensory
    potentials in the rat. Electroencephalography and Clinical

DISCUSSION

DR. VERRILLO: How do you answer the criticism of McBurney (1974, 1976) and others, that because pain is not on a continuum with the other sensations that precede pain, it is not legitimate then to use Signal Detection Theory which requires that the noise and signal be on the same continuum.

DR. HARKINS: I do not. What I say is that the individual's ability to discriminate between suprathreshold noxious events can be studied using Signal Detection Theory. If you can show, especially using a zero (pain) level intensity, that the d' changes between zero and some suprathreshold level, then one can infer that you have modulated the system.

DR. PERL: I might point out, Dr. Verrillo, that it is only an assumption that pain is not on the same continuum. We do not know what the continuum for pain is, nor that for most of the somatic senses, which makes it hard to compare pain with other sensations. Let me raise another issue. The underlying assumption in Dr. Harkins' study is that tooth pulp stimulation evokes an afferent message interpreted solely as pain, a proposal dating back over thirty years (Brookhart et al., 1953; Goetzl et al., 1943; Hardy et al., 1952). The idea that pain is the only sensory experience one can get from electrical stimulation of the teeth has not been universally accepted, particularly with stimulation done in the way Dr. Harkins used. Even in the case of electrodes inserted so that just the tooth pulp is activated, it has been claimed that a sort of innocuous sensation is evoked as well, a sensation said to be masked by the electrical stimulation. The first stage in addressing your observations on the evoked potentials is that underlying assumption. What evidence do you have that your stimulation does not initiate another kind of input which would show gradation, for whatever reason, in the fashion you have shown to exist?

DR. HARKINS: There are pre-pain sensations from teeth in response to electrical stimuli of the type that I use. This is an observation that I have made, and Mumford and Bowsher have proven it. I am not sure how to respond to that other than to say that the level of stimulation for the pre-pain sensation is very narrow, it is not observable in all subjects, does not seem to be graded, there seems to be a jump from the sensation of "something" to a very faint pain, and when individuals try to describe the sensation, it is very difficult. I found, unless one gives the instruction, "Judge when you first feel something", versus "when you first feel pain", you generally get a pain response and not the "something". I am not sure how this underlying problem limits the interpretability of the evoked response and, perhaps, the signal detection data. I assume that this pre-pain sensation is not graded, although the pain sensation is graded.

DR. POULOS: Along a similar line I was curious, especially at the higher levels, how well localized was the sensation and with particular reference to a paper presented by (Kenneth V. Anderson et al. 1977). Physiological and Anatomical Studies Revealing an Extensive Transmedian Innervation of Feline Canine Teeth, In: Pain in the trigeminal region, (Anderson and Matthews, Eds.) Elsevier/ North-Holland Biomedical Press, 1977 pp 149-160. I would remind you of discussions that took place at the Bristol symposium about bilateral primary afferent input in that system. Do you see anything like that and how well localized is the pain?

DR. HARKINS: It is very badly localized. As to the projection system, I cannot comment.

DR. JÄRVILEHTO: It seems to me that you have quite strong faith in the neural origin of these potentials. I presume that the pain sensation is associated with several kinds of reflex responses which might contribute to the potential measurements. How do you exclude possible extra-cranial sources of these potentials, especially when you measure responses to pain?

DR. HARKINS: The reflexive activities would be in the first 80 to 100 msec after the stimuli. In the case of these pain evoked potentials we are looking at the earliest positive component at about 100 msec. The possible myogenic contaminants that could come in have been studied extensively by (Chatrian et al, 1975) and his group. Under different conditions, there is one early component that appears at about 60 msec that may be myogenic in origin, coming from neck muscle, but the stimulus artifact tends to obscure these earlier responses.

DR. JÄRVILEHTO: There is one response that has the same latency as the negative component, namely the blink response. How do you exclude that?

DR. HARKINS: During the series of trials we have our very well instructed subjects fixate - eyes open and fixate. We limit our recording sessions, for any one series, to 64 shocks, on the average. Plenty of time is allowed for the subjects to blink, if they need to, between trials. Within trials - it is very easy to interact with the subject and determine when he is going to have to blink.

DR. JÄRVILEHTO: But, have you measured eye movement?

DR. HARKINS: Yes, we have looked at eye movement and found that it does not contribute to that negative potential.

DR. STOWELL: May I comment on the problem of artifacts, particularly, eye blink, eye movement artifacts, and myogenic artifacts. There are routine controls for this in all evoked potential work and I would entirely agree with Dr. Harkins that for average evoked potentials to non-noxious and noxious stimulation we can rule out non-neural components both in the early and the later time course of the evoked response. This is for averages. When you start to look at single trial evoked potentials, there is another story, but I have no story to tell at the moment on this (Stowell, H., 1979). There is a very big problem here in elucidating how much interference we are getting on the single trial but if you average 16, 32, or more trials then I think you can rule interference out. Do you agree with that?

DR. HARKINS: Yes.

DR. PERL: Dr. Stowell, did you report that C-fiber input evokes cortical potentials? If so, I should be interested in hearing about that, relative to the present work.

DR. STOWELL: No, I do not think I have ever dared to state that these were C-fiber evoked potentials. No, I would not make the jump from the skin to the scalp. Not quite so quickly. One might make some interpretation from latencies and say that at about 500 msec for the finger stimulation one might estimate, for a 1 m or 110 cm conduction path, one would not expect anything earlier than 500 msec in the evoked potential for a C-fiber. I would not claim any C-fiber activity in these late evoked potentials. Aδ-fibers is as far as we can go at the moment.

DR. ZOTTERMAN: There are a few C-fibers in the man but as far as I have heard recently the majority are Aδ-fibers. They were first recorded by Pfaffman, you know, in Adrian's laboratory in 1939.

DR. STOWELL: I would like to ask Dr. Harkins if he would agree with me that the late component, negative about 130 msec, positive 200 or 180 to 250 msecs is the vertex component in evoked potential?

DR. HARKINS: Yes, I think it is a vertex component. Chatrian's work has shown that it is maximal in central vertex (Chatrian, G. E., Canfield, R. C., Knauss, T. A., and Lettich, E. 1975).

DR. STOWELL: In that case, can we say anything about its possible cerebral origin? Since the vertex component is very widespread, where does it come from?

DR. HARKINS: I do not know where it comes from. I think it is cerebral in origin. If you look at the vertex response to auditory stimulation and the vertex response to dental stimulation they appear very similar.

DR. STOWELL: Have you been able to replicate the amplitude measurements and correlate them with psychophysical respones when recording at the specific site, the hypothetical SI site, the dental area.

DR. HARKINS: We have not tried that.

REFERENCES

Adair, E. R., Stevens, J. C., & Marks, L. E. Thermally induced pain, the doe scale, and the psychophysical power law. American Journal of Psychology, 1968, 81, 147-164.

Anderson, K. V., Rosing, H. S., & Pearl. G. S. Physiological and anatomical studies revealing an extensive transmedian innervation of feline canine teeth. In D. S. Anderson & B. Mathews (eds.), Pain in the trigeminal region. Amsterdam: Elsevier Pub. Co., 1977.

Brookhart, H. M., Livingston, W. K., & Haugen, F. P. Functional characteristics of afferent fibers from tooth pulp of cat. Journal of Neurophysiology, 1953, 16, 634-642.

Chatrian, G. E., Canfield, R. C., Knauss, T. A., & Leftich, E. Cerebral responses to electrical tooth pulp stimulation in man. An objective correlate of acute experimental pain. Neurology, 1975, 25, 745-757.

Goetzl, F. R., Burrill, D. Y., & Ivy, A. C. A critical analysis of algesimetric methods with suggestions for a useful procedure. Quarterly Bulletin Northwestern University Medical School, 1943, 17, 280-291.

Hardy, J. D., Wolff, H. G., & Goodell, H. Pain sensations and reactions. Baltimore: Williams & Wilkins, Co., 1952.

McBurney, D. H. Acupuncture, pain and signal detection theory. Science, 1974, 189, 66.

McBurney, D. H. Signal detection theory and pain. Anesthesiology, 1976, 44, 356-358.

Stowell, H. Single-epoch somatosensory evoked potentials at vertex: a time window specified for electro-ocular monitoring. Electroencephalography and Clinical Neurophysiology, 1979, 46, 220-223.

BURNING AND SECOND PAIN: AN ALTERNATIVE INTERPRETATION

S. Croze and R. Duclaux

Laboratoire de Neurophysiologie sensorielle, Université

Claude Bernard, Faculté de Médecine Lyon Sud, B.P. 12,

69600 OULLINS, France

In most studies using heat as a painful stimulus the sensation of second pain is defined as the occurrence of a burning sensation. From the results obtained in reaction time measurements and in nerve block experiments it has been assumed that burning or second pain is caused by the activation of polymodal nociceptors innervated by slowly conducting afferent fibers of the C type (Price and Dubner, 1977). It follows from this assumption that any painful thermal stimulus that activates C-polymodal nociceptors will evoke a burning or a thermal pain sensation. In order to verify or invalidate this assumption we studied, in human subjects, the effect of the stimulus area on the quality of the pain sensation evoked by very hot or very cold stimuli.

METHODS

Naive subjects were asked for the sensation they felt after a very brief application of six stimuli on the back of the hand. The subjects ignored which of the six stimuli was being applied. The stimuli consisted of a needle, three copper cylinders of the same area, one at $+60^\circ C$ and the others at $-40^\circ C$ and $+20^\circ C$, a von Frey hair of 1.65 mg and an air puff. Only the former three stimuli were immediately painful. The latter three were used as control and distractors. The area of the copper cylinders was varied from 1 to 100 mm^2 with intermediary steps of 3.5, 10, 25, 38, and 78 mm^2. Each of the six stimuli was randomly applied ten times to each of five subjects.

RESULTS

The sensation evoked by the needle was one of pricking in 99 percent of the trials. In 1 percent of the cases, the subjects reported a sensation of burning after needle application.

The sensation evoked by the very hot and the very cold stimuli depended on the surface area of the stimulus, as shown in Fig. 1. For 1 mm^2 stimuli the sensation was almost always one of pricking with no recognition of the thermal character of the stimulus (Fig. 1).

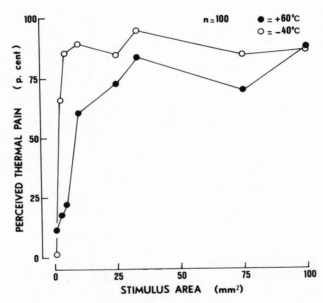

Fig. 1. Percent of judgements of thermal pain after the application of very hot (+ 60 °C) and very cold (-40 °C) stimuli on the back of the hand, as a function of the area of the stimuli. The thermal character of the stimuli was not recognized when punctate stimuli (1 mm^2) were used. In order to obtain a recognition in most of the stimulus applications, the area of the stimuli must reach 5 mm^2 and 25 mm^2 for cold and hot, respectively.

As the surface of stimulation was increased the percent of judgements of thermal pain increased. Judgements of thermal pain were either "burning" or "pricking plus warm" for the very hot stimuli. They were either "freezing", "burning" or "pricking plus cold" for the very cold stimuli.

Judgements of thermal pain for the very hot stimuli reached 73 percent of the trails for a stimulation area of 25 mm^2. For larger surfaces up to 100 mm^2, thermal pain was perceived in 75 to 90 percent of the applications (Fig. 1). Thermal pain was more readily perceived after the application of a very cold stimulus. For a 5 mm^2 stimulator thermal pain was perceived in 86 percent of the applications and from 5 mm^2 up to an area of 100 mm^2 thermal pain was perceived in 85 to 95 percent of the stimuli.

DISCUSSION

The present study shows that a punctate (1 mm^2) very hot or very cold thermal stimuli evoke only a pure pricking sensation with no burning or thermal pain sensation. Since C-polymodal nociceptors are readily activated by temperatures higher than -42°C (Bessou and Perl, 1969; Croze, Duclaux, and Kenshalo, 1976), the present results indicate that these receptors cannot give rise to a burning or thermal pain sensation. However, C-polymodal nociceptors may be responsible, together with Aδ-mechano-thermal nociceptors, for the **pure** pricking sensation obtained with both mechanical (needle) or punctate thermal stimuli. The activity of these receptors would result in a unique sensation of pain, that of pricking, whatever the physical nature of the stimulus, hot, cold or heavy pressure. Yet, the sensitivity of these noci-ceptors to very cold stimuli has to be proved in order to make this assumption acceptable.

Which receptors are at the origin of thermal pain sensation? The present results show that thermal pain is a complex sensation that associates a pricking pain sensation and a thermal sensation. We have seen that thermal pain cannot be due to the activity of the polymodal nociceptors. It may therefore originate the specific thermoreceptors. This assumption seems to be confirmed by the re-sults shown in Fig. 1. Here, the frequency of judgements of thermal pain reached its maximum for a stimulus area of 5 mm^2 with cold, and 25 mm^2 with hot. This discrepancy may be correlated with the fact that cold receptors are more numerous, more sensitive and closer to the skin surface than warm receptors (Hensel, 1974). The thermal character of the pain sensation would occur after specific thermoreceptors have been activated by a diffusion of heat or cold from the thermode.

The present results show that a clear distinction must be made between second pain and thermal pain sensations. When the skin is heated or cooled the occurrence of a thermal pain sensation must not be taken as a signal for the occurrence of second pain since the thermal character of pain may not be due to the activity of nociceptors but to that of specific thermoreceptors.

SUMMARY

In most studies using heat as a painful stimulus the sensation of second pain is defined as the occurrence of a burning sensation. It has been assumed that burning or second pain is caused by the activation of polymodal nociceptors innervated by slowly conducting C-afferent fibers. Therefore any painful thermal stimulus that activates C-polymodal nociceptors should evoke a burning or a thermal pain sensation. In order to test this hypothesis we studied, in humans, the effect of the stimulus area on the quality of the pain sensation evoked by very hot or very cold stimuli.

A punctate hot (+ 60 °C) or cold (- 40 °C) painful stimulus of 1 mm^2, applied to the back of the hand, induces a pure pricking pain sensation which is systematically mistaken with the pain evoked by a needle. These results show that skin nociceptors are mechanothermal, but cannot discriminate the thermal character of a painful thermal stimulus. However, when the stimulation area is increased to 23 mm^2 for heat and to 5 mm^2 for cold, pain is felt, respectively, as burning and freezing.

These results show that punctate hot stimuli, although they can readily activate C-polymodal nociceptors, do not give rise to a burning or thermal pain sensation. Activation of C-polymodal nociceptors results only in a pure pricking pain sensation. Thermal pain sensations probably originate in the specific thermoreceptors activated by a diffusion of heat from the thermode. Burning pain must be clearly distinguished from second pain, since burning does not result from the activation of nociceptors but from that of specific thermoreceptors.

ACKNOWLEDGMENTS

This work was supported by the Centre National de la Recherche Scientifique (C.N.R.S.).

REFERENCES

Bessou, P. & Perl, E. Response of cutaneous sensory units with unmyelinated fibers to noxious stimuli. Journal of Neurophysiology, 1969, 32, 1025-1043.
Croze, S., Duclaux, R., & Kenshalo, D. R. The thermal sensitivity of the polymodal nociceptors in the monkey. Journal of Physiology (London), 1976, 263, 539-562.

Hensel, H. Thermoreceptors. *Annual Review of Physiology*, 1974,
     36, 233-249.
Price, D. D. & Dubner, R. Neurons that subserve the sensory-dis-
     criminative aspects of pain. *Pain*, 1977, 3, 307-388.

DISCUSSION

DR. PERL: I would like to use the Chairman's prerogative and ask
a question. Thomas Lewis (1942) noted that simple mechanical
pricking or sudden pinch elicits two pain sensations, particularly
from distal portions of the limbs; many people have confirmed this,
especially from the feet. As a matter of fact, we have tried this
from time to time on ourselves and on students. The report,
frequently but not uniformly, is a double sensation from a single,
localized, mechanical noxious stimulation. Lewis disagreed with
Professor Zotterman (1933) and later workers (Bishop & Landau,
1958), who considered the two sensations to have different sensory
qualities; Lewis argued that they had similar qualities, and that
the later sensation did not necessarily have a burning quality.
Without getting into the details of this argument, how could you
account, in your scheme of things, for the double sensory experience that noxious mechanical stimulation provokes in many
human beings?

DR. DUCLAUX: You mean, to which receptors can we try to impute
these two sensations?

DR. PERL: Yes, that; or else the question of whether they actually
exist, because you have done another series of experiments pertinent to that. Lewis and Pochin (1937) used a thermal stimulus
to show the effect of distance from the central nervous system on
the two pain sensations; however, they also mentioned the double
sensation and its apparent relation to the distance of conduction
with mechanical stimulation.

DR. DUCLAUX: As far as the sensation is concerned we only asked
the subject for the whole experience. We did not ask the subject
to separate what they felt first and then later. They just said,
"that is pricking, that is burning, that is freezing, etc." Maybe we missed something, I am not sure. As far as the receptors
are concerned, I think our experiments show clearly that when you
excite mechanothermal nociceptors with either mechanical or thermal
stimuli, they give the same sensation. Dr. Zotterman and Dr.
Iggo have both said that here. They said that even if receptors
respond to more than one form of stimulus energy they always give
one sensation--always the same sensation.

DR. PERL: So, if I interpret you correctly, it is that you have
not dealt with first and second pain, but rather with the pricking
versus the burning sensation. This then was related to first and
second pain only to the extent that the previous literature has
related it?

DR. DUCLAUX: You are quite right. In literature you find usually the painful stimulus used is thermal and usually the second pain is described as a burning pain but that is not always the case because, as Dr. Zotterman showed us the first day, when you block the nerve fibers and when you stimulate mechanically you get a late pain that is not burning.

DR. ZOTTERMAN: Yes, it is.

DR. DUCLAUX: It is?

DR. PERL: Not only did Professor Zotterman describe that, but Bishop and Landau (1958) have also described the same burning sensation.

DR. ZOTTERMAN: I think this presentation was very interesting be-cause you are quite right in the analysis of the warm and cold pain sensation. I used only a needle prick, as I showed the other day, and all the subjects reported that the second pain had quite another character than the first, which is pricking pain. That is my own experience, too. First of all, the experience you have with the second pain in my experiments, after 20 min of arrested blood flow, is very nasty.

DR. LINDBLOM: Have you tried to measure the reaction times? That would perhaps clear up the issue of whether the pricking pain was always the first pain or sometimes could be the second pain, or the C-fiber mediated pain. It is possible that when the first pain is abolished, the second pain does not retain its quality. I can refer to a series of pain patients who were investigated in Stockholm last year, first by Dr. Verrillo and me, who measured the reaction times for pain elicited by mechanical stimuli. These reaction times were short and were compatible with A-fiber mediated pain. Later, Dr. Fruhstorfer from Marburg and I measured the reaction time of thermally evoked pain. The pain sensation did not have the deep burning quality but was rather pricking, or biting in character and occurred at a reaction time that un-doubtedly indicated C-fiber mediation. So, the pricking pain may be late. Another observation in these patients, who had an ab-normal and exaggerated type of response, was that they could re-port simultaneous burning with the pricking pain, or as you say, first a short pricking pain and then a burning afterimage. Some-times the pain was sustained and overwhelmed the burning sensation. So the two sensations could interplay but basically they started simultaneously.

DR. HENSEL: You mentioned the relative number of warm and cold spots. I think this whole business must be thoroughly reinvesti-gated because I think that some of the warm spots might have been

missed by the small thermal stimuli. It depends very much on their
depth in skin, because of the three-dimensional heat flow which
means that only a small fraction of the external temperature
actually will reach the receptor. A cold receptor is localized
very superfically so we found that even when having a cold wire of
50μm in diameter, that is the diameter of a human hair, and you
approach the skin with this wire the cold receptor might start
firing before the wire touched the skin just by cold radiation.
This is never the case with warm receptors. This is to say, that
in my opinion, all these measurements are very unreliable.

DR. DUCLAUX: You would say that the difference in discrimination
between warm and cold is perhaps due to the depth of the receptors.

DR. POULOS: One problem that I have with pricking pain plus
thermal on the cold side is, at least in the monkey nervous system,
that we get a complete block, other than a very brief dynamic response, to temperatures as low as 15°C. I would predict that your
40°C would surely block any activity in specific cold receptors.
One other observation I would like to make, but for which I have
absolutely no explanation, is that the thermal sensations associated with the pain system can be very complicated. For example, in collaboration with Richard Lende (Lende & Poulos, 1970)
we examined a group of patients who had undergone cordotomies for
relief of intractable pain. On sensory examination, these patients
very frequently would report ice cubes and cold test tubes as
warm, but were insensitive to pin prick. While I have no explanation for the observation it forbodes quite a complicated system.

DR. IGGO: I would like to bring into the discussion the fact that
there is a spinal cord interpolated between the skin and the
sensorium. We now know, starting with experiments of Christensen
and Perl (1970), that there are in the superficial part of the
spinal cord, neurons that appear to be specifically excited by
noxious stimulation. It is also known that these send projecting
axons across the cord up into the thalamus. In some work done in
the laboratory in Edinburgh, mostly on the cat, but also some on
the monkey, there is evidence that these nociceptor driven, lamina
I cells fall into two kinds, one that is excited only by the Aδ
afferent fibers and by mechanical stimulation or pricking and the
other excited by both mechanical and thermal stimulation. The
thermal stimuli are mediated through the nonmyelinated afferent
fibers. So here is a system where there is a preservation of a
difference that exists in the periphery that may match the reports
of first and second pain. At least the two kinds of input are kept
separate. There seems to be a pathway for the so-called pricking
sensible, mechanical sensitive nociceptors and another pathway in
which there is convergence of both the mechanically sensitive

nociceptors and the thermally sensitive nociceptors. So perhaps
you need to bear that in mind in your interpretation.

DR. DUCLAUX: I will only make a comment about sensation. In
preliminary experiments that we are doing now, it is obvious that
the subjects cannot recognize the nature of the stimulus. The
sensation produced by the very hot, very cold, and needle stimuli,
seems to be exactly the same. If you ask a subject which stimulus
was applied to the skin, in 50 per cent of the trials with a hot
stimulus, he will say, "needle." In 50 per cent of the trials he
will say, "you applied the cylinder." So that means that the
sensation produced by the two forms of stimulation is the same.
My hypothesis is that the cells must be the same somewhere.

DR. IGGO: I am not trying to suggest that these nociceptor pathways are preserving any sensory quality of the stimulus. They are
presumably dealing with what finally gets interpreted as pain and
as we have been hearing in this meeting, there are simultaneous
inputs along other channels that may provide information about the
quality of the stimulus, as you are suggesting.

DR. TOREBJÖRK: You have not given us any alternative interpretation for the first and second pain, but you have indicated to us
that we should not associate, as frequently as we perhaps may do,
the first pain with pricking and the second pain with burning.
This is especially true, as you have shown, when stimulating with
such small contact areas that presumably activate only a few receptors which mediate the sensation of pain.

DR. DUCLAUX: I agree with you. It is the same thing that Dr.
Perl was talking about before, but in most of the papers dealing
with first and second pain the finding exists. The scientists say
first is pricking and the second is burning pain.

DR. HENSEL: Just a short comment on Dr. Poulos' observation. I
think that you are right in assuming that cold fibers under thermode
would be blocked but you have to take into consideration the horizontal spread of cold, which might be quite considerable. I
remember when Yngve Zotterman (Hensel and Zotterman, 1951)
and I did this work on the persisting cold sensation, the whole
sensation comes from the spread of cooling outside the area of the
thermode and using such a cold object you would have considerable
cooling around the thermode and this might be the cause of your
additional cold sensation.

DR. DUCLAUX: May I ask a question of the audience? As you saw
in some cases we had reports of burning for very cold stimuli.
Does anybody have an explanation of that?

DR. PERL: I might point out there will probably be almost as many explanations as there are people in the room. But at least one could fall back on Professor Iggo's comment, to the effect that somewhere between the input and perceptual recognition there lies a nervous system.

REFERENCES

Bishop, G. H. & Landau, W. M. Evidence for a double peripheral
        pathway for pain. Science, 1958, 128, 712-713.
Christensen, B. N. & Perl, E. R. Spinal neurons specifically ex-
        cited by noxious or thermal stimuli: the marginal zone of the
        dorsal horn. Journal of Neurophysiology, 1970, 33, 293-307.
Hensel, H. & Zotterman, Y. The persisting cold sensation. Acta
        Physiologica Scandivavica, 1951, 22, 106-113.
Lende, R. A., & Poulos, D. Functional localization in the trigeminal
        root. Journal of Neurosurgery, 1974, 40, 504-513.
Lewis, T. Pain. New York: MacMillan, 1942.
Lewis, T. & Pochin, E. E. Double pain response of the human skin
        to a single stimulus. Clinical Science, 1937, 3, 67-76.
Zotterman, Y. Studies in the peripheral nervous mechanism of pain.
        Acta Medica Scandivavica, 1933, 80, 185-242.

GENERAL DISCUSSION

(Editor's note: Following the formal paper sessions, an informal discussion was held on topics of acute interest to the participants. Dr. Iggo's comments were made on the afternoon before, occasioned by the necessity of an early departure. They are, however, included here in the general discussion that follows).

<u>DR. IGGO</u>: I would like to take the opportunity to make one or two comments about the meeting as I have seen it so far, and I hope that some of these points would perhaps be taken up in some of the general discussion tomorrow. First, it has been quite striking at this meeting, the extent to which the physiological function of receptors seems to have dominated the approaches that have been adopted by so many different workers, both in the psychological and in the physiological areas. This is quite a contrast to the situation in the previous meeting held here in Tallahassee (Kenshalo, 1968). At that time it was still possible to have arguments and discussions about the input to the central nervous system from the skin, an input carried in array of non-specific cutaneous receptors and to try and account for the various perceptions on the basis of some kind of analysis carried out by the central nervous system. Since that meeting and in fact, even before that meeting, it was already becoming quite clear that a great deal of analysis occurred in periphery. This makes this particular meeting very interesting. So much emphasis is now being placed on the existence of specific peripheral cutaneous receptors. In fact, I might even be tempted to suggest that we have leapt so to speak, from the morpho-psychological fallacy, as Brain described it in 1952, (where we tried to account for all sorts of psychological events in terms of the receptor morphology to a kind of afferent-unit-psychological fallacy in which we try to account for the whole system in terms of the physiological characteristics of the afferent units, and I think that is perhaps something to bear in mind, and perhaps talk about. This may be equally misleading.

A second aspect relates to the remarkable new technology of recording in conscious human subjects from efferent units in the peripheral nerve, by poking an insulated wire through the skin. This appears to be remarkably simple and desperately easy, so why are we not all doing it? Well, we all know why we are not doing it. It is not easy! But, we need to remember that there is the possibility of a bias in the sample. This bias is partly related to the point that Åke Vallbo was dealing with right at the end of his presentation--the possibility that the recording method selects the afferent units that are being examined, where only the larger myelinated and non-myelinated afferent fibers are being sampled. In fact, Roland Johansson knows perfectly well that about half of the myelinated fibers in the human median nerve have diameters less than about 6 μm. If you accept the conduction velocity records obtained by stimulating the nerve electrically, almost none of the published samples have come from that 50 percent of the myelinated afferent fibers in the nerve. And this should cause us to be rather cautious about assuming that the available sample obtained from human subjects, so far, is a true and unbiased sample. For example, one receptor type that seems to have been left out in the cold is Burgess' F receptor (Burgess & Perl, 1973). Nobody has yet mentioned it and we should, at least now, mention it even if we are not too sure of what it is. It is supposed to have large myelinated axons. People in this room have been recording from the larger myelinated fibers and the puzzle is, what happened to it? Furthermore, all the thermoreceptor work has been concerned with the nonmyelinated warm fibers rather than with the cold fibers which have axons of 1 to 2 μm diameter and which are myelinated.

There is another topic that impressed me throughout the course of the meeting, and that is the question of terminology. You might say that is a pretty sterile kind of thing to be wasting your time with, but in fact, we have to communicate with one another and, so far as possible, we should try to use expressions that we can agree upon. It would be sensible if all the people in this area could reach a common view on what terms to use. Here I refer specifically to the expression "modality." In the original psychological literature, modality, as I understand it, referred to the specific senses of taste, vision, hearing and smell. Common sensibility lumps all the remaining sensibilities together. We have been talking about common sensibility which in that terminology is a single modality. But in fact, listening to the presentations today, we have had people talking about the PC modality, as the high frequency modality of mechanical stimulation where the expression is transferred to the stimulus. It is necessary, however, to try to avoid confusion. Part of the difficulty is that the term 'mode' can be used to refer to the characteristics of a population. There may be a bimodal distribution as, in fact, there is in the axon diameters of myelinated fibers in the median nerve. I do not have a solution, but we should be aware of what we are up to. Herbert Hensel, for example, at times, I thought, was getting on very nicely when he was talking about qualities. Then, quite suddenly, he would use the expression 'modality' and, I think, meant the same thing. He seemed to use quality and modality as synonyms. If we are going to do that, we should be absolutely clear as to what we are talking about. It means we have abandoned the original definition of modality as relating to the different senses. We could have a contrast between the modality of taste and one of the qualities of common sensation, the quality of touch.

Otherwise, we are going to start dividing everything up into a lot of very fine modality divisions that will not help the discussion in the long run. Well, I do not know whether anybody feels that is as important as I do, but I really felt that I should raise the issue.

DR. PERL: I want to comment on the question of modality, because Professor Iggo has made a very important point, though he has perhaps also taken some liberty with the history. To know what we are talking about, we should indeed define our topic in some reasonable fashion. As I read the history, the use of the term modality has a derivation different from what you suggest. It originates partly in the classification of the senses by the ancient Greek philosophers, and partly in Weber's (1846) emphasis, in the mid-nineteenth century, on a common sensibility from the body. The term modality can represent either, as you suggest, some fraction of a population or, alternatively, a specific type of sense. We have heard it used this afternoon in an entirely acceptable way; that is, to distinguish the perceptual response of a human being to vibration from that provoked by another form of mechanical stimulation. In this usage, the reference is to the result of stimulation. It would be a terrible trap to return to the old common sensibility notion, which suggested that every sensory experience from the body, all the somatic senses, were essentially one and the same. Your warning against going to the other extreme, however, is important. We do not want to divide experience solely on the basis of a physical parameter that defines the stimulus, and to presume that that is a psychophysical entity.

DR. IGGO: Would you like to put on the record the fact that there is the central problem of sensational percept and the peripheral problem of defining, as accurately as possible, the stimulus condition?

DR. PERL: We are in agreement. We must distinguish between defining the physical stimulus and defining the perceptual recognition.

DR. HENSEL: I used the term modality mostly in the classical sense you suggested. On the other hand it is not very easy, because this is essentially a matter of definition. Even when going back in history to the time Johannes Müller (Müller, J. 1840) who brought up the concept of sensory specificity and modality, was talking at his time, of a common sense of feeling including warmth, cold, pain and so on. Even at his time the discussion had already started as to whether this concept was correct.

DR. IGGO: This is partly what the discussion is about. We do have

this term related to the percept, and there is a strong tendency
for people to use the expression modality with respect to a
specified narrow band of peripheral stimulus conditions which, as
Dr. Hensel made very clear in this talk, are biophysical parameters.
This is a confusion that is arising. One should be careful, just
because we have established that there may be certain kinds of
mechanoreceptors responsive to a particular range of parameters of
stimulation, to avoid using the expression 'modality' with respect
to them. We are perhaps safer if we restrict the use of the term
to the sensory function.

DR. ZOTTERMAN: How would you define the function?

DR. IGGO: One must start to talk in terms of temperature sensitivity and the ranges of temperature sensitivity, and units that
respond to increases of temperature or decreases of temperature
etc. I recognize it is cumbersome.

DR. VERRILLO: I have some points that I would like to make,
reflecting my own bias, about things that have happened at this
conference. The first, is that everyone should be very careful
about precise definitions of the stimuli that they use. This is
a persistent theme in the talks that I give, but I am sometimes
distressed (I have not been as distressed this time as I have at
others) about the precision with which the stimuli are defined. I
maintain that if you do not know what the stimulus is, then you
do not know what the response means. With technology where it is
today, we are beyond the point where we can continue to use
wooden sticks and similar crude methods and still maintain that we
precisely define stimulus.
        There should be more standardization of the units used. We
have a particular bias; we use a decibel scale. I would like to
see that used more extensively because it allows a more direct
comparison of data, not only within a single modality, but across
modalities. I realize that thermal stimuli will provide difficulties. However, the receptor responds to the energy delivered.
Thinking in terms of the energy that the stimulus is giving to the
receptor, it clarifies and simplifies a lot of the data that,
heretofore, may have been very difficult to interpret. There are
a number of experiments that lead one to believe that energy is
the significant parameter of the stimulus to which the receptor
responds, such as the 3 dB curves that we get in various experiments.
        Now, I speak as a psychophysicist and urge investigators to
standardize the psychophysical methods that are used. I am
particularly sensitive to the methods that are used in what is
called magnitude estimation or magnitude production. The curves
and the slopes that we obtain may be meaningless, unless we employ
the same methods. There are, for example, many experiments in the

literature that show that slopes can vary as a function of the
standard used. The use of the standard or modulus was discontinued
by the Stevens group, who originated the method, many years ago
because it injected a bias. Yet it is still being used. Why
introduce a bias when it is not necessary? Also there are other
ways to measure thresholds, for instance, than the ways that are
most often used today. There are more precise ways to measure
responses to within one or two decibels, which the other methods
do not permit.

I was struck by the contrast between the first symposium on
skin (Kenshalo, 1968) that was held here in Tallahassee and the one
that we have today. At that time the psychophysicists and
physiologists were quite a distance apart. It was difficult to
talk to each other. I did not see that this time. We seem to be
moving out of the era when psychologists were trained not to
dabble in physiology. I echo the statement made by Prof. Zotterman
that psychophysics provides us with very powerful methods of
measuring sensation. In the history of the investigation of
sensory mechanisms many phenomena were discovered and measured
first by psychophysical methods. This provides hunches for
physiological investigations. But, this is not a one way street.
A lot of ideas come from reading the physiological literature.

The last point relates to all the above points, and that is,
it would be gratifying to see more combinations of logic and data.
Logic means a synthesis of information. If you have only logic
you can gaze at perfect but empty spheres. On the other hand, if
you use only data, you can gaze at a full, but very shapeless
universe.

DR. HENSEL: With reference to your first point, concerning the
definition of the stimulus, this is a very difficult question, and
these questions cannot be solved, for example, by using decibel
units. Any physical stimulus we use is arbitrarily in correlation
with sensation, because physics defines its basic units without
regard of human sensation. They are arbitrarily defined, so it is
not surprising that they will not fit sensation. Our task, with
the so-called psychophysics, is to find out the correlation between
the arbitrarily defined physical units and sensation. Furthermore,
there are many areas of sensation where a decibel scale cannot be
used, take, for example, the static temperature sensation. The
The physical temperature scale starts with 0° Kelvin and has only
warmth, no cold. Temperature sensations start at 307° Kelvin, that
is the zero point on the sensation scale. It is a bipolar scale
with warm and cold. It has temperature, as well as the first
derivative to time, which is not the case in the physical scale.
So, one must be very careful in the starting with any definition
of the stimulus.

DR. STEVENS: The decibel scale was originally used as a measure
of power losses in transmission along telephone lines and involved
tremendous ranges of power.

   So the usefulness of the decibel scale proves itself when
enormous ranges of stimulus intensity are involved. In hearing,
vision, and vibration it seems to be a very useful notation but,
in temperature, I do not see that it is very useful, because
starting from physiological zero we cover such a very small range
that it would only make things difficult to have to go through
logarithmic transformations.

DR. VERRILLO: I hope you did not interpret what I said to mean you
should force people working with temperature and any kind of
sensation into using a particular scale. I said in the beginning
that I realized the difficulties.

DR. PERL: I think Celsius forced us into a scale a long time ago.
But I would like to make a comment on the decibel scale. I am not
sure that your point is well taken, Dr. Stevens, when you argue for
enormous differences in quantitative scales for vision and hearing, compared to some of the other senses. There are arguments
that the total range is greater for certain sensory modalities
than for others, but that is not necessarily so when it is placed
in terms of energy, as was proposed by Professor Hensel. What one
really should do to make a basis for comparisons would be to
calculate the amount of energy contained in stimuli from threshold
through saturation. I think it is safe to say that for mechanical
stimuli we deal with three to four log unit ranges between the
threshold for the most sensitive sensory units and saturation of
the least sensitive ones. I do not recall the values for temperature, but Professor Hensel may be able to describe the range of
temperature sense.

DR. HENSEL: Even speaking in terms of energy you might run into
difficulties. Take a cold or warm receptor that is firing with a
temperature field that is constant in time and constant in space.
There is no transfer of external thermal energy. You could speak
of a chemical energy of the receptor pulses, but this is not known,
so you have difficulties in defining your stimulus in terms of
energy.

DR. LaMOTTE: I have two comments to make. First, instead of
standardizing variables, one might show relationships between one
variable and another. For example, we measured surface skin
temperature during radiant heating, but one can also model what is
happening underneath the skin, as Dr. Hensel has done, to try to
show how surface skin temperature is related to the temperature of
deeper layers. With studies of mechanically evoked pain, one would

have to study not only displacement of the skin as a relevant
physical variable, but to look also at how displacement changes
with force. One might control the force of the stimulus in some
experiments and measure the resulting displacement due to relaxation of the skin, or control displacement and observe the force
required to produce that displacement. My second comment is that
psychophysical functions, such as those obtained by the method of
magnitude estimation, are influenced not only by choice of
stimulus parameters, but also by cognitive or judgemental variables
(Poulton, 1968). Correlative peripheral nerve recordings might
reveal the extent to which a variable (e.g. the range of stimuli
chosen) is reflected in first order neural events, as opposed to
higher order events in the central nervous system.

DR. ZOTTERMAN: In working on the skin, we are in a more difficult
position than other sensory physiologists. The eye and the ear
receptors are protected; they are kept in a very good condition,
protected from damage from the outside. But, the skin changes so
much in different parts of the body and depends on the individual
uses of the skin. The skin on my hand and the worker in the field,
for example, is quite different. The horny layer is two to three
times as thick in such a worker. We have to be aware that we are
not in that favorable position when we make our estimations of the
stimulus. We always have to take into account the particular
state of the skin and its physical properties, which makes it
much more difficult.

DR. JOHANSSON: It is not only of interest to consider the intensity aspects, which may be measured in decibels, but what about
the spatial aspects? I think these are very important. In the
tactile system the intensity aspect in terms of energy delivered
to the skin, may be of less importance than all the spacial integration, inhibition, differentiation, and so on, probably occurring
in the CNS.

DR. VERRILLO: You can add to that the various stimuli we used on
the skin. There is also a power spectrum of the stimulus that is
not very often reported. Because you put square pulses to the skin
does not mean that is what the receptor is receiving, it is important to know the frequency distribution of the energy in that
stimulus, which may be quite different from a single pulse, for
instance. Now there are methods available to do this with the fast
Fourier analysis and a computer.

DR. LINDBLOM: I would like to add here that the temporal aspect
is also important, the rate at which a certain stimulus is applied.

DR. PERL: We have probably exhausted this topic, not because we

have solved the problem, but because we created it. I have one
final plea, in company with Dr. Verrillo, which is that whenever
we describe our stimuli, let us be sure to do so in such terms
that other people, even if they cannot replicate them exactly,
will understand what they were. At least then we shall have a
possibility of comparing future work with past efforts in some
rational way. That has been done to some extent in certain
psychophysical studies and some of the more modern physiological
studies. Where their measurements have been comparable, the
results permit us to correlate the activity of neural elements
with other measures.

DR. POULOS: I think it is important to readers of volumes
emanating from symposiums to have a summary of a consensus, if
that is possible, for certain problems that have woven themselves
throughout the presentations. There are two I would suggest that
we attempt to obtain some consensus for. One is the differences
observed in the human recording as to fiber type and those
observed in animal studies. The second is, how secure the participants feel that the single fibers recorded from in the psychophysical studies are the fibers providing the information of the
perception reported. Here we should consider the importance of
parallel channels, and so on. Perhaps we could start with Dr.
Vallbo who addressed these questions.

DR. VALLBO: I will give a short comment on the first point about
fiber diameters in animals and man. In a very broad sense the
higher up you look in the phylogenetic scale, more of the fibers are
myelinated. Moreover, when you go from proximal areas to distal
areas of the extremities, more of the fibers are myelinated. On
the other hand, it is not true that the diameters, of the myelinated
fibers in general, are larger in man than e.g. in cats. Actually,
it often appears to be the other way around.
     The other point was how convinced I am that the fiber recorded
from really is essential for the sensation. I must emphasize that
this is not always a claim. It is very important to differentiate
between two kinds of situations, the one when you record from a
single unit and you assume that this very unit is the essential
one for the sensation. That has to be proved in the particular
experiment. Whether that can be done, and how it can be done
varies from one experiment to the other, as well as how high a
probability can be reached at that point. A difficult point
is whether you can exclude that parallel lines are activated or not.
On the other hand, in most experiments of this kind, when you record from a single unit, this unit represents a group of units
which are, or are assumed to be, essential for the sensation.
The conscious human subject offers a wealth of possibilities because you can control what you activate and at the same time study

the sensations associated with the stimulus. You can design stimuli that are very particular for the kind of input that you want to create, and insure that you have been successful. It seems from what has come out of some of the comments here that it might be possible to activate, for instance, a single cold unit, (we have been stimulating what we think are single tactile units) would be interesting to see more studies of that kind.

DR. PERL: There is some published data that indicates the probability of a bias in the human sample. I am rather surprized no one has brought this up. The evidence from other primates, along with Hensel and Boman's (1960) work on man, proves the presence of cooling-type thermoreceptors with thin myelinated fibers. So one should suspect something when a new technique misses a probable part of a population. When microelectrodes were first used to record from primary fibers, in a large series of experiments that yielded many elements per experiment, Burgess and his associates (Burgess et al., 1968) compared the population of fibers they recorded from with the distribution that one would expect to find based upon histological measurements of the same nerves. They found a good correspondence between the distribution of conduction velocities and the distribution of fiber diameters in a given nerve for the larger elements of the population, but a much poorer fit for the smaller diameter, more slowly conducting group. Recordings with microelectrodes of even very small tip diameters (under 0.5 μm) definitely bias the sample toward the more rapidly conducting elements. The sample included elements with all the conduction speeds expected for myelinated fibers, so the entire population was represented, but the proportion was significantly skewed toward the more rapidly conducting elements. That result came with the smallest type of microelectrode so far used in such experiments.
     What we learn from the work on man is quite different. In those studies, rather large metal microelectrodes (which would look like crowbars in the electron microscopic pictures, compared to the glass capillary electrodes) are used to record from single C-fibers or from rapidly conducting myelinated fibers. For some reason, they rarely record well from single slowly conducting myelinated fibers, so elements from that population are usually passed over. We can only speculate on the possible mechanisms at work. One might be Dr. Torebjörk's suggestion, which is based upon the known anatomical vagaries of the distribution of the peripheral nerve C-fibers, running from one Schwann cell sheath to another. Perhaps by a chance combination of receptive field selection and recording site, the electrode happens into the circumstance of recording from a single C-fiber activated effectively by natural stimuli, while other fibers in that particular Schwann bundle have different responsive fields. Therefore you see a unitary C-fiber potential.

But Dr. Torebjörk has given us another idea: he suggested that his
action potentials came from extracellular recordings of activity
produced by fibers that were without nodes of Ranvier to limit the
loci from which current fields are produced. Dr. Vallbo commented
on this too. Through such peculiar selection, we may look at
only the slowest or the most rapidly conducting fibers, completely
missing the population that may make up the largest proportion of
myelinated fibers. A combination of speculation and evidence
suggests that there is a major population that has been completely
missed heretofore, or at least sampled so rarely that we have no
clear idea about what it comprises.

DR. HENSEL: First, I would take Dr. Poulos' general question and
make a general comment on my impression of this symposium. My
impression is that during the period when we were working only with
animals and drawing more vague conclusions from animals to man we
were much more optimistic than during the time when we started to
make direct comparisons in humans with neural activity and sensation.
This is a good progress, that we have become more critical about
these analogies and parallels. Now we can make the direct comparisons.
      The point that Dr. Vallbo has made is very important. It is
very difficult to say whether the unit, or even the population
that we are recording from, is the same as that involved in sensory experience. There might be several exceptions and you
mentioned, for example, the cold spot. The cold spot is an example
where it might be possible to record from the single fiber, because we have now enough morphological material to say that each
cold spot, at least in the cat, is served by one single fiber.
Since the cold spots are not very densely distributed, it is
rather easy to stimulate a single cold spot without stimulating
others. The same will hold for the warm spots. For the mechanoreceptors, it is more difficult because they are very densely
distributed and it is difficult to decide whether you stimulate
one or a few of the receptors.

DR. JOHANSSON: I have thought a bit of the problem brought up by
Dr. Iggo yesterday and Dr. Perl, today, concerning the bias in the
human sample. There are three factors that I would like to discuss
which may account for the bias. One factor which has been touched
on, is the possibility of spatial segregation within the peripheral
nerve trunks. We have studied morphologically the median nerve
at the level of the wrist and counted the number of myelinated
fibers and also measured the diameters in order to establish a
fiber spectrum. The fiber spectrum is strictly bimodal with 50
percent large myelinated fibers (Vallbo and Johansson, 1978).
The dividing line is about 7 μm. There is absolutely no spatial
segregation between the thick and thin myelinated fibers, which

would suggest that the thinner fibers are less available for the
electrode tip. Another factor, which was brought up by Dr. Vallbo
and also by Dr. Perl, is that it might be more difficult to record
from the thinner myelinated fibers as they are smaller and you
probably have to impale the myelin with the electrode.

The third factor, which I think accounts for the fact that
only few Aδ units have been recorded from during the searching
procedures. This was also discussed by Dr. Konietzny yesterday
when he answered a question after his communication.

Has anyone really designed a searching procedure for cold
units or pain prick sensitive units which account for the majority
of the thin myelinated unit population in the distal parts of the
limb? The Aδ units that we have found by "accident" when searching
for mechanoreceptive units were not spontaneously active.

DR. POULOS: The cold units should be spontaneously active under
most conditions.

DR. JOHANSSON: Perhaps other people have that opinion, but the
cold units we have found are not spontaneously active when you
have the blood flow and everything regulated by the conscious
organism. Have you other opinions?

DR. PERL: We did some experiments searching for units responsive
to electrically initiated volleys in a conscious human subject;
all of us can guess at the problem with this technique. When
the electrical stimulus is strong enough to excite the slowly
conducting myelinated fibers, every time a volley is initiated the
subject has a brief moment of discomfort. Most subjects will not
tolerate this for long. One must stimulate very infrequently, to
avoid summation of effect and the subject's subsequent dissatis-
faction with the experimental situation. Yet this still seems to
me the only way to determine systematically that every unit
contacted by the electrode is recognized. It is an unacceptable
experiment when the afferent activity can reach the central
nervous system, and one way around the problem may be that old
trick, used since the 1930's, of blocking conduction in a nerve
centrally with a local anaesthetic, then looking for units by
electrical excitation of the distal nerve. Such a procedure would
eliminate discomfort and permit a specific search for slowly
conducting myelinated fibers. Our own experience in animal
experiments was that the high threshold mechanical nociceptors
went largely unseen until it was decided to pass over all rapidly
conducting fibers encountered in the search. Only then was the
selection bias of the electrodes overcome; in the initial work we
estimated that only some 20 percent of the Aδ fibers present were
sampled. Since about 80 percent of that group in cat consists of
low threshold mechanically excitable units, the resulting sample

was skewed enough to hide the mechanical nociceptors with myelinated
fibers.

DR. JOHANSSON: I would like to comment on one more point concerning the possibilities of recording from A δ-units and C-units.
As we heard from Dr. Torebjörk this morning, his main cue, which
you would not have if you were going to record from A δ-units, is
the ongoing impulse activity in the small bundles of C-units.
This activity directs him to the appropriate part of the nerve.
Another point is that there are quite a few units that can be
recorded from, but whose receptive field we have not been able to
find. We know that they are myelinated fibers because of the
shape of the action potential. If we record from the median
nerve at the wrist, for instance, they should be afferent fibers.
These might be fibers, which we have no searching procedure for.

DR. POULOS: I would like to make one comment on your comments on
segregation in peripheral nerve, which implies a functional
segregation. This has become an important clinical point. In the
trigeminal system, for example, where some neurosurgeons still
believe pain and temperature are segregated in a particular
portion of the main sensory root. Richard Lende and I studied
this rather extensively in both the root and the trigeminal
ganglion. Lende, R. A., and Poulos, D. A., (1970); Pelletier, V. A.,
Poulos, D. A. and Lende, R. A. (1974); Poulos, D. A. (1976). Our
experience was one that you all have reported, in a sense, and
that is, you can isolate in a given electrode penetration a
particular functional type and the probability of encountering
another unit of that type close by is quite high. But, the
important point that should be made is, while there is what we
called a micro-localization these groupings of cells appear
throughout the distribution of that body part's representation.
I think this is an important point that should be made. When we
talk about functional segregation it is important that we do not
imply that all of the pain and temperature fibers are isolated in
one portion of the peripheral nerve.

DR. PERL: I agree with Dr. Poulos, but it is true that just before the fibers enter the central nervous system, there is another
segregation based on size. This has been known for 80 years and
was recently documented once again in the primate, including man
(Sindou et al., 1974; Snyder, 1977). The debate over whether
small diameter fibers are segregated in the lateral division of
the dorsal root was finally ended by Snyder's (1977) work at the
electron microscopic level. Ranson and Billingsley (1916) were
probably right in proposing the lateral and medial divisions in the
cat, but for the wrong reason. In cat, the segregation occurs not
in the root itself, but after entry into the cord (Earle, 1952;

Kerr, 1975; Snyder, 1977). In primates, on the other hand, congregation of fine afferent fibers in the lateral division of the root itself does seem to occur. Thus, there is a segregation by size, but the receptive classes do not segregate completely. Only to the extent that fiber diameter and functional class correlate may this relate to sensibility.

DR. HENSEL: I would like to make a brief comment on spontaneous activity. According to our experience in cat and monkey, all specific cold fibers should be spontaneously active at normal skin temperature. There might be other fibers around and we also are looking for possible cold fibers in the very low temperature range that might have other properties.

DR. VALLBO: I would like to emphasize that the examples that you have mentioned about the segregation of fibers according to specificity within a nerve, all refer to points close to the central nervous system. Am I right? It seems reasonable that the fibers sort themselves out according to the portion of the spinal cord they go to which might be related to modality. Whereas, the farther out you go towards periphery, it seems reasonable that the fascicles are more mixed because there are fibers of all kinds going to any skin area.

DR. POULOS: Dr. Perl was referring to the root entry zone. In the trigeminal system they are still quite mixed just as the root enters medulla. Once it is in the root entry zone proper, there is a segregation.

DR. PERL: I believe the evidence points to three types of segregation. The first is the regional segregation close to the peripheral termination point. There, everything from a given area of the skin or from a given portion of the muscle comes together in peripheral nerve bundles. A second segregation was referred to earlier; this occurs some distance from the peripheral termination, along the pathway of the nerve. If you dissect a peripheral nerve or sample unitary potentials with a microelectrode, you will encounter a given kind of unit with remarkable frequency in some part of the nerve. This suggests that by a rearrangement within the peripheral nerve, some grouping of the elements has taken place. At the spinal cord entrance zone, there is a third kind of segregation, which sorts the dorsal root fibers according to diameter. In short, it looks as if there is a topographical combination most peripherally, an intermediate or mixed arrangement more centrally in the nerve (grouping by regions as well as by receptor types), and then a grouping by receptor type and fiber size right at the spinal cord entry zone.

    Thus, at least three segregations appear to exist. The

segregation by type of sense organs is very difficult to document, however. Many people who have done surveys of afferent fiber categories at one or another location along the primary afferent pathway recognize, or have commented on, the tendency to find groups of similar units. I suppose the only way to prove the existence of the sensory type of congregation would be to mark individual fibers indelibly and demonstrate the relative location of fibers sharing similar functional characteristics.

There are some other issues that need to be brought up. In reference to Professor Iggo, we owe him the courtesy of discussing the "modality" issue, or at least trying to define the nature of the problem. Let me start by pointing out that the word "modality" is established in common English usage, and I suspect its equivalent appears in common usage in most languages. To assign a narrow definition to it at this state would simply fly in the face of common understanding. When we speak of modes of energy, we mean several things: the way the distribution goes, or the kind of event itself. It seems foolish to argue that use of the word "modality" must be limited to describing only the sensation or else just the stimulus. No matter what terminologies we employ in our work, we are all obliged to state clearly what it is the terms are being used to describe. Let us unambiguously define whether we refer to the product of perception or the result of the defined stimulus.

We ran into this difficulty many years ago, when we tried to name the peculiar high threshold receptors that respond to several kinds of cutaneous stimulation: mechanical, heat, and chemical (the last has had relatively little attention in this conference). The problem was how to label these sensory units in a distinctive fashion that would give a clue to their features. We decided to create a hybrid word, deliberately combining Latin and Greek roots to set it apart from names others were using, while yet describing its multiple responsiveness. The chemical responsiveness interested us particularly, because there were possibilities that heat and mechanical stimuli alone would excite other cutaneous sensory units. By choosing the word "polymodal" we were describing the variety of types of effective stimuli, not the eventual perceptual reaction. Whatever linguistic mistakes were made in assembling it, the term is now widely used for describing a kind of cutaneous sensory receptor that has been found in many beasts, including man, and that has a common set of characteristics in several species.

The unresolved issue I see still before us is how this kind of cutaneous receptor relates to perceptual experience. We have heard some of the questions about this. Thus, I think we do need to worry about which end of the process we are talking about when we speak of modality. The third criterion is coincidence. That means that you can experience two modalities at the same time and the same place. Some item can be both green and heavy, but it cannot be green and red at the same time and in the same space. Applying these criteria to the skin, we must confess that we have to speak of different modalities and different senses. You can feel warmth, and hot, and pain at the same time, so it would be justified not to speak of one cutaneous modality, as Johannes Müller did, but to speak of different modalities or senses of the skin.

Now talking of the term polymodal or multimodal, it is not too dangerous to use this term. I would understand that it means mode or kind of, and we will not confuse this with a sensory modality. I suggest that we keep the term polymodal and multimodal and if we know what we are talking about then it is all right. But what is very important is to discern between a modality in the sense of a phenomenon and in the sense of a physical unit.

DR. ZOTTERMAN: Well, we are in rather a dilemma because if we describe properly in physical terms what you call a polymodal nociceptive fiber, for instance, that is a high threshold mechanoreceptive fiber, for instance, that is a high threshold mechanoreceptive fiber as well as a high threshold thermal fiber. Those are its mode of stimulation. But it does not mediate mechanical or tactile sensation or thermal sensation. It mediates pain. The question is do you want to express these things either in the sensory way or by the mode of stimulation to which they are sensitive? You have to describe both of them. But that is a very long description and you must have some kind of nice abbreviations for everyone. For practical use polymodal nociceptors we described in the beginning means the high threshold mechanoreceptor and high threshold thermal receptor that mediates pain. That is a very long story. You cannot write that but once in a paper.

DR. PERL: I am not sure, Professor Zotterman, that everyone will agree that polymodal sensory units must mediate pain. Some of us side with you, and others might find they still need more convincing on the issue. I hope we can at least agree that it is probably better to stick with a nomenclature that is understood and to make sure that we now utilize it consistently. Our descriptions have emphasized that sensory units called polymodal are strongly responsive to a number of different stimuli.

DR. TUCKER: Professor Hensel's comments are very clarifying for me. In the chemical senses we think of olfaction as one modality, taste as another modality, and in taste there are sweet, salt, sour, and bitter qualities. Then at the very end, he undid it all for me, by referring to a unit that has polymodal qualities. Then Dr. Zotterman put his finger right on the problem, there. So, to you people in this area, who keep up with each other's work, you know what you mean but to the outsiders, it may not be so clear.

DR. PERL: Several sets of investigators, over the years, tried to define the responsiveness of cutaneous sensory units to chemical stimuli. They report substantial discrepancies. That is, different kinds of sensory units can be excited by chemical agents applied to the general circulation, applied by close arterial injection, and in some cases when applied to the skin itself. Recently Szolcsanyi (unpublished) has been using the rabbit ear, a classic preparation in which you can control the vascular inflow and outflow for a limited region supplied by a long nerve. Threshold quantities of chemical substances (including some producing itch in smaller quantities and pain in larger) consistently excite polymodal nociceptors. Very small amounts of bradykinin (1/10 of what others report using in muscle), capsaicin (the irritant extract of red pepper), and organic irritants (like xylol) regularly activate only this kind of cutaneous unit at very low concentrations. Stinging nettle, which at low concentrations evokes itch and at higher concentrations evokes pain, also selectively excites such units at low concentrations. This kind of C-fiber unit is one of several types that give an ongoing discharge when exposed to substances associated with inflammation, producing prolonged tissue and vascular changes, which revives the old theory of Rothman (1943) and Shelley and Arthur (1959): that itch results from weak activation of the same sensory apparatus responsible for pain. The evidence suggests that the point is worth exploring. Any eventual answer will probably come from analyses of the sensory units in man, because only man easily differentiates the several sensory experiences associated with aversive circumstances. Those who record from afferent C-fibers in man have the option of examining this interesting question. Part of the problem is whether the quality of the itch sensation is the same as the quality of pain. So far, no one has found a sensory element that responds preferentially to the chemical irritants but lacks the other qualities of a nociceptor, namely, the capacity to signal systematically the presence of tissue-damaging stimuli and to grade its response systematically at tissue-damaging intensities or stimulation.

DR. ZOTTERMAN: During the summer I used to burn my forearms so much that after 5 days the skin peeled off. At that period I would get a frightful itch, and I wondered what it could be. While I was with Thomas Lewis for eight months in 1926 working on the skin, at that time we thought of liberation of histamine and such things. But, the itch comes exactly at the time when the skin is peeling off. I had two ideas about it. One was that during the peeling off, you could watch under a microscope to see movements in the skin. When it peels off it must break up, and it could be a mechanical stimulus for some fibers. If you have low threshold C-fibers, which I believed at that time there could be, we do not know, yet we have them in the cat, anyhow, that could be a stimulus. The funny thing is that I could stop this itch by putting a hand on the skin with strong pressure and the itch absolutely stopped. I thought it might be the pressure that inhibited this kind of peeling from the skin. That was one idea. Then later on I had another explanation. The mechanical stimulation of the skin may bring up some inhibition. Perhaps today you could believe that the mechanical stimulation brings about a release of opiate polypeptides, centrally, which would stop the itch.

DR. HENSEL: There might be one experimental possibility to study this in animals using the scratching behavior of the animal. Perhaps combining this behavioral response with some neurophysiological work it might be possible also to get an experimental approach to the question of itch in animals.

DR. PERL: A comment, from an old Sherrington reader: one sees scratching behavior under circumstances that might be more akin to tickle than to itch.

DR. TOREBJÖRK: I am glad you have made a distinction between tickling and itch, because itch has a much more protopathic or pain-like character. In a paper called "Afferent C-units responding to mechanical, thermal and chemical stimuli in human non-glabrous skin." Torebjörk, H. E. (1974) I described the low frequency activity which you can elicit in the C-units by von Frey hair, by itch powder, or by a nettle leaf, correlated with the sensation of itch. These experiments were made without selective blocking of A-fibers and, hence, I could not say, for sure, that the neural activity in C-fibers actually, in itself alone, correlated with the itch sensation. I did draw attention to the fact that they might contribute to that sensation. Since then, I have tried several times to make selective blocking of A-fibers and by the same means to induce itch sensations. I found that sensations of itching pain can still be felt after blocking of A-fiber impulses. The C-fibers may thus contribute to itch, but the itch sensation could be more complicated than that. So, I do not exclude the contribution from other fibers or receptors, as well.

DR. PERL: Yes, I knew of your work and it figured in the interpretation I just suggested. An additional bit of evidence from Szolcsanyi's (unpublished) work on the rabbit ear is that a remarkable differentiation of the responsiveness to small quantities of the irritant chemicals exists among cutaneous sense organs. The high threshold mechanoreceptors, for example, do not respond to itch-producing substances. Some years ago, Fjällbrant and

Iggo (1961) noted slowly adapting cutaneous receptors that responded to a variety of intravascularly injected substances; but these receptors were not excited even by concentrations ten times greater than what excited the C-fiber polymodal nociceptors.

DR. STEVENS: While at a cocktail party I got into a conversation with a VIP dermatologist in the Yale School of Medicine and he asked me how much we know about itch and I said I do not think there is very much known about it, but people often tried to relate it to low level pain. He said that what he really wanted to know was whether aspirin relieved it. I said, "Are you asking me?" I am now asking you. Does anybody know the answer to that question?

DR. PERL: Aspirin does not relieve itch in the clinical situation. Whether it would at threshold in the normal individual who happens to have a bite from an insect, I think each person could answer for himself. In my case it does not.

DR. STOWELL: Has anyone succeeded in producing itch with any parameter of electrical stimulation, percutaneous, transcutaneous, etc?

DR. PERL: There are descriptions in the literature of itch-like sensations produced by weak electrical stimulation of the skin. Both Thomas Lewis (1942; Lewis et al., 1927) and George Bishop (1944) mention itch from cutaneous electrical stimulation.

REFERENCES

Bishop, G. H. The peripheral unit for pain. Journal of Neuro-
    physiology, 1944, 7, 71-80.
Brain, R. Presidential address. In C. A. Keele & R. Smith (Eds.),
    The assessment of pain in man and animals. London: Living-
    stone, 1962.
Burgess, P. R., Petit, D., & Warren, R. M. Receptor types in cat
    hairy skin supplied for myelinated fibers. Journal of Neuro-
    physiology, 1968, 31, 833-848.
Burgess, P. R. & Perl, E. R. Cutaneous mechanoreceptors and noci-
    ceptors. In A. Iggo (Ed.), Somatosensory system, Vol. II,
    Handbook of sensory physiology. Berlin: Springer Verlag,
    1973.
Earle, K. M. The tract of Lissauer and its possible relation to
    the pain pathway. Journal of Comparative Neurology, 1952, 96,
    93-111.
Fjällbrant, N. & Iggo, A. The effect of histamine, 5-hydroxytrypta-
    mine and acetylcholine on cutaneous afferent fibers. Journal
    of Physiology (London), 1961, 156, 578-590.

Hensel, H. & Boman, K. A. Afferent impulses in cutaneous sensory
     nerves in human subjects. Journal of Neurophysiology, 1960,
     23, 564-578.

Kenshalo, D. K. The skin sense. Springfield: Charles C. Thomas,
     1968.

Kerr, F. W. L. Neuroanatomical substrates of nociception in the
     spinal cord. Pain, 1975, 1, 325-356.

Lende, R. A. & Poulous, D. A. Functional localization in the tri-
     geminal ganglion in the monkey. Journal of Neurosurgery,
     1970, 33, 336-343.

Lewis, T. Pain. New York: MacMillan, 1942.

Lewis, T., Grant, R. T., & Marvin, H. M. Vascular reactions of the
     skin to injury. Part X. The intervention of a chemical
     stimulus illustrated especially by the flare. The response
     to faradism. Heart, 1927, 14, 139-160.

Müller, J. Handbuch der physiologie des Menschen. Koblenz, 1840.

Pelletier, V. A., Poulos, D. A., & Lende, R. A. Functional locali-
     zation in the trigeminal root. Journal of Neurosurgery, 1974,
     40, 504-513.

Poulos, D. A. Functional and anatomical localization in the tri-
     geminal root: In support of Frazier. In T. P. Morley (Ed.),
     Current controversies in neurosurgery. Philadelphia: W. B.
     Saunders, 1976.

Poulton, E. C. The psychophysics: Six models for magnitude esti-
     mation. Psychological Bulletin, 1968, 69, 1-19.

Ranson, S. W. & Billingsley, P. R. The conduction of painful affer-
     ent impulses in the spinal nerves. American Journal of Phy-
     siology, 1916, 40, 571-584.

Rothman, S. The nature of itching. Research Publication, Asso-
     ciation for Research in Nervous and Mental Diseases, 1943, 23,
     110-122.

Shelley, W. B. & Arthur, R. P. The peripheral mechanism of itch
     in man. In G. E. W. Wolstonholme & M. O'Connor (Eds), Pain
     and itch. Nervous Mechanisms. London: Churchill, 1959.

Sindou, M., Quoex, C., & Baleydier, C. Fiber organization at the
     posterior spinal cord-rootlet junction in man. Journal of
     Comparative Neurology, 1974, 153, 15-26.

Snyder, R. The organization of the dorsal root entry zone in
     cats and monkeys. Journal of Comparative Neurology, 1977,
     174, 47-70.

Torebjörk, H. E. Afferent C units responding to mechanical, thermal
     and chemical stimuli in human non-glabrous skin. Acta Phy-
     siologica Scandinavica, 1974, 92, 374-390.

Vallbo, Å. B. & Johansson, R. S. Tactile sensory innervation of the
     glabrous skin of the human hand. In G. Gordon (Ed.), Active
     touch, the mechanism of recognition of objects by manipulation.
     Oxford: Pergamon Press, 1978.

Weber, E. H. Der tastsinn und das gemeingefühl. In. R. Wagner
     (Ed.), Handwörterbuch der physiologie, Vol. 2, Part 2. Biewig:
     Braunschweig, 1846.

CONTRIBUTORS AND INVITED PARTICIPANTS

Allen B. Chatt
Department of Neurology
Yale University
School of Medicine
New Haven, CONNECTICUT

James C. Craig
Department of Psychology
Indiana University
Bloomington, INDIANA

Gernot S. Doetsch
Sensory Neurophysiology Lab
Central State Hospital
Milledgeville, GEORGIA

Duane A. Dreyer
Department of Physiology
University of North Carolina
Chapel Hill, NORTH CAROLINA

Roland Duclaux
Laboratoire de Physiologie
Université Claude Bernard
U.E.R. Medicale Lyon Sud-Ouest
69600 Oullins, FRANCE

Dexter M. Easton
Department of Biological
   Sciences
Florida State University
Tallahassee, FLORIDA

Ove C. Franzén
Department of Psychology
University of Uppsala
S-752 20 Uppsala, SWEDEN

George A. Gescheider
Department of Psychology
Princeton University
Princeton, NEW JERSEY

Barry G. Green
Department of Psychology
Princeton University
Princeton, NEW JERSEY

Heikki Hämäläinen
Department of Psychology
University of Helsinki
SF-00170 Helsinki, FINLAND

Stephen W. Harkins
Department of Psychiatry
University of Washington
Seattle, WASHINGTON

Herbert Hensel
Institute of Physiology
University of Marburg
Deutschhausstrasse 2
D-355 Marburg, WEST GERMANY

Ainsley Iggo
Department of Physiology
Faculty of Veterinary Medicine
University of Edinburgh
Edinburgh EH 9 1QH, SCOTLAND

Timo V. Järvilehto
Department of Psychology
University of Helsinki
SF-00170 Helsinki, FINLAND

William M. Jenkins
Department of Psychology
Florida State University
Tallahassee, FLORIDA

Roland S. Johansson
Department of Physiology
University of Umeå
S-901 87 Umeå, SWEDEN

Dan R. Kenshalo, Jr.
Marine Biomedical Institute
200 University Boulevard
Galveston, TEXAS

Jacob H. Kirman
Department of Psychology
CUNY Queens College
Flushing, NEW YORK

Frithjof G. Konietzny
Institute of Physiology
University of Marburg
Deutschhausstrasse 2
D-355 Marburg, WEST GERMANY

Albert T. Kulics
Department of Pharmacology
University of Pittsburgh
School of Medicine
Pittsburgh, PENNSYLVANIA

Robert M. LaMotte
Department of Anesthesiology
Yale University
School of Medicine
New Haven, CONNECTICUT

Susan J. Lederman
Department of Psychology
Queens University
Kingston, CANADA

Ulf F. Lindblom
Department of Neurology
Huddinge Hospital
S-141 86 Huddinge, SWEDEN

Mary M. Luck
Department of Neuroscience
University of Florida
College of Medicine
Gainesville, FLORIDA

Helen H. Molinari
Department of Psychology
Florida State University
Tallahassee, FLORIDA

Edward R. Perl
Department of Physiology
University of North Carolina
Chapel Hill, NORTH CAROLINA

Dennis A. Poulos
Department of Neurosurgery
Albany Medical College
Albany, NEW YORK

Rebecca B. Price
Department of Biological
    Science
Florida State University
Tallahassee, FLORIDA

Richard H. Ray
Department of Physiology
Medical College of Georgia
Augusta, GEORGIA

Arnold Starr
Department of Neurology &
    Psychobiology
University of California
Irvine, CALIFORNIA

Joseph C. Stevens
John B. Pierce Foundation
290 Congress Avenue
New Haven, CONNECTICUT

Hilton Stowell
Sensory Neurophysiology Lab.
Central State Hospital
Milledgeville, GEORGIA

Erik Torebjörk
Department of Clinical Neuro-
    physiology
Academic Hospital
S-750 14 Uppsala, SWEDEN

Daniel L. Trevino
Department of Physiology
University of North Carolina
Chapel Hill, NORTH CAROLINA

Donald Tucker
Department of Biological
    Science
Florida State University
Tallahassee, FLORIDA

Åke B. Vallbo
Department of Physiology
University of Umeå
S-901 87 Umeå, SWEDEN

Ronald T. Verrillo
Institute for Sensory Research
Syracuse University
Syracuse, NEW YORK

Charles J. Vierck, Jr.
Department of Neuroscience
University of Florida
College of Medicine
Gainesville, FLORIDA

Barry L. Whitsel
Department of Physiology
University of North Carolina
Chapel Hill, NORTH CAROLINA

Yngve Zotterman
Wenner-Gren Center
Sveavagen 166
S-113 46 Stockholm, SWEDEN

AUTHOR INDEX*

Reference pages are underlined.

*Index prepared by Daniel Linehan

419

SUBJECT INDEX